Pediatric Dentistry with Case Studies

Pediatric Dentistry with Case Studies

Editor: Carly White

AMERICAN
MEDICAL PUBLISHERS
www.americanmedicalpublishers.com

AMERICAN
MEDICAL PUBLISHERS
www.americanmedicalpublishers.com

American Medical Publishers,
41 Flatbush Avenue,
1st Floor, New York,
NY 11217, USA

Pediatric Dentistry with Case Studies
Edited by Carly White

ISBN 979-8-88740-652-7 (Hardback)

Contents

Preface

This book has been a concerted effort by a group of academicians, researchers and scientists, who have contributed their research works for the realization of the book. This book has materialized in the wake of emerging advancements and innovations in this field. Therefore, the need of the hour was to compile all the required researches and disseminate the knowledge to a broad spectrum of people comprising of students, researchers and specialists of the field.

Pediatric dentistry, also known as pedodontics, is a branch of dentistry that focuses on the dental care and oral health of infants, children and adolescents. One of the major aspects of pediatric dentistry is the monitoring of the growth and development of the teeth and jaws of children. This involves the evaluation of the eruption of primary teeth and the development of permanent teeth, as well as the identification of any orthodontic abnormalities. It is also involves the administration of preventative dental care which helps in the promotion of good oral health from an early age. This encompasses dental cleanings, dental sealants, and dental check-ups. This book contains some path-breaking studies in the field of pediatric dentistry. The various studies that are constantly contributing towards advancing treatment modalities and evolution of this field are examined in detail. This book is a resource guide for experts as well as students.

At the end of the preface, I would like to thank the authors for their brilliant chapters and the publisher for guiding us all-through the making of the book till its final stage. Also, I would like to thank my family for providing the support and encouragement throughout my academic career and research projects.

Editor

1

Oligodontia and Facial Phenotype Associated with a Rare Syndrome

Fatima Ezzahra Zidane and Mustapha El Alloussi

College of Health Sciences, International Faculty of Dental Medicine, BioMed Unit, International University of Rabat, Technopolis Parc, Rocade of Rabat-Salé, Sala-Al Jadida 11100, Morocco

Correspondence should be addressed to Fatima Ezzahra Zidane; fatima-ezzahra.zidane@uir.ac.ma

Academic Editor: Tommaso Lombardi

Introduction. Oligodontia is a dental abnormality in which the patient is missing teeth. It is a hereditary disorder characterized by agenesis of more than six primary or permanent teeth, excluding the wisdom teeth. Oligodontia is often related with an abnormal size of teeth, conical shape, taurodontism, frequent enamel abnormalities, and delayed eruption. Oligodontia may be clinically isolated or associated with ectodermal dysplasia, a large group of rare diseases, and other syndromes. *Patient Information.* Dental characteristics of a six-and-a-half-year-old Moroccan boy with oligodontia and in apparent good health were described. *Clinical Findings.* Three syndromes associated with oligodontia have been discussed. Above all, based on the facial phenotype, Dubowitz syndrome has been retained as the most likely diagnostic hypothesis. This case could be the first reported case described in Morocco, but a thorough examination with genetic analysis must be carried out. *Conclusion.* Oligodontia could clinically be isolated or associated with ectodermal dysplasia, a large group of rare diseases, and other syndromes.

1. Introduction

Agenesis of teeth is the most common developmental dental anomaly in human beings. Several terms have been used to describe the congenital absence of teeth. Oligodontia implies agenesis of at least six definitive teeth, excluding wisdom teeth. Often teeth absent are the terminal teeth of a series [premolars (32–15%), maxillary lateral incisors (27%), and third molars (25%)] [1]. Oligodontia is a rare anomaly with a prevalence of 0.3% in permanent teeth and less in the primary dentition. The pathology can be isolated or can be associated with other ectodermal abnormalities and syndromes, such as ectodermal dysplasia, cleft lip, and palate [2]. Moreover, different epidemiological studies have shown a varying prevalence of oligodontia, depending on ethnic origin, with an average ranging from 0.1 to 0.2% [3]. Besides agenesis, other anomalies of size and shape can also be observed, such as rotation of the teeth, delayed dental development, and eruption [4]. Furthermore, hypo-development of the jaws and alveolar bone with modification of the facial structures and functional consequences were noticed. Optimally, agenesis should be detected earlier during childhood. Multiple dental agenesis is most frequently discovered fortuitously. The diagnosis can only be confirmed by the orthopantogram (the absence of the dental follicle is a sign of agenesis). Oligodontia is most frequently associated with syndromes and may be one of the signs to enhance the early diagnosis of these syndromes. The aim of this report was to describe the dental characteristics of a six-and-a-half-year-old Moroccan boy with oligodontia; this case might be the first reported case of Dubowitz syndrome (DS) described in Morocco, but a thorough examination with genetic analysis must be carried out.

2. Patient Information

A six-and-a-half-year-old Moroccan boy presented to the dental office for pain as a reason for consultation. The diagnosis of oligodontia has not been made previously.

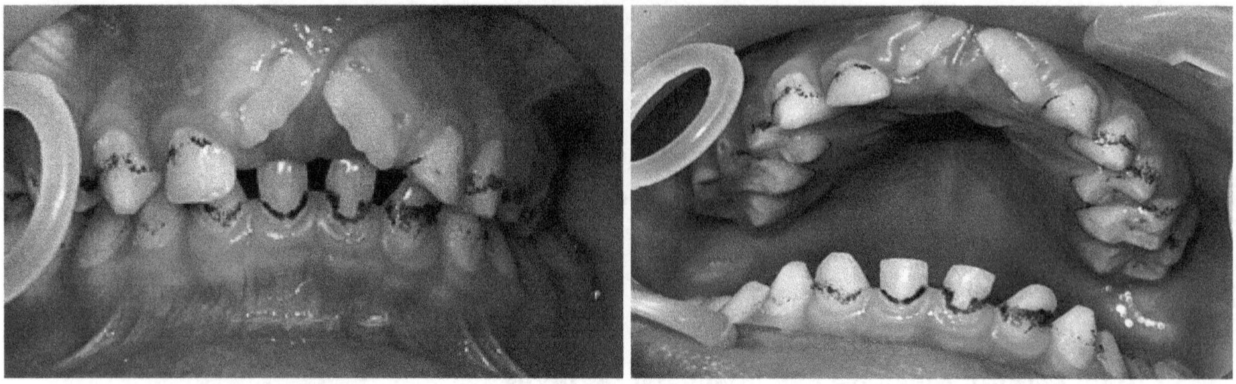

Figure 1: Chromogenic bacteria, rotation of the lower incisors, and a high narrow palate.

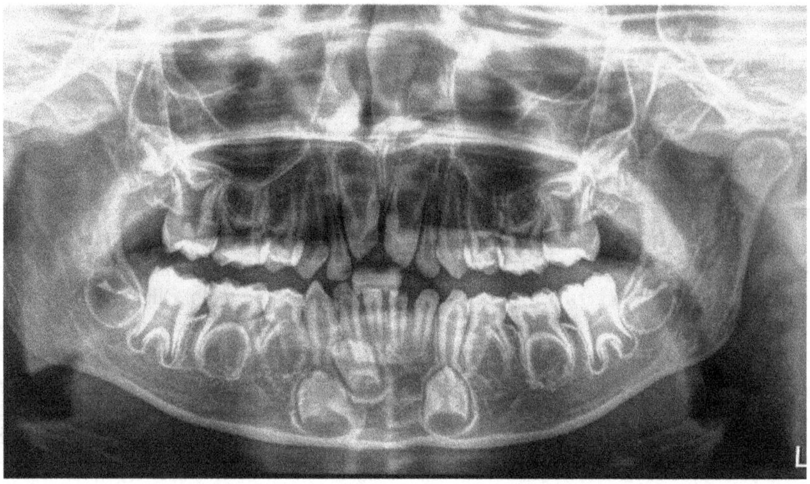

Figure 2: Panoramic radiographic view demonstrating oligodontia, chronologically delayed eruption, and taurodontism.

3. Clinical Findings

During the dental examination, the patient had a high-pitched voice and mild mental retardation (no test was assessed to quantify it). In the extraoral examination, clinical anomalies including a triangular face, small head, little frontal bossing, low-set ears, saddle nose, and eczema were found. The intraoral examination revealed mixed dentition, chromogenic bacteria, rotation of the upper incisors, and a high narrow palate (Figure 1).

The panoramic radiograph showed absence of teeth germ of teeth #15, #14, #13, #12, #22, #23, #24, #25, #35, #34, #32, #31, #41, #44, and #45. Chronologically delayed eruption and taurodontism on the first molars (Figure 2) were detected. In addition, profile radiography of the patient's skull showed skeletal class II (Figure 3).

4. Discussion

Oligodontia is a polygenic inheritance influenced by environmental factors and may be associated with other symptoms affecting ectodermal structures, a large group of rare diseases, such as ectodermal anhidrotic syndrome, Down syndrome, or DS [5]. Several signs of the patient are part of the clinical picture of several syndromes including fetal alcohol syndrome (FAS), Bloom syndrome (BS), and DS [6].

FAS is a condition in a child that results from alcohol exposure during the mother's pregnancy, and it causes brain damage and growth problems. The problems vary from child to child. Physical defects may include distinctive facial features (small eyes, thin upper lip, short upturned nose, small head circumference, and brain size).

Brain and central nervous system problems, heart defects, and problems with kidneys are also found in children with FAS [7]. Even if the symptoms expressed in the patient were similar to FAS, the patient's mother did not drink alcohol. BS is a rare chromosome disruption syndrome characterized by marked genetic instability associated with pre- and postnatal growth retardation, predisposition to cancer, pigmentary lesions, eye disorders, and oligodontia. Only people with BS have red and purple patches on their skin caused by blood vessels [8], a thing that was not notified in this case. All the patient's signs were closest to DS. DS was described in 1965, in a girl with intrauterine growth retardation and distinctive facies: large low set ears, retrognathia, ptosis, eczema, and short stature [6, 8]. Microcephaly, varying degrees of developmental and motoric delay, and a variety of minor anomalies, intelligence varies

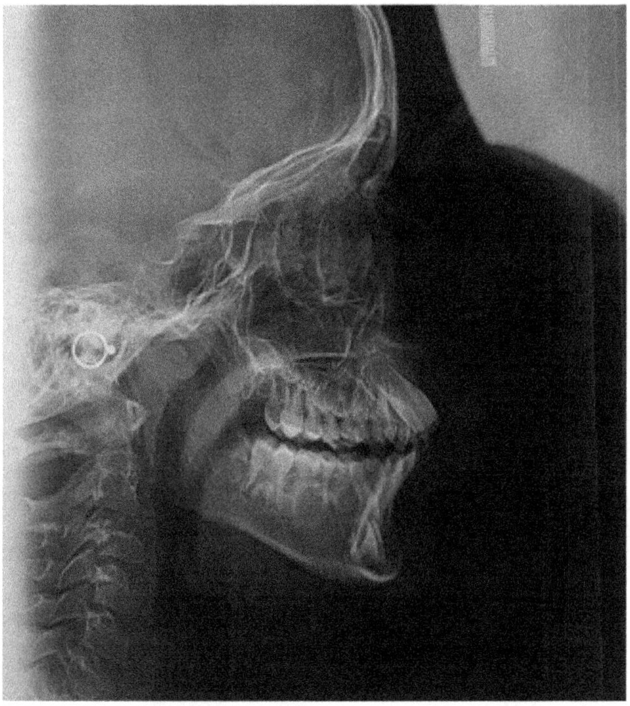

FIGURE 3: Lateral radiographic view showing skeletal class II.

from severe retardation to average levels, delayed speech (60%), and hyperactivity (40%) were reported in litterature [6, 8, 9]. Aplastic anemias [6, 10], neoplasms, leukemia, lymphoma, and neuroblastoma associated with DS were reported [11]. This syndrome is associated with common physical characteristics: small stature, slow growth, microcephaly, intellectual disability, eczema, triangle shaped face, high sloping forehead, ptosis, blepharophimosis, large ears, and sparse hair [12, 13]. All these characteristics were notified in the patient besides ptosis and blepharophimosis.

DS is an autosomal recessive condition, but the specific gene mutation responsible has not yet been identified [11, 13]. It appears to affect both sexes and all ethnicities equally. The overall incidence of DS is very rare. Approximately 150 cases have been reported in the literature, with various other associated anomalies [6, 8]. Most of these cases have been reported in the USA, Europe, Middle East, Russia, and Japan [14]. This case might be the first case of DS with dental findings from the country, but a thorough examination with genetic analysis must be carried out.

In 141 individuals with DS, facial anomalies and microcephaly were present in 112 patients and blepharophimosis in 60. A prominent round nose tip was considered as especially characteristic of DS at a young age. Multiple dental carious lesions, retarded eruption, microdontia, malocclusion, diastema, and fusion of dental elements were found [6, 14]. In 1990, velopharyngeal insufficiency was described for the first time [15]. Oral features include a thin upper lip border, small oral cavity, prominent philtrum, narrow and deep palate, micrognathia, prognathism, and retrognathism [6]. The patient presented alterations of thin upper lip border, micrognathia, retarded eruption, and malocclusion.

Growth retardation, which is due to growth hormone (GH) deficiency, could be due to gene mutations [16, 17]. DS is accompanied with a deficiency in the GH, which may be caused by genetic mutations, malformations of the hypothalamus, or pituitary gland during development; GH deficiency also correlates with low levels of IgG antibodies, a condition found in Dubowitz patients [17]. DS has autosomal recessive inheritance [18]. Affected siblings have been described in nine families, with both sexes affected.

5. Conclusion

Oligodontia may be isolated or associated with syndromes, such as Down syndrome, BS, or DS. The diagnosis of DS is usually based on the characteristic facial appearance, growth data, and medical history. Because of the risks, early diagnosis is essential to avoid complications.

Authors' Contributions

Fatima Ezzahra Zidane contributed to conception, design, data acquisition, and interpretation; performed all statistical analyses; and drafted and critically revised the manuscript. Mustapha El Alloussi contributed to conception and design, and critically revised the manuscript. Both authors gave their final approval and agreed to be accountable for all aspects of the work.

References

[1] I. B. O'Dowling and T. G. McNamara, "Congenital absence of permanent teeth among Irish school-children," *Journal of the Irish Dental Association*, vol. 36, no. 4, pp. 136–138, 1990.

[2] T. Shimizu and T. Maeda, "Prevalence and genetic basis of tooth agenesis," *Japanese Dental Science Review*, vol. 45, pp. 52–58, 2009.

[3] N. Worsaae, B. N. Jensen, B. Holm, and J. Holsko, "Treatment of severe hypodontia-oligodontia–an interdisciplinary concept," *International Journal of Oral and Maxillofacial Surgery*, vol. 36, no. 6, pp. 473–480, 2007.

[4] B. Rune and K. V. Sarnäs, "Tooth size and tooth formation in children with advanced hypodontia," *Angle Orthodontist*, vol. 44, no. 4, pp. 316–321, 1974.

[5] A. H. Al-Ani, J. S. Antoun, W. M. Thomson, T. R. Merriman, and M. Farella, "Hypodontia: an update on its etiology, classification, and clinical management," *BioMed Research International*, vol. 2017, 2017.

[6] V. Dubowitz, "Familial low birthweight dwarfism with unusual facies and a skin eruption," *Journal of Medical Genetics*, vol. 2, no. 1, pp. 12–17, 1965.

[7] M. Mathieu, P. Berquin, S. Epelbaum, C. Lenaerts, and C. Piussan, "Le syndrome de Dubowitz. Un diagnostic à ne pas méconnaître [Dubowitz syndrome. A diagnosis not to be missed]," *Archives Francaises de Pediatrie*, vol. 48, no. 10, pp. 715–718, 1991.

[8] R. M. Winter, "Dubowitz syndrome," *Journal of Medical Genetics*, vol. 23, no. 1, pp. 11–13, 1986.

[9] K. T. Moller and R. J. Gorlin, "The Dubowitz syndrome: a retrospective," *Journal of Craniofacial Genetics and Developmental Biology Supplement*, vol. 1, pp. 283–286, 1985.

[10] J. M. Opitz, R. A. Pfeiffer, J. P. Hermann, and T. Kushnick, "Studies of malformation syndromes of man XXIV B: the Dubowitz syndrome. Further observations," *Zeitschrift fur Kinderheilkunde*, vol. 116, no. 1, pp. 1–12, 1973.

[11] B. Modell, M. W. Darlison, H. Malherbe et al., "Congenital disorders: epidemiological methods for answering calls for action," *Journal of Community Genetics*, vol. 9, no. 4, pp. 335–340, 2018.

[12] I. Kondo, K. Takeda, K. Kuwajima, and T. Hirano, "A Japanese patient with the Dubowitz syndrome," *Clinical Genetics*, vol. 31, no. 6, pp. 389–392, 1987.

[13] A. Ballini, S. Cantore, D. Tullo, and A. Desiate, "Dental and craniofacial characteristics in a patient with Dubowitz syndrome: a case report," *Journal of Medical Case Reports*, vol. 27, no. 5, p. 38, 2011.

[14] A. Hamosh, A. F. Scott, J. Amberger, D. Valle, and V. A. McKusick, "Online Mendelian inheritance in man (OMIM)," *Human Mutation*, vol. 15, no. 1, pp. 57–61, 2000.

[15] A. Ahmad, A. Amalfitano, Y. T. Chen, P. S. Kishnani, C. Miller, and R. Kelley, "Dubowitz syndrome: a defect in the cholesterol biosynthetic pathway?," *American Journal of Medical Genetics*, vol. 86, no. 5, pp. 503504, 1999.

[16] S. Lyonnet, G. Schwartz, G. Gatin, Y. de Prost, A. Munnich, and M. Le Merrer, "Blepharophimosis, eczema, and growth and developmental delay in a young adult: late features of Dubowitz syndrome?," *Journal of Medical Genetics*, vol. 29, no. 1, pp. 6869, 1992.

[17] T. Hirano, I. Izumi, and K. Tamura, "Growth hormone deficiency in Dubowitz syndrome," *Acta Paediatrica Japonica*, vol. 38, no. 3, pp. 267–269, 1996.

[18] T. Lerman-Sagie, P. Merlob, A. Shuper et al., "New findings in a patient with Dubowitz syndrome: velopharyngeal insufficiency and hypoparathyroidism," *American Journal of Medical Genetics*, vol. 37, no. 2, pp. 241–243, 1990.

2

Anxiolysis in the Surgical Management of a Compound Odontoma in a Pediatric Patient

Pier Paolo Poli,[1] Luca Creminelli,[2] Emma Grecchi,[2] Silvia Pieriboni,[1] Gregorio Menozzi,[2] and Carlo Maiorana[3]

[1]*Department of Biomedical, Surgical and Dental Sciences, University of Milan, Via Commenda 10, 20122 Milan, Italy*
[2]*Oral Surgery Department, Maxillofacial Surgery and Odontostomatology Unit, Fondazione IRCCS Cà Granda Maggiore Policlinico Hospital, University of Milan, Via Commenda 10, 20122 Milan, Italy*
[3]*Oral Surgery and Implantology Departments, Maxillofacial Surgery and Odontostomatology Unit, Fondazione IRCCS Cà Granda Maggiore Policlinico Hospital, University of Milan, Via Commenda 10, 20122 Milan, Italy*

Correspondence should be addressed to Silvia Pieriboni; silvia.pieriboni24@gmail.com

Academic Editor: Maria Beatriz Duarte Gavião

Among odontogenic tumors, odontoma is the most frequent. The common treatment contemplates a conservative approach. While this procedure is generally accepted and tolerated, some difficulties may be encountered in the case of pediatric patients. Indeed, negative feelings of tension, apprehension, nervousness, and fear are likely to occur. The present report is aimed at discussing the management of a compound odontoma in a pediatric patient under anxiolysis with diazepam on an outpatient basis. The surgery was carried out without complications, and the discharge was completed safely. Oral premedication with diazepam should be considered to avoid more invasive sedation procedures in anxious pediatric patients.

1. Introduction

Odontomas are benign calcifying odontogenic tumors of the oral cavity. Generally, odontomas are considered to be hamartomatous developmental malformations of dental tissues rather than true neoplasms, as both epithelial and ectomesenchymal components have morphologically normal cells with defective structural arrangement [1]. Two basic types of odontoma can be identified: complex and compound. The complex type is characterized by unorganized dental tissue with dysplastic dentin covered by enamel, resulting in haphazard amorphous calcifications. The compound odontoma forms multiple disordered and irregular tooth-like elements [2]. Complex odontomas most frequently occur in the posterior molar regions, whereas compound odontomas tend to develop in the anterior maxilla [3]. The incidence of odontogenic tumors is low, ranging from 0.002% to 0.1%, with the odontoma representing the most common entity, accounting for 20% to 67% of all odontogenic neoplasms [4]. The multifactorial etiology of odontomas is still debated. Local trauma in the primary dentition period, infection growth pressure, hereditary anomalies, family history, and developmental influences have been suggested as possible causes [5]. Most lesions are detected on routine radiographs as a consequence of their slow and painless growth. Eruption disturbances including impaction, delayed eruption, or retention of primary or permanent teeth are common clinical findings [6]. While these lesions can be diagnosed at any age, it is worthy of note that odontomas are considered to be the most common types of odontogenic tumors in the pediatric population [3]. Pediatric dentistry often involves patients with high levels of anxiety and fear. Currently available evidence suggests that approximately 6% [7] to 40% [8] of children exhibit anxiety with respect to dental treatment. Furthermore, anxiety is exacerbated by invasive and long-lasting procedures including surgical interventions [9]. Anxious patients are likely to express subjective feelings of tension, apprehension, nervousness, and fear that might compromise dental treatment. For such reasons, anxiolysis has been used to facilitate dental care for anxious and uncooperative pediatric dental patients with successful results [10]. In view of the above, this report is aimed at presenting a case of compound odontoma surgically managed in association with anxiolysis protocol in a pediatric patient on an outpatient basis.

2. Case Report

A 7-year-old healthy Caucasian boy was referred by the orthodontist to investigate the edentulous space between the first and second primary upper left molars, together with an unusual swelling in the same region. After an interview with the parents, a noncontributory medical history was confirmed.

The intraoral clinical examination revealed mixed dentition with no decayed teeth. A 6 mm edentulous space between the two primary upper left molars was observed. In addition, expansion of the cortical bone was present on the vestibular aspect of the right hemi-maxilla. The bony hard swelling was firm and asymptomatic. The overlying mucosa was normal and nontender on palpation. Second-level radiological investigation was performed by means of the cone-beam computed tomography (CBCT) scan, which confirmed the presence of an irregular radiopaque mass located by the roots of the primary molars (Figure 1).

In more detail, the well-corticated lesion was characterized by multiple radiopaque structures encapsulated within a radiolucent cavity. Moreover, the lesion progressed in a vestibular direction so that the permanent second premolar germ resulted dislocated palatally. As a matter of fact, the germ could be palpated on the palatal aspect of the edentulous ridge. The clinical and radiographic presentations led to an initial diagnostic hypothesis of compound odontoma. The suggested treatment plan consisted of surgical removal of the lesion under oral sedation of the patient on an outpatient basis. After discussing the aforesaid surgical procedure, an informed consent signed by the parents was obtained.

Before the surgery, the following vital parameters were recorded: arterial blood pressure (systolic/diastolic pressure ratio: 85/50 mmHg), peripheral capillary oxygen saturation (SpO2: 99%), and heart rate (84 bpm). The weight and height of the patient were also registered (26 kg and 126 cm, respectively). At this point, the anxiolysis protocol used in the department in the case of pediatric patients was adopted (Table 1).

In this specific case, premedication consisted of oral administration of 15 drops of diazepam [11] 3 mg/ml (Valium®, Roche Pharmaceuticals, Monza, Italy) and topical application of 15% lidocaine spray (OGNA Pharmaceuticals, Muggiò, Italy). A fingertip pulse oximeter was used during the entire procedure to monitor the oxygen saturation of the patient.

Local anesthesia was induced with infiltrations of mepivacaine hydrochloride 3% (Optocain® 30 mg/ml, Molteni Dental Srl, Milan, Italy). Crestal incision with vertical releasing incisions located at the mesial and distal aspects of the first and second primary molars, respectively, was performed to raise a trapezoidal mucoperiosteal flap. The odontoma was accessed by removing the thin overlying cortical layer with a round bur mounted on a straight surgical handpiece under copious irrigation of sterile saline (Figure 2).

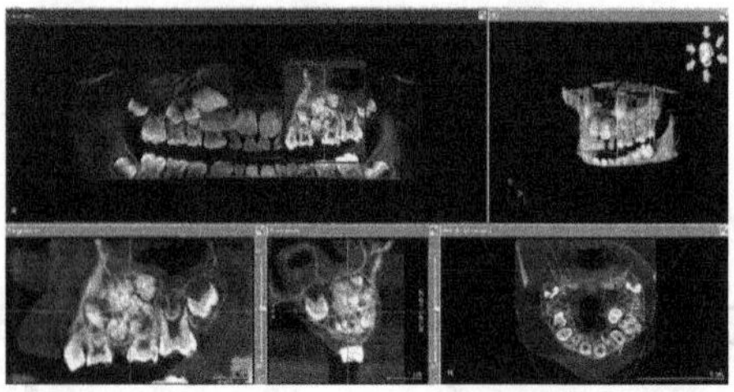

FIGURE 1: Cone-beam computed tomography showing radiopaque calcified structures with irregular margins characterized by a tooth-like configuration enclosed in radiolucent peripheral borders. The entire lesion measures approximately 12 × 15 × 19 mm.

TABLE 1: Anxiolysis protocol adopted in the case of pediatric patients.

N_2O/O_2 [a]
OR midazolam 0.50-0.75 mg/kg oral administration (maximum: 20 mg) or 0.2 mg/kg intravenous medication (maximum: 10 mg)[b] ± N_2O/O_2 *
OR diazepam 0.2-0.5 mg/kg oral administration (maximum: 10 mg)[b] ± N_2O/O_2 *
OR hydroxyzine oral solution 0.5 mg/kg ± N_2O/O_2 [a]

[a]Medical nitrous oxide/oxygen mixture. The percentage of N_2O is titrated for each patient during every procedure; [b]the drug used as benzodiazepines antagonist is flumazenil 0.01 mg/kg (maximum: 0.2 mg) followed if necessary by additional 0.01 mg/kg every minute up to five times (maximum tolerated cumulative dose: 1 mg).

The denticles were subsequently exposed and removed in a total of 14 pieces (Figure 3).

All harvested samples were sent for histopathological analysis. The surgical site was debrided and irrigated to remove any remnants, and the integrity of the maxillary sinus walls was checked. First intention sealing of the surgical wound was finally achieved with a 4/0 resorbable suture (Polysorb™, Covidien, Dublin, Ireland).

The time elapsed between the premedication and the end of the surgical procedure was 90 minutes. The vital parameters recorded immediately after the surgery were as follows: arterial blood pressure (systolic/diastolic pressure ratio: 80/50 mmHg), peripheral capillary oxygen saturation (SpO2: 100%), and heart rate (82 bpm).

The patient was prescribed antibiotic therapy consisting of 7.5 ml amoxicillin clavulanate pediatric suspension (Augmentin® pediatric suspension, GlaxoSmithKline, Verona, Italy) 3 times daily for 6 days and analgesics according to the patient needs. The rationale for antibiotic administration was to reduce the risk of infection of the blood clot during the immediate postoperative period in view of the considerable size of the lesion.

Postoperative care instructions included soft warm diet for 48 hours, 0.2% chlorhexidine mouthwash 2 times daily up to suture removal, topical application of ice, and refrainment from mechanical plaque removal of the primary molars

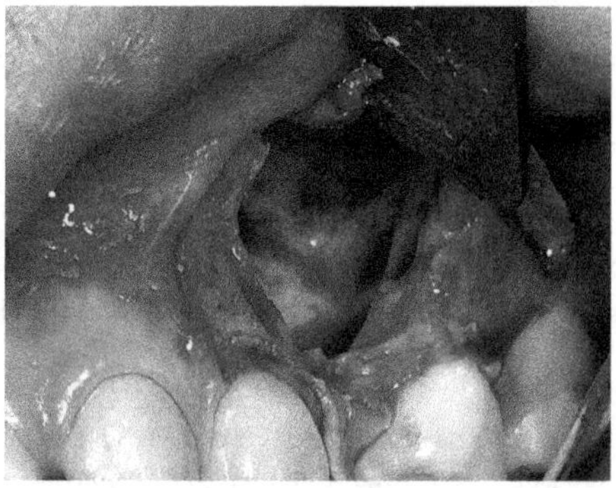

Figure 2: Intraoral clinical photograph of the surgical access showing the residual bone cavity after removal of the odontoma, with preservation of the adjacent maxillary sinus walls.

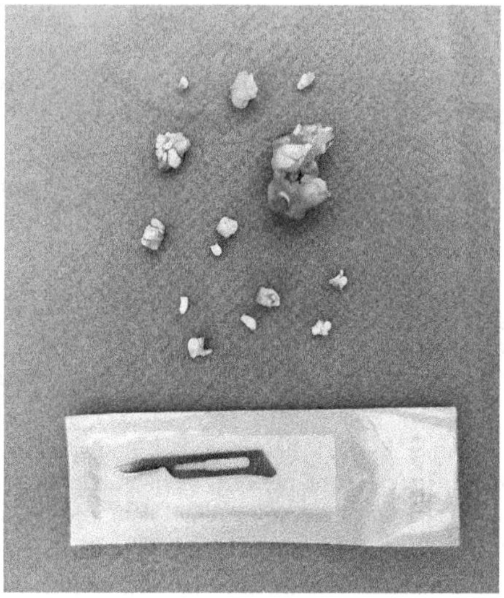

Figure 3: Clinical view of the compound odontoma surgically removed in multiple mineralized pieces resembling tooth structures.

for 7 days. The patient was discharged in stable conditions 90 minutes after the end of the surgical procedure. The healing proceeded uneventfully, and sutures were removed after 7 days. The histopathological report provided by the Department of Anatomic Pathology confirmed the diagnosis of compound odontoma (Figure 4).

3. Discussion

The present report described the surgical management of a compound odontoma detected in a pediatric patient with in-office sedation. Heterogeneity can be found among data reported from the literature with respect to the epidemiology of the disease. The present case is consistent with other studies reporting that compound odontoma is more frequently diagnosed in male subjects [6, 12] during the first two decades of life [13] in the premaxillary region [14]. Also, the clinical and radiological characteristics of the odontoma diagnosed in the present case resemble those commonly encountered for this type of lesion. Clinically, a firm bony

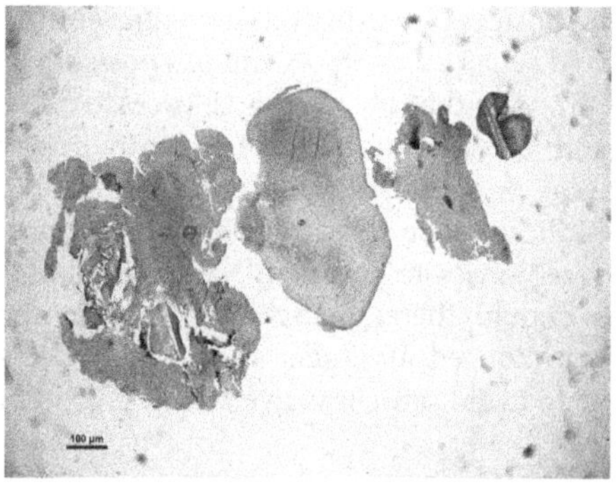

Figure 4: Low-power magnification of a resected specimen showing dental tissue, dentin, cement, and nonmineralized oral tissue composed of connective tissue typical of dental pulp, partially surrounded by a connective fibrous tissue capsule (hematoxylin and eosin staining; original magnification: ×10).

swelling of the oral vestibule covered by normal mucosa with no signs of inflammation can be appreciated [15]. Although they are commonly asymptomatic, clinical manifestations may occur, such as retention of deciduous teeth, noneruption of permanent teeth, and tooth displacement [13]. These clinical findings, if recognized, might explain the early diagnosis achieved in the present report. Dentition anomalies, and in particular the retention of the permanent second premolar, have led to a radiological second-level investigation which confirmed the suspect of compound odontoma. As a matter of fact, the CBCT exams showed multiple radiopaque tooth-like structures of various sizes surrounded by a radiolucid halo, compatible with compound odontoma at an advanced stage of development [13]. It is noteworthy that the mean age of patients at diagnosis of odontoma is normally between 20 and 30 years [4, 16, 17], with a mean age reported for compound odontoma of 20.5 years [17]. Conservative surgical enucleation and curettage were performed as the treatment of choice [3]. As mentioned above, extended dental treatments such as oral surgery procedures may cause deterioration of the pediatric patient behavior associated with dental fear and dental anxiety [9]. In particular, dental anxiety indicates an excessive and unreasonable negative emotional state that might jeopardize the outcome of the procedure [18]. In such cases, anxiolysis, better known as *minimal sedation*, might be advocated to induce a state of a minimally depressed level of consciousness with ventilatory and cardiovascular functions unaffected [19]. In the present report, this effect has been positively exploited to minimize the psychological trauma and to control behavior and movements of the pediatric patient. Among benzodiazepines, diazepam has been used for many years successfully. It has been claimed that diazepam represents the safer drug for anxiety management in dentistry if compared to midazolam due to its pharmacological profile [20]. Other authors observed no differences between the behaviors of children premedicated with oral diazepam or oral midazolam [21]. Conversely, emerging evidence provided better results for oral midazolam with respect to oral diazepam when the behavioral parameters including sleep, crying, movement, and overall behavior were compared [22]. In the present case, the immediate postoperative period was uneventful, and the patient was discharged safely 90 minutes postsurgery. It must be noted however that postdischarge excessive somnolence, nausea, and emesis have been frequently reported after oral sedation in pediatric dental patients [23]. Anxiolysis with oral administration of diazepam induced positive psychological responses to treatment and safe discharge. This procedure should therefore be considered in the case of potentially prolonged surgical interventions in pediatric dental patients to avoid more invasive sedation procedures.

References

[1] P. Gonzalez-Alva, H. Inoue, Y. Miyazaki et al., "Podoplanin expression in odontomas: clinicopathological study and immunohistochemical analysis of 86 cases," *Journal of Oral Science*, vol. 53, no. 1, pp. 67–75, 2011.

[2] F. Prætorius and A. Piattelli, "Odontogenic tumours," in *WHO Classification of Tumours Pathology and Genetics of Head and Neck Tumours*, L. Barnes, J. W. Evenson, P. A. Reichart, and D. Sindransky, Eds., IARC Press, Lyon, France, 2005.

[3] J. M. Abrahams and S. A. McClure, "Pediatric odontogenic tumors," *Oral and Maxillofacial Surgery Clinics of North America*, vol. 28, no. 1, pp. 45–58, 2016.

[4] P. Boffano, E. Zavattero, F. Roccia, and C. Gallesio, "Complex and compound odontomas," *Journal of Craniofacial Surgery*, vol. 23, no. 3, pp. 685–688, 2012.

[5] C. Gervasoni, A. Tronchet, S. Spotti et al., "Odontomas: review of the literature and case reports," *Journal of biological regulators and homeostatic agents*, vol. 31, no. 2, Supplement 1, pp. 119–125, 2017.

[6] G. Isola, M. Cicciù, L. Fiorillo, and G. Matarese, "Association between odontoma and impacted teeth," *Journal of Craniofacial Surgery*, vol. 28, no. 3, pp. 755–758, 2017.

[7] J. Olak, M. Saag, S. Honkala et al., "Children's dental fear in relation to dental health and parental dental fear," *Stomatologica*, vol. 15, pp. 26–31, 2013.

[8] V. Colares, C. Franca, A. Ferreira, H. A. Amorim Filho, and M. C. A. Oliveira, "Dental anxiety and dental pain in 5- to 12-year-old children in Recife, Brazil," *European Archives of Paediatric Dentistry*, vol. 14, no. 1, pp. 15–19, 2013.

[9] Z. Jamali, E. Najafpour, Z. Ebrahim Adhami, A. Sighari Deljavan, N. A. Aminabadi, and S. Shirazi, "Does the length of dental procedure influence children's behavior during and after treatment? A systematic review and critical appraisal," *Journal of Dental Research, Dental Clinics, Dental Prospects*, vol. 12, no. 1, pp. 68–76, 2018.

[10] R. K. Pandey, S. K. Bahetwar, A. K. Saksena, and G. Chandra, "A comparative evaluation of drops versus atomized administration of intranasal ketamine for the procedural sedation of young uncooperative pediatric dental patients: a prospective crossover trial," *Journal of Clinical Pediatric Dentistry*, vol. 36, no. 1, pp. 79–84, 2011.

[11] G. Manani, C. Bacci, G. Zanette, and E. Facci, "Compound Odontoma in Anterior Mandible—A Case Report," *Dental Cadmos*, vol. 80, no. 7, pp. 357–369, 2012.

[12] E. Uma, "Compound odontoma in anterior mandible-a case report," *Malaysian Journal of Medical Sciences*, vol. 24, no. 3, pp. 92–95, 2017.

[13] R. Gedik and S. Muftuoglu, "Compound odontoma: differential diagnosis and review of the literature," *West Indian Medical Journal*, vol. 63, no. 7, pp. 793–795, 2014.

[14] B. H. De Oliveira, V. Campos, and S. Marcal, "Compound odontoma-diagnosis and treatment: three case reports," *Pediatric Dentistry*, vol. 23, no. 2, pp. 151–157, 2001.

[15] A. Kalra, E. C. Sheehy, J. Johnson, and F. McDonald, "A bag of marbles: a fascinating compound odontoma of the maxilla," *Pediatric dentistry*, vol. 40, pp. 140–142, 2018.

[16] C. Bereket, N. Cakir-Ozkan, I. Sener et al., "Complex and compound odontomas: analysis of 69 cases and a rare case of erupted compound odontoma," *Nigerian Journal of Clinical Practice*, vol. 18, no. 6, pp. 726–730, 2015.

[17] P. W. Kammerer, D. Schneider, E. Schiegnitz et al., "Clinical parameter of odontoma with special emphasis on treatment of impacted teeth—a retrospective multicentre study and literature review," *Clinical Oral Investigations*, vol. 20, no. 7, pp. 1827–1835, 2016.

[18] G. Klingberg and A. G. Broberg, "Dental fear/anxiety and dental behaviour management problems in children and adolescents: a review of prevalence and concomitant psychological factors," *International Journal of Paediatric Dentistry*, vol. 17, no. 6, pp. 391–406, 2007.

[19] "Practice guidelines for moderate procedural sedation and analgesia 2018: a report by the American Society of Anesthesiologists Task Force on Moderate Procedural Sedation and Analgesia, American Association of Oral and Maxillofacial Surgeons, American College of Radiology, American Dental Association, American Society of Dentist Anesthesiologists, and Society of Interventional Radiology," *Anesthesiology*, vol. 128, no. 3, pp. 437–479, 2018.

[20] G. Manani, E. Facco, L. Favero et al., "Comparison by means of bispectral index score, between anxiolysis induced by diazepam and sedation induced by midazolam," *Minerva Stomatologica*, vol. 60, no. 7-8, pp. 365–381, 2011.

[21] T. R. Vetter, "A comparison of midazolam, diazepam, and placebo as oral anesthetic premedicants in younger children," *Journal of Clinical Anesthesia*, vol. 5, no. 1, pp. 58–61, 1993.

[22] P. Tyagi, S. Tyagi, and A. Jain, "Sedative effects of oral midazolam, intravenous midazolam and oral diazepam in the dental treatment of children," *Journal of Clinical Pediatric Dentistry*, vol. 37, no. 3, pp. 301–306, 2013.

[23] A. Huang and T. Tanbonliong, "Oral sedation postdischarge adverse events in pediatric dental patients," *Anesthesia Progress*, vol. 62, no. 3, pp. 91–99, 2015.

3

Unusual Maxillary First Molars with C-Shaped Morphology on the Same Patient: Variation in Root Canal Anatomy

Naji Kharouf,[1] Youssef Haïkel,[1,2] and Davide Mancino[1,2]

[1]*Inserm UMR_S 1121, Biomaterials and Bioengineering, Strasbourg University, 11 Rue Humann, 67085 Strasbourg, France*
[2]*Faculty of Dental Medicine, Department of Endodontics, Strasbourg University, 8 Rue Sainte Elisabeth 67000 Strasbourg, France*

Correspondence should be addressed to Davide Mancino; mancinodacidendo@gmail.com

Academic Editor: Gianrico Spagnuolo

A maxillary first molar should be considered a four-canal tooth until proved otherwise; however, a clinician should also be aware of the possibility of the presence of C-shaped root canal configuration with or without possibility of splitting into two or three canals. The two clinical cases reported in this paper describe the endodontic treatment of two maxillary first molars, on the same patient, with uncommon anatomy: the first case is about a maxillary first molar with only one C-shaped root and one oval canal with a large buccolingual diameter, a C1 type according to Fan's classification; the second case, about the contralateral maxillary first molar, is probably the first case documented of a maxillary first molar with a C-shaped root canal and C-shaped root with complete fusion of the three roots, having a C3 configuration.

1. Introduction

Human maxillary first molars are usually considered as three-rooted teeth with four root canals for the presence of a second canal in the MB root (MB2). In addition, lateral ramifications and apical delta of the root canal system may frequently occur, increasing the probability of leaving untreated spaces after the root canal therapy [1].

Back in 1925, Hess pointed out the complexity of the root canal system of maxillary molars [2]. Later on, many articles have been published concerning the canal configurations of the maxillary first molars and of maxillary molars in general [3, 4].

Probably, a maxillary first molar is the tooth with the wider range of anatomical variations [5, 6]. Many of these anatomical variations are confirmed in literature, and the incidence of four root canals in three roots for the presence of MB2 ranges from 25% to 96.1% [3, 7].

A literature review on 8399 maxillary first molars showed that the MB root had two or more canals in 56.8% of cases [8]. The incidence of three root canals in three roots ranges from 32.14% [3] to 75% [4]. The incidence of two root canals in two roots ranges from 1.85% to 0.3% [9]. Indeed, the incidence of four roots or one root and one canal as well as the existence of C-shaped root morphology and C-shaped root canal is very rare.

According to De Moor [10], the probability of observing a C-shaped canal in a maxillary first molar was as low as 0.091%.

The C-shaped canal system is an anatomic variation occurring mostly in mandibular second molars, especially in Asian populations, although it can also occur in maxillary and other mandibular molars. A tooth is qualified as having a C-shaped root canal if it has the following features: fused roots, a longitudinal groove on the lingual or buccal surfaces of the root, and at least one cross-section of the canal that belongs to the C1, C2, or C3 configuration [11]. A C-shaped root, which always contains a C-shaped canal, results from the failure of Hertwig's epithelial sheath to develop or fuse in the furcation area in the developing stage of the teeth [12].

The C-shaped root morphology should not be confused with the taurodont root morphology, even though both are caused by an inward folding of the tooth wall [12].

The C-shaped morphology constitutes one of the most important anatomic variations without any association with

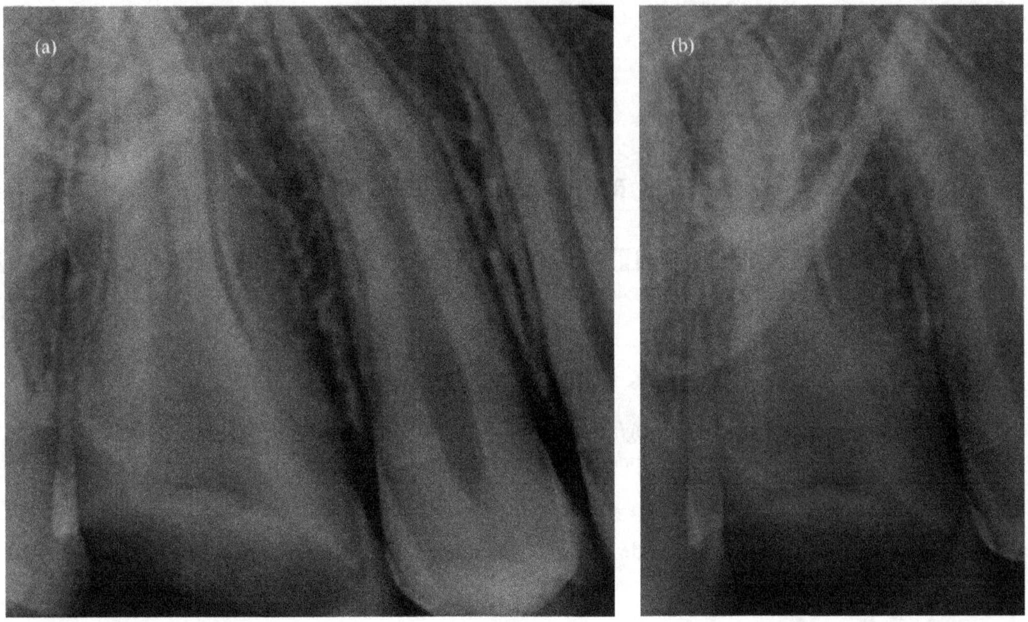

(a) (b)

FIGURE 1: (a) Preoperative orthoradial X-ray; (b) preoperative distal angulated X-ray.

genetic malformation, whereas taurodont root morphology has been found to occur as an isolated trait with familial tendency or as a feature in a wide variety of multiple-system malformation syndromes, and it does not exhibit any cross-section of the canal that belongs to the C1, C2, or C3 configuration.

The two clinical cases reported below describe the endodontic treatment of two maxillary first molars, on the same patient, with uncommon anatomy: the first case is about a maxillary first molar with only one C-shaped root and one oval canal with a large buccolingual diameter, a C1 type according to Fan's classification [13]; the second case is about the contralateral maxillary first molar with a C-shaped root and 3 root canals, a C3 type according to Fan's classification.

2. Case Reports

A 13-year-old Caucasian female was referred to the Clinic of Endodontics of Dental School, University of Strasbourg. Her medical history found no outstanding findings that would contribute to treatment problems. The 13-year-old Caucasian female was referred by his general dentist to the Clinic of Endodontics of Dental School, University of Strasbourg, for endodontic treatment on the right and left maxillary first molars, both with symptomatic irreversible pulpitis.

All procedures were done in conformity with current state of the art practices in endodontic. These included effective local anesthesia, rigorous clinical and radiographic preaccess analysis, appropriate tooth restoration to insure watertight rubber dam installation, and surgical microscopic manipulations for precision (Leica M320). The endodontic treatments were performed in one session.

2.1. Maxillary Right First Molar. Two preoperative radiographs were taken, with different angles: the first, with an orthoradial projection; the second, a distal angulated projection. They showed the presence of one wide canal and the presence of a deep mesial groove (Figure 1). After a careful study of the preoperative radiographs, the cementoenamel junction (CEJ) was identified by performing a circumferential probing with a periodontal probe. This allowed to have a three-dimensional view of the pulp canal system before starting the treatment [14]. Probing identified the presence of two middle deep grooves in the distal and mesial aspects of the tooth. After the rubber dam placement, the endodontic access cavity preparation was started with a # 012 cylindrical diamond drill and enlarged with a Start X1 ultrasonic tip (Dentsply Sirona, York, USA). The pulp chamber was localized, and the access cavity preparation was refined with the same tip. Only one oval orifice, with a large buncolingual diameter, was localized. Then, keeping the pulp chamber constantly flooded with 6% sodium hypochlorite, root canal shaping was performed, using a step down technique without initial manual scouting [15]:

(1) Initial preflaring

(2) Apical scouting

(3) Glide path

(4) Shaping

The initial mechanical preflaring was performed at first with Proglider (Dentsply Sirona) until 2/3 of estimated radiographic working length (WL) applying an in and out movement, using an endodontic engine (300 rpm/5 Ncm). After the initial preflaring, a #25 NiTiflex K-file (Dentsply

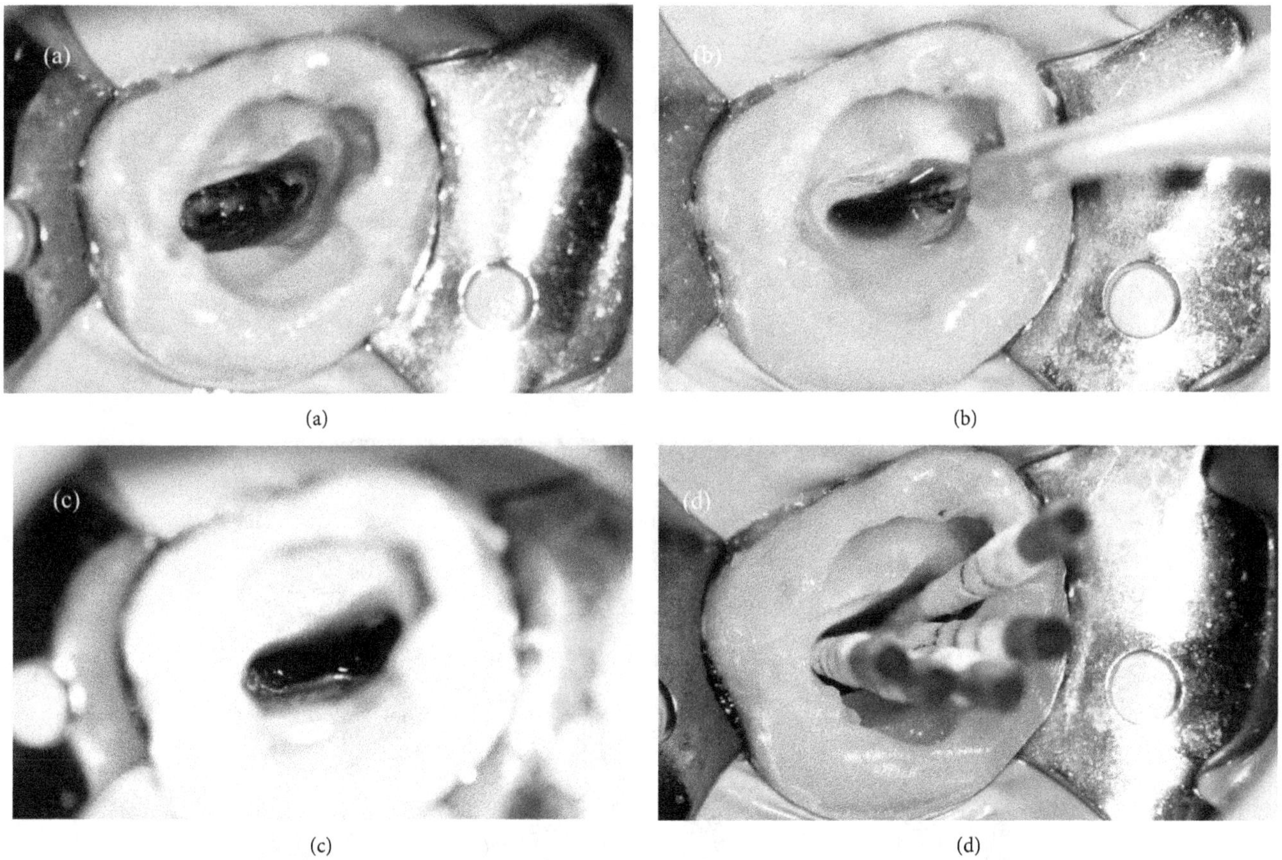

Figure 2: (a) Root canal system at the end of shaping procedure. (b, c) Root canal system during final rinse. (d) Canal drying using five sterile paper points.

Sirona) easily scouted the canal until WL + 0.5 mm. Length determination, on the buccal and palatal poles of the root canal, was taken using an electronic apex locator (Root ZX; J Morita Co., Kyoto, Japan).

Then, a mechanical glide path using Proglider at working length was performed. The tooth was shaped, as if it had two canals, buccal and palatal. Root canal shaping was performed by preparing the root canal system until the WL with ProTaper Next X1, X2, and X3 (operating at 300 rpm and torque of 5 N/cm). The foramen, on the buccal pole, was gauged introducing a # 60/02 NiTi hand file, which was snug at working length, using the pecking technique [16]. Indeed, the minor diameter on the palatal pole was gauged introducing a # 70/02 NiTi hand file.

The isthmus between the buccal and palatal poles was shaped using a bended sonofile #15 K-file (Satalec, France).

After the shaping procedure (Figure 2(a)), in order to assure proper three-dimensional cleaning of the root canal system, the final rinse solutions were activated using EndoUltra (Micro-Mega, Besançon, France): at first, an aqueous solution of EDTA 17% was activated inside the canal for 120 seconds. After rinsing with physiological saline, an aqueous solution of NaOCl 6% was activated inside the canal for 240 seconds (Figures 2(b) and 2(c)). The canal was dried three times using five sterile paper points, arranged in accordance with its palatal-buccal axis (Figure 2(d)).

In order to perform a tridimensional filling, the tooth was filled using a bioceramic material, MTA Biorep (Itena, Paris, France), creating an apical plug of 4 mm thickness (Figure 3(a)). It was mixed according to the manufacturer's instructions and delivered to the apical portion of the canal using the MAP System (Produits Dentaires, Vevey, Switzerland). The NiTi tip chosen for this case was the yellow 0.90 mm diameter instrument. After the positioning of the MTA Biorep apical plug, the bioceramic material was adapted to the canal walls using at first the yellow NiTi Machtou hand plugger, followed by the red hand plugger. The remaining part of the root canal was filled with thermoplastic gutta-percha, using EQ-V fill (Meta Biomed, Chungcheongbuk-do, Republic of Korea) in association with a canal sealer (Figure 3(b)). The final radiographs showed a well-obturated canal of this single-rooted maxillary first molar, with a large buccopalatal diameter (Figures 3(c) and 3(d)).

2.2. Maxillary Left First Molar. One week later, the contralateral maxillary first molar was treated too. Two preoperative radiographies were taken, with different angulations. The radiographs showed the presence of a deep pulp chamber floor with an unusual anatomy; two canals were clearly detectable (Figure 4). After a careful study of the preoperative radiographs, the cementoenamel junction (CEJ) was identified by performing a circumferential probing with a

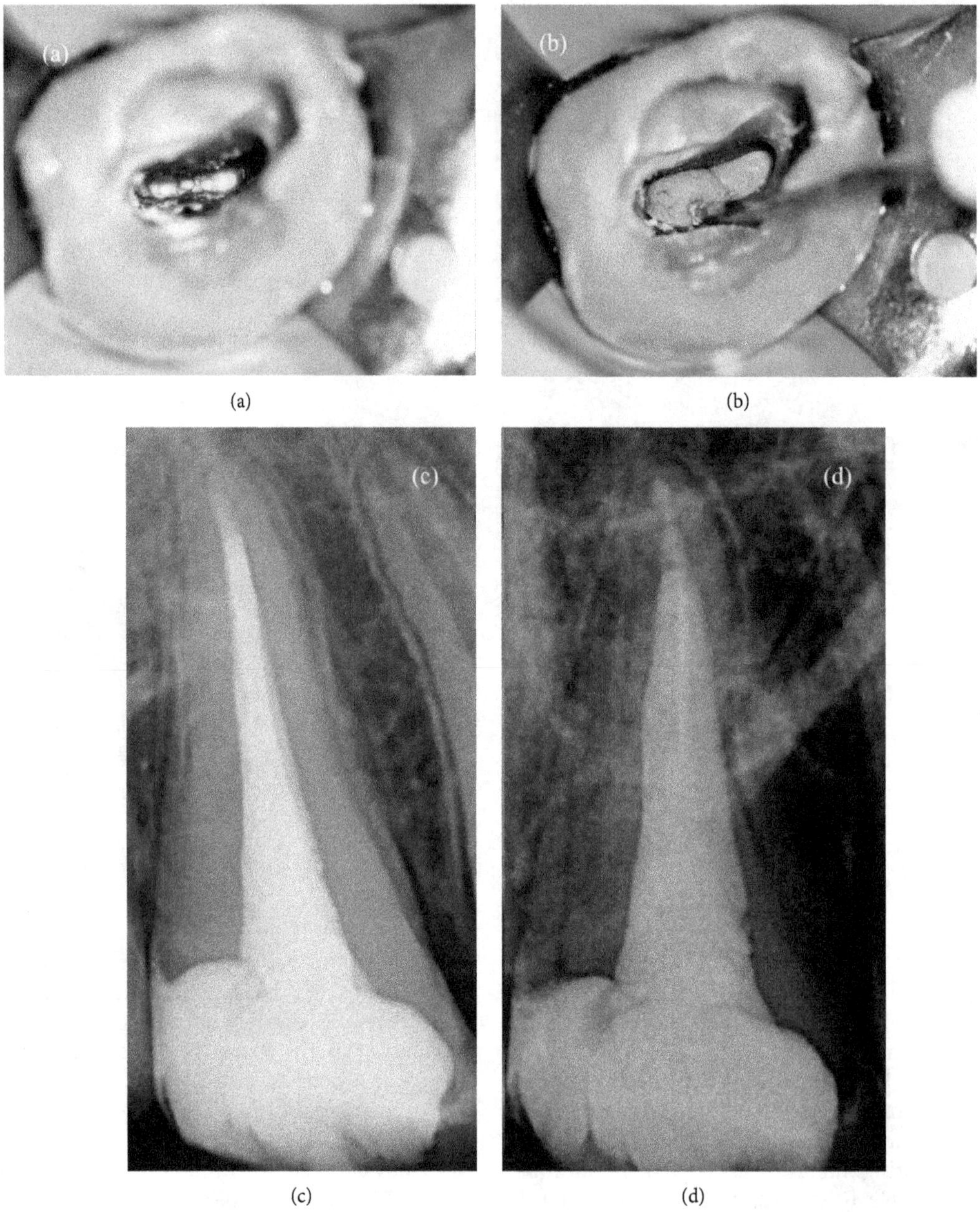

FIGURE 3: (a) Visualization of the apical plug. (b) Backfilling of the root canal system using thermoplastic gutta-percha. (c) Postoperative orthoradial X-ray. (d) Postoperative angulated X-ray.

periodontal probe. The probing identified the presence of one middle deep groove in the buccal aspect of the tooth, a feature of the C-shaped canal system. Then, for the rubber dam placement, the endodontic access cavity preparation was started with a # 012 cylindrical diamond drill and enlarged with a Start X1 (Dentsply Sirona) ultrasonic tip.

An oval MB orifice, a distal circular orifice, and a ribbon palatal orifice were easily localized with the same tip, under microscopic examination. P canal and D canal were separated by a deep isthmus (Figure 5).

The root canals were shaped with the same technique used in the first case, performed in the order: initial preflaring, apical scouting, glide path, and shaping using for the P canal PTX1, PTX2, and PTX 3 until WL and for the MB and D canal PTX1 and ProFile 25/04 until WL. MB and D canal were shaped in a minimally invasive way in order to avoid any risk of stripping. The isthmus was shaped using a bended sonofile #15 K-file.

The cleaning step was managed in the same way as the first case for the D canal, including the isthmus management, whereas for the distal and MB canal, the irrigation solutions were activated using EQ-S (Meta Biomed, Chungcheongbuk-do, Republic of Korea) with a white tip (15/02) at WL-0.5 mm.

Then, the canals were dried using sterile paper points. After having applied a drop of the AH Plus root canal sealer (Dentsply Sirona) with a coated paper point in the entrance

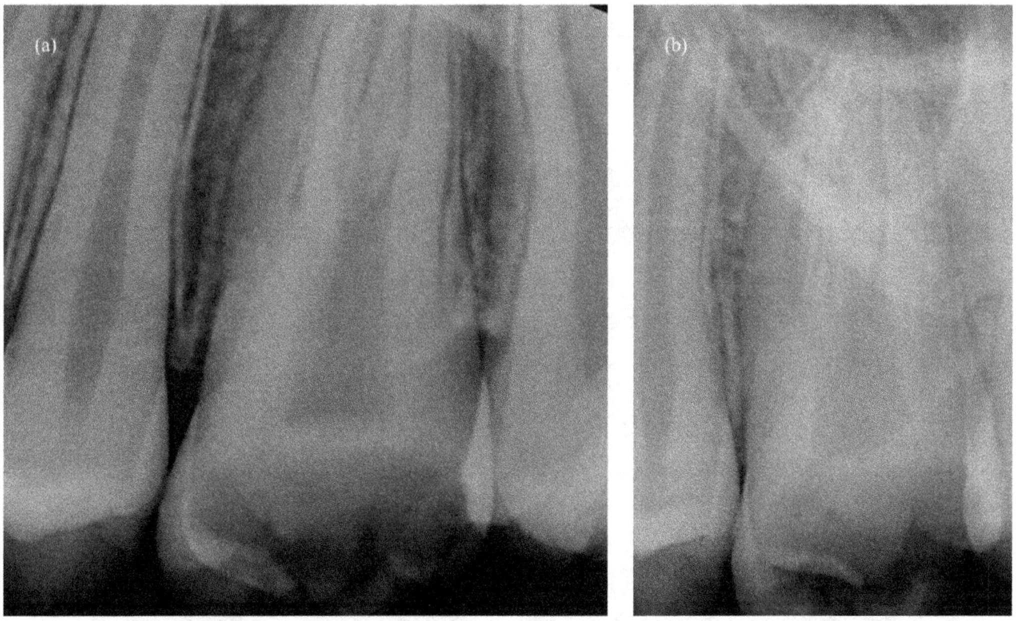

(a) (b)

Figure 4: (a) Preoperative orthoradial X-ray; (b) preoperative distal angulated X-ray.

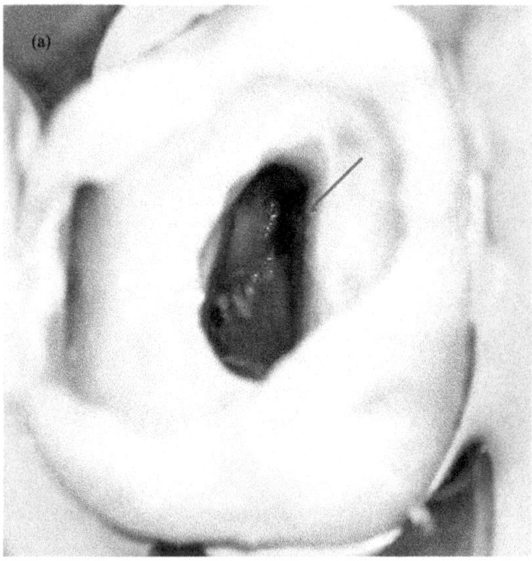

(a)

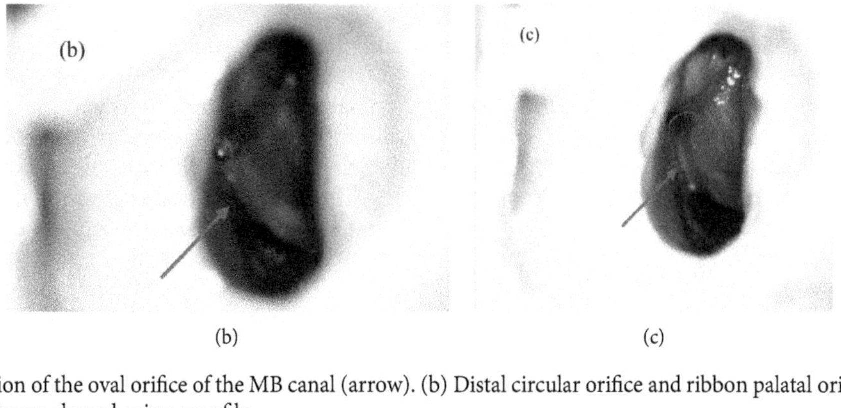

(b) (c)

Figure 5: (a) Visualization of the oval orifice of the MB canal (arrow). (b) Distal circular orifice and ribbon palatal orifice separated by a deep isthmus (arrow). (c) Isthmus shaped using sonofile.

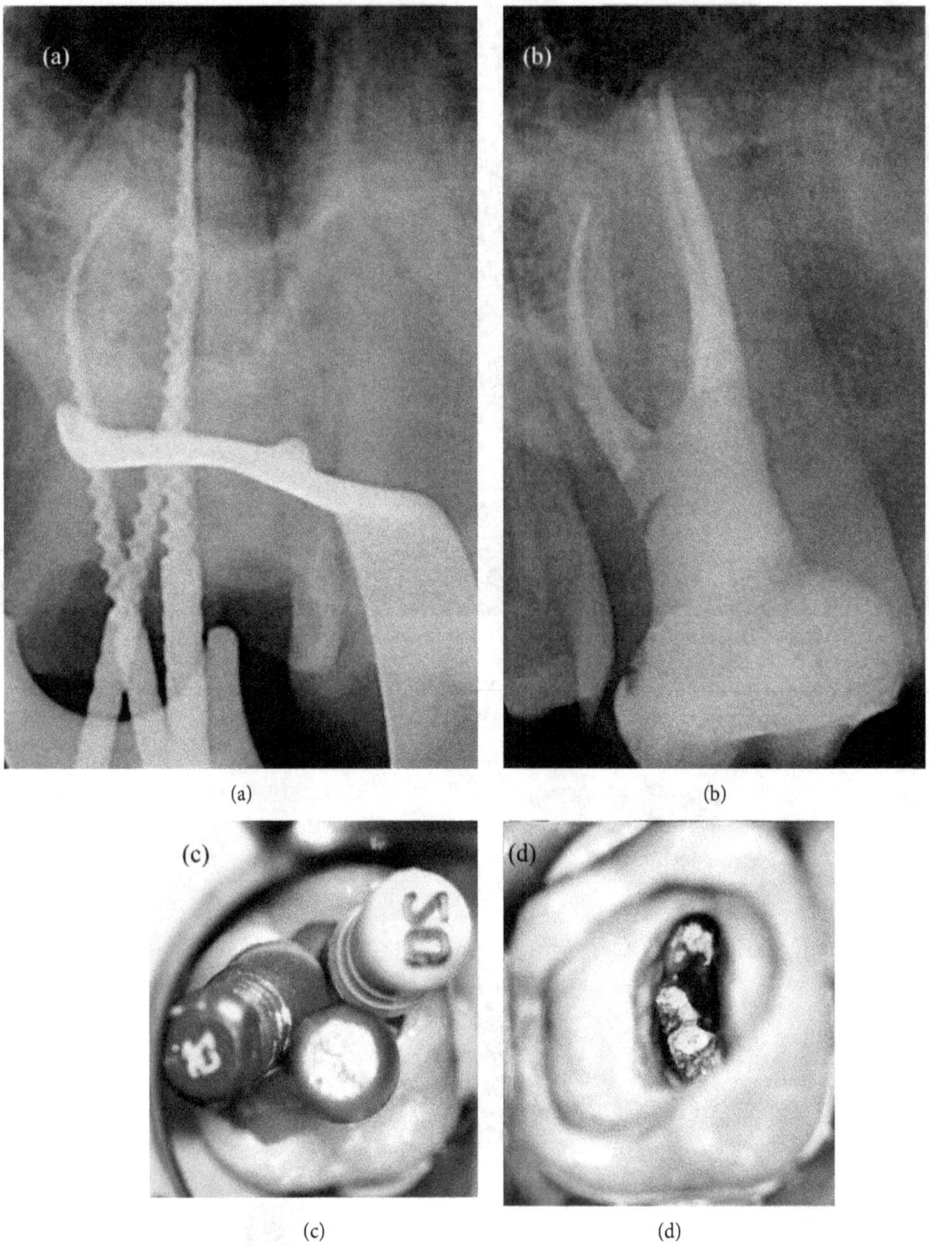

FIGURE 6: (a) Intraoperative orthoradial X-ray using verifiers. (b) Postoperative angulated X-ray. (c) Intraoperative photo with verifier. (d) Intraoperative photos after Thermafil filling.

of each canal, MB and D canals were filled with Thermafil 25 and P canal with Thermafil 35.

The carrier-based technique used in this case should be able to fill in a tridimensional way the D and MB canals shaped with a small taper as well as the isthmus between the P and D canals without any risk of root fracture (Figure 6).

3. Discussion

The maxillary first molar is a tooth that presents a high risk of missing canals, and it should be considered a four-canal tooth until proved otherwise. However, the clinician should also be aware of the possibility of the presence of C-shaped root and C-shaped root canal configuration with or without possibility of splitting into two or three canals. A limited number of reports have described the existence of C-shaped canals in maxillary first molars [11, 17–19].

The two clinical cases reported describe the endodontic treatment of two maxillary first molars, on the same patient, with C-shaped morphology.

Coronal anatomy and dimensions of both maxillary first molars were within normal limits and provided no indication of the unusual root and root canal configuration.

But, as these cases show, a painstaking preaccess analysis of the preoperative radiographs, the systematic identification

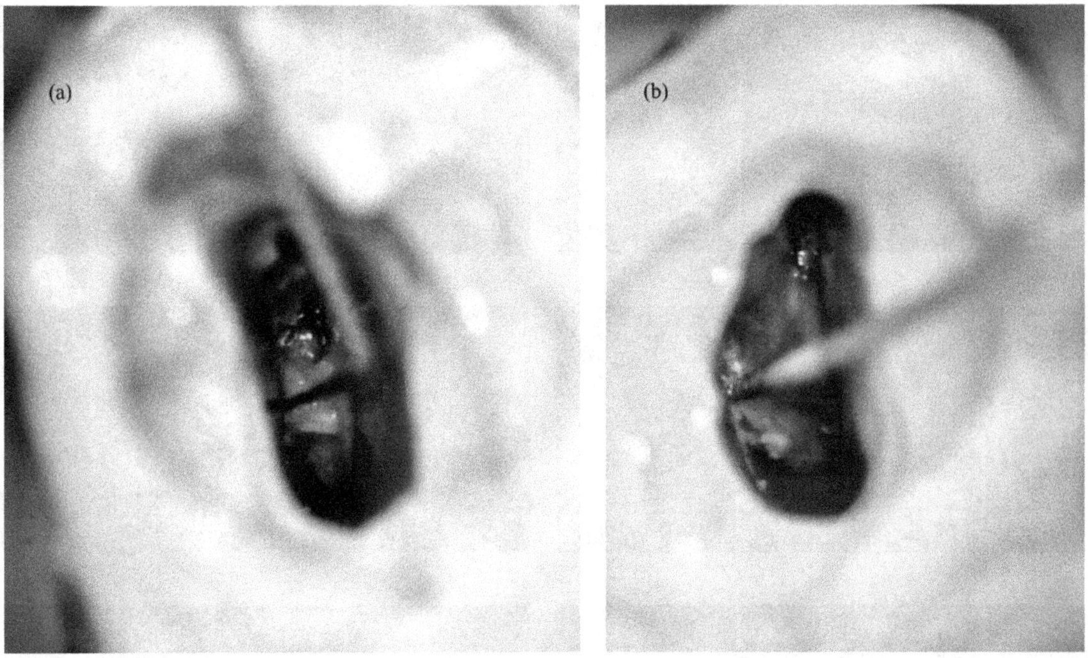

(a) (b)

FIGURE 7: (a) First case: the canal portion between the buccal and the palatal poles was shaped using a bended sonofile #15 K. (b) Second case: the isthmus between P and D canals was shaped using a bended sonofile #15 K.

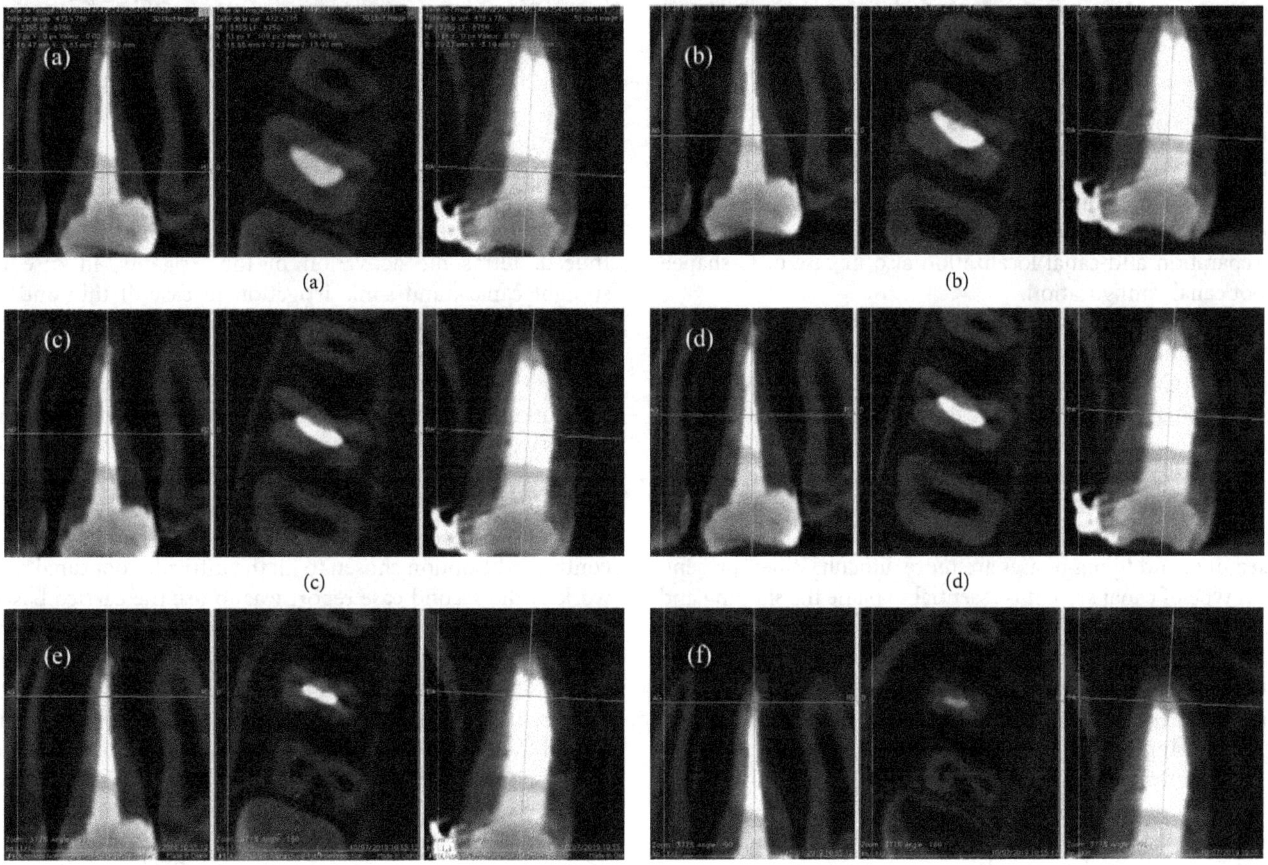

(a) (b) (c) (d) (e) (f)

FIGURE 8: (a–f) CT images of the tooth at different level display, without any doubt, the C1 configuration of this maxillary right molar.

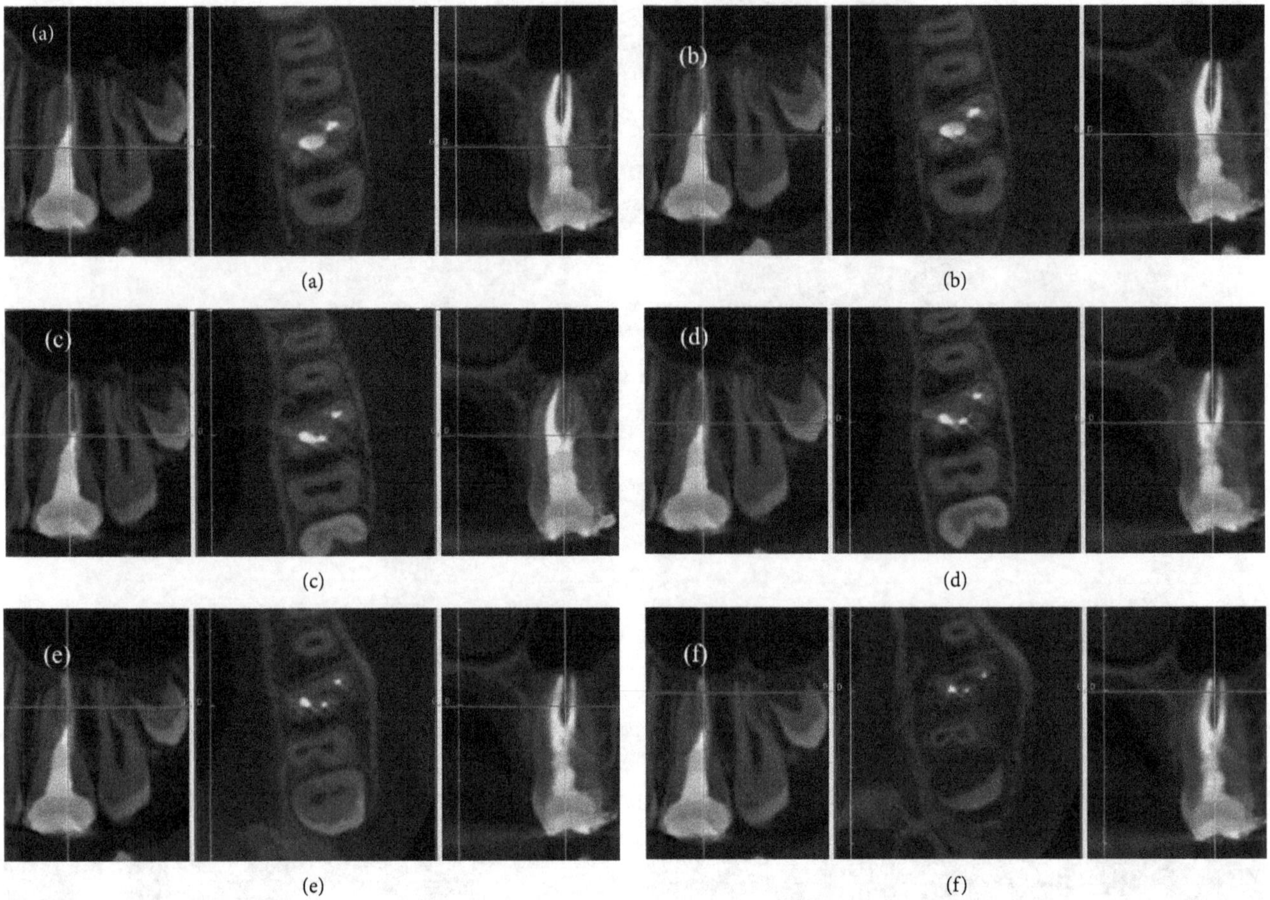

Figure 9: (a–f) CT images of the tooth at different level display, without any doubt, the C3 configuration of this maxillary left molar.

of the CEJ, using a periodontal probe, and the use of a surgical microscope coupled with the use of specific endodontic ultrasonic tips allow a high accuracy of the access cavity preparation and canal localization also in case of C-shaped root canal configuration.

On the one hand, in this case, in accordance with the AAE position statement, conventional intraoral radiography, and not CBCT, was the imaging modality of choice [20], considering the young age of the patient too. On the other hand, it is evident that if an intraoperative CBCT were needed it would be taken using limited FOV.

It is all too evident that in cases of C-shaped root canal configuration, like these maxillary first molars, the shaping, cleaning, and filling phases are more difficult. When present, this type of canal system is essential to plane the shaping and cleaning procedure.

Hence, in a C-shaped root, the first step before starting the shaping procedure is the localization of the groove, where the thickness of the dentin is smaller, in order to avoid any risk of stripping.

Therefore, in the first case report, the canal portion between the buccal and the palatal pole was shaped using a bended sonofile #15 K, as well as the isthmus between P and D canals in the second case report (Figure 7). For the same reason, in the second case, the MB and D canals were shaped in a very conservative way, using a ProFile 25/04.

Moreover, the efficacy of irrigation should be enhanced in order to improve the chemical digestion, cleaning, and disinfection of the irrigants in these irregular canal areas. Indeed, ultrasonic activation of the irrigants, in case of straight canals, and sonic irrigation in case of thin and/or curved canals should be used. These procedures allowed to obtain a tridimensional cleaning without enlarging the apical foramen and the root canal taper. The last goal was to obtain a tridimensional filling. Obviously, two different filling techniques were used to manage these two maxillary first molars. For the first case, the unique option to fill in a tridimensional way this oval canal with a very large buncolingual diameter was to use a bioceramic material, like MTA Biorep. On the contrary, the option chosen to fill the intricate root canal network of the second case report was to use the carried based technique. Five months later unawares, the young patient came back to the Clinic of Dental Surgery of Dental School, University of Strasbourg, to take a CBCT in order to plane the surgical extraction of third molars. Based on an examination of the CBCT, we could visualize the exact configuration of these maxillary first molars. Therefore, the first case reported in this paper is, without any doubt, a rare case of a maxillary first molar with one root canal and C-shaped morphology, a C1 type according to Fan's classification (Figure 8), whereas the second case is probably the first case documented of a maxillary first molar with a C-shaped root

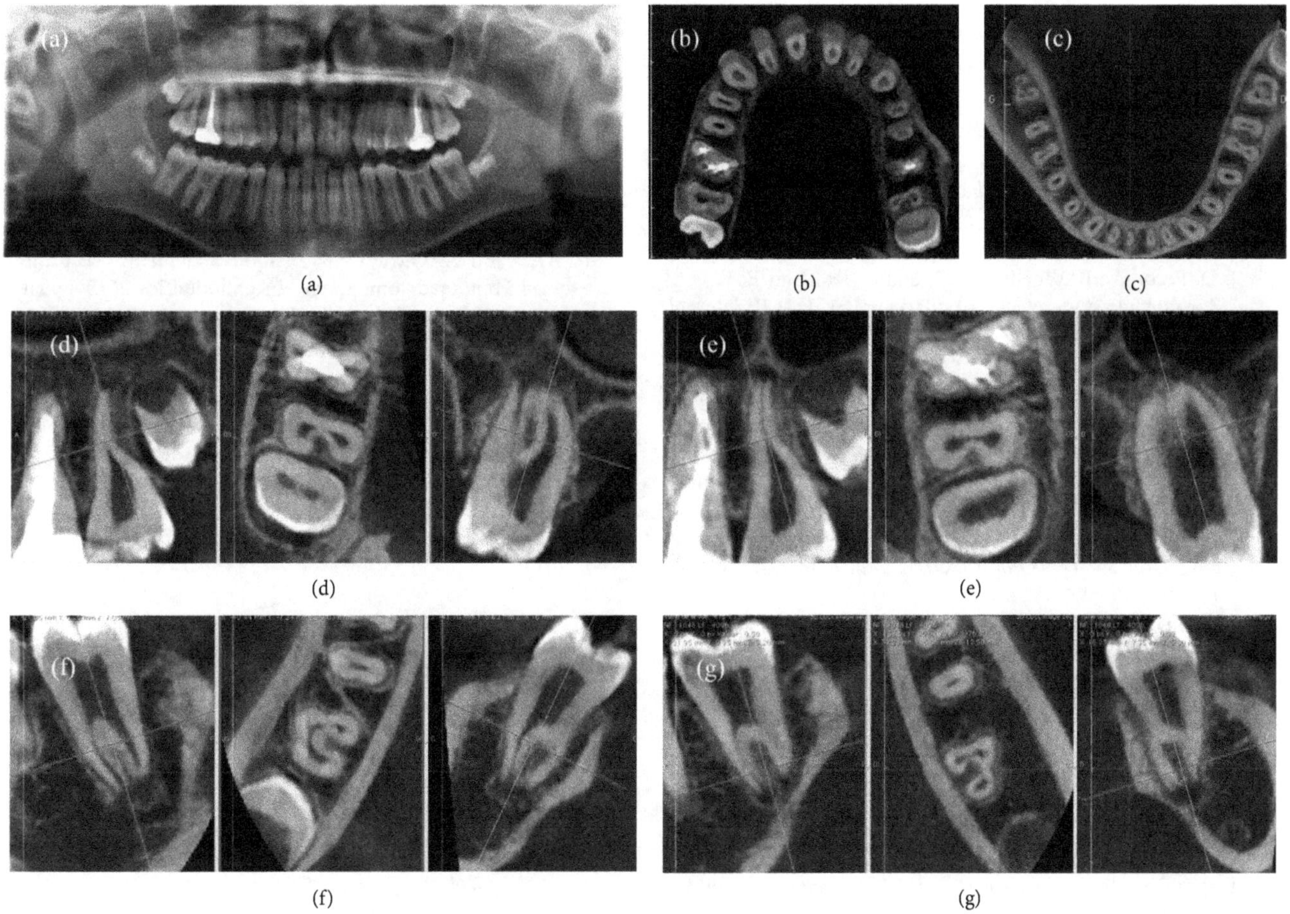

FIGURE 10: (a) Panorex; (b) CT-image of maxillary arch; (c) CT-image of mandibular arch; (d) CT images of the maxillary right second molar showing the C-shaped anatomy; (e) CT images of the maxillary left second molar showing the C-shaped anatomy; (f) CT images of the mandibular right second molar showing the C-shaped anatomy; (g) CT images of the maxillary left second molar showing the C-shaped anatomy.

canal and C-shaped root with complete fusion of the three roots, having a C3 configuration (Figure 9). It presented one independent oval MB canal and one C-shaped root canal that apically splits into two canals, whereas the cases reported by Moor presented a C-shaped root canal for the fusion of the D and P canals without the fusion of the three roots.

In general, tooth morphology is bilaterally symmetrical. According to Sabala et al., when present on one side, a C-shaped canal may be found in the contralateral tooth in over 70% of individuals [21]. Nevertheless, this convincement, that anatomical variations appear frequently contralaterally, can be partially confirmed in the present cases. Indeed, if it is true that the two first maxillary molars have both a C-shaped anatomy, it is equally true that the right maxillary first molar presents a C-shaped anatomy with only one oval root canal and the left maxillary first molar presents a C-shaped anatomy with a deep pulp chamber floor and three root canals.

Moreover, it was possible to highlight the C-shaped root morphology on both mandibular and maxillary second molars too (Figure 10). No doubt, reports of cases with unusual root and root canal anatomy have an important didactic value. Their documentation in case reports may facilitate the identification and successful management of equivalent cases, if they need an endodontic treatment.

4. Conclusion

Even if a maxillary first molar is considered a four-canal tooth, the clinician should be aware of the possibility of the presence of fewer canals with a C-shaped root canal configuration.

Therefore, the cases reported showed that the C-shaped canal system is an anatomic variation also occurring in maxillary first molars.

If conventional radiograph in these cases of C-shaped root canal for some clinicians is not clear enough, it would be better to take intraoperative CBCT, only if needed, especially on young patients.

Indeed, as these cases show, also in the case of C-shaped root canal configuration, the clinician's knowledge of the endodontic anatomy, a painstaking preaccess analysis of the preoperative radiographs, the systematic identification of the CEJ, using a periodontal probe, and the use of a surgical microscope coupled with the use of specific endodontic ultrasonic tips allow a high accuracy of the access cavity preparation and canal localization.

References

[1] B. B. Marroquin, M. A. El-Sayed, and B. Willershausen-Zonnchen, "Morphology of the physiological foramen: I. Maxillary and mandibular molars," *Journal of Endodontics*, vol. 30, no. 35, pp. 321–328, 2004.

[2] W. Hess, *The Anatomy of the Root Canals of the Teeth of the Permanent Dentition, Part 1*, William Wood and Co, New York, 1925.

[3] J. D. Pecora, J. B. Woelfel, M. D. Sousa Neto, and E. P. Issa, "Morphologic study of the maxillary molars. Part II: internal anatomy," *Brazilian Dental Journal*, vol. 3, no. 1, pp. 53–57, 1992.

[4] P. Neelakantan, C. Subbarao, R. Ahuja, C. V. Subbarao, and J. L. Gutmann, "Cone-beam computed tomography study of root and canal morphology of maxillary first and second molars in an Indian population," *Journal of Endodontics*, vol. 36, no. 10, pp. 1622–1627, 2010.

[5] F. J. Vertucci, "Root canal anatomy of the human permanent teeth," *Oral Surgery, Oral Medicine, Oral Pathology*, vol. 58, no. 5, pp. 589–599, 1984.

[6] G. Cantatore, E. Berutti, and A. Castellucci, "Missed anatomy: frequency and clinical impact," *Endodontic Topics*, vol. 15, no. 1, pp. 3–31, 2006.

[7] J. C. Kulild and D. D. Peters, "Incidence and configuration of canal systems in the mesiobuccal root of maxillary first and second molars," *Journal of Endodontics*, vol. 16, no. 7, pp. 311–317, 1990.

[8] B. M. Cleghorn, W. H. Christie, and C. C. Dong, "Root and root canal morphology of the human permanent maxillary first molar: a literature review," *Journal of Endodontics*, vol. 32, no. 9, pp. 813–821, 2006.

[9] J. J. Stropko, "Canal morphology of maxillary molars: clinical observations of canal configurations," *Journal of Endodontics*, vol. 25, no. 6, pp. 446–450, 1999.

[10] R. J. G. De Moor, "C-shaped root canal configuration in maxillary first molars," *International Endodontic Journal*, vol. 35, no. 2, pp. 200–208, 2002.

[11] H. Jafarzadeh and Y. Wu, "The C-shaped root canal configuration: a review," *Journal of Endodontics*, vol. 33, no. 5, pp. 517–523, 2007.

[12] A. Kato, A. Ziegler, N. Higuchi, K. Nakata, H. Nakamura, and N. Ohno, "Aetiology, incidence and morphology of the C-shaped root canal system and its impact on clinical endodontics," *International Endodontic Journal*, vol. 47, no. 11, pp. 1012–1033, 2014.

[13] B. Fan, G. S. Cheung, M. Fan, J. L. Gutmann, and Z. Bian, "C-shaped canal system in mandibular second molars: part I—anatomical features," *Journal of Endodontics*, vol. 30, no. 12, pp. 899–903, 2004.

[14] P. Krasner and J. Rankow, "Anatomy of the pulp-chamber floor," *Journal of Endodontics*, vol. 30, no. 1, pp. 5–16, 2004.

[15] D. Mancino and N. Kharouf, "Root canal treatment of dilacerated second maxillary premolars: planning the shaping procedure," *Journal of Clincal and Experimental Dentistry*, vol. 10, no. 6, pp. e624–e627, 2018.

[16] M. Amato, A. Iandolo, G. Pantaleo et al., "The IG- file use to gauge the apical diameter in endodontics: an *in vitro* study," *Open Dentistry Journal*, vol. 12, pp. 638–646, 2018.

[17] E. Dankner, S. Friedman, and A. Stabholz, "Bilateral C shape configuration in maxillary first molars," *Journal of Endodontics*, vol. 16, no. 12, pp. 601–603, 1990.

[18] C. W. Newton and S. McDonald, "A C-shaped canal configuration in a maxillary first molar," *Journal of Endodontics*, vol. 10, no. 8, pp. 397–399, 1984.

[19] Z. Yılmaz, B. Tuncel, A. Serper, and S. Calt, "C-shaped root canal in a maxillary first molar: a case report," *International Endodontic Journal*, vol. 39, no. 2, pp. 162–166, 2006.

[20] "AAE and AAOMR Joint Position Statement: use of cone beam computed tomography in endodontics 2015 update," *Journal of Endodontics*, vol. 41, no. 9, pp. 1393–1396, 2015.

[21] C. L. Sabala, F. W. Benenati, and B. R. Neas, "Bilateral root or root canal aberrations in a dental school patient population," *Journal of Endodontics*, vol. 20, no. 1, pp. 38–42, 1994.

4

Management of a Complex Dentoalveolar Traumatic Injury with Multiple Avulsions

Anita Thakur and Seema Thakur

Department of Pediatric and Preventive Dentistry, H.P Government Dental College and Hospital Shimla, Himachal Pradesh, India

Correspondence should be addressed to Seema Thakur; cima2009@hotmail.com

Academic Editor: Andrea Scribante

Background. Dentoalveolar trauma is a major cause of tooth loss in children. Avulsion, luxation, crown, and root fracture are the injuries to primary and permanent dentition. The incidence of trauma for maxillary anterior teeth ranges for 4%-91%. Many case reports have been published regarding the treatment of trauma to anterior teeth; however, case reports comprising multiple avulsions including canines and premolars are rare in literature. *Method.* After mouth rinsing was done with 2% betadine solution, the luxated teeth numbers 31 and 42 were repositioned into the tooth socket and were secured with the composite resin-wire splint. Tooth number 32 was extracted because it was disarticulated from the socket, and the socket was disrupted because of the alveolar fracture. The maxillary avulsed teeth could not be reimplanted because of the alveolar socket damage which was due to the alveolar bone fracture. *Results.* The patient was reevaluated for the removable prosthesis in recall visits; the patient was well adapted to the appliance with no complaints regarding mastication and speech. The patient was advised to report periodically for further adjustments in the prosthesis and for radiographic evaluation. *Conclusions.* This case report includes proper history taking, diagnosis, and treatment of a complex dentoalveolar trauma along with short-term prosthetic rehabilitation for improvement of aesthetics, phonetics, and mastication of growing child.

1. Background

Dentoalveolar trauma is one of the main causes of tooth loss in pediatric population. The trauma can lead to tooth loss via variety of ways like untreated avulsion, root resorption, or extraction due to acute injury [1]. These injuries of the teeth and supporting structures to the children can pose a major challenge to the practitioner because of the dynamic state of occlusal development [2–4]. Avulsion, luxation, crown, and root fracture are the injuries to primary and permanent dentition. Injury to deciduous teeth may damage the underlying permanent tooth; however, if trauma occurs to the permanent teeth, it may compromise their long-term prognosis [3]. The most common cause of dental injury was fall, followed by sports [5]. The incidence of trauma for maxillary anterior teeth and premolars is reported in between 4%-91% and 0.6%, respectively. The incidence reported for luxation injury is 26%, for alveolar fracture 5.5%, for soft tissue injury 47%-58%, and 4%-22% for avulsion in the literature [6–9]. This great variation in reporting rates could be attributed to many factors including type of study, trauma classification, study size and population, geographical area, and different cultural behaviours [10]. Many case reports have been published describing the treatment of avulsed permanent incisors but the treatment following multiple avulsions including canines and premolars has been rarely found in the literature. This case report includes history taking, diagnostic considerations, and immediate treatment plan followed by transitional prosthetic rehabilitation for young child.

2. Case Report

An 11-year-old male child was referred to the Department of Pediatric and Preventive Dentistry, Himachal Pradesh Govt Dental College and Hospital (HPGDC) Shimla, India, following severe dentoalveolar trauma along with soft tissue injuries. The parents reported that when the child was returning from the school, he got hit by a motorcycle and fell on the ground. At the time of the injury, the child spat out many permanent and deciduous teeth of both the arches. The patient had two episodes of vomiting and history of oral bleeding at the time of the traumatic injury. There was no history of loss of consciousness, seizures, and bleeding from ear and nose. The mother collected the knockedout teeth in an empty box, and the child was taken to the nearby regional hospital. The soft tissue wounds were debrided, and lacerated wounds were sutured by the physician attending the child, and the patient was referred to Indira Gandhi Medical College and Hospital (IGMC), Shimla. The patient was attended in the emergency department of the medical hospital and further referred to HPGDC for additional care because of the severity of dentoalveolar trauma.

The patient arrived in the Department of Pediatric and Preventive Dentistry 24 hr after the trauma. On extraoral examination, the face was apparently symmetrical with diffuse swellings present with respect to the upper lip and chin regions. Sutures were present on the right side of upper lip extending beyond the vermilion border and chin region. Mandibular movements were restricted, and tenderness on palpation was present with respect to chin region and bilateral lower molar region (Figure 1(a)).

Intraoral examination revealed deranged occlusion with inadequate mouth opening, and sutures were present on the right side of the upper and lower lips. Multiple bruises and lacerations were also visible. There was an avulsion of teeth numbers 11, 12, 21, 22, 23, 24, 65, and 41. Tooth number 32 was disarticulated from the tooth socket along with the fracture of labial and lingual cortical plates. Teeth numbers 31 and 42 were luxated from the tooth socket (Figures 2(b) and 2(c)). Extensive intraoral damage to the soft tissue was noted in the maxillary area with multiple abrasions and lacerations. Sutures were present in the maxillary alveolar ridge area which was placed after compressing and approximating the tooth socket area in the regional hospital (Figure 1(b)). The dentoalveolar fracture with multiple avulsions was clearly evident from the computed tomography (CT) scan (64 Slice MDCT scanner Light Speed VCT-XTE GE Healthcare, Grandview Blvd. Waukesha, WI, U.S.A) of the patient which was performed in the IGMC (Figures 3(a)–3(c) and 4).

An informed verbal and written consent was taken from the patient and parents, respectively. The patient was taken to the minor operating theatre for the treatment under local anaesthesia. The mouth rinsing was done with 2% betadine solution (Cipladine, Cipla Ltd. Mumbai, India) before the procedure. The parents were informed about the risks, benefits, and poor prognosis of the proposed treatment. The luxated teeth numbers 31 and 42 were repositioned into the tooth socket and were secured with the composite resin-wire splint [1] (Figure 2(a)). Tooth number 32 was extracted because it was disarticulated from the socket, and the socket was disrupted because of the alveolar fracture (Figures 3(a)–3(c)). The maxillary avulsed teeth could not be reimplanted because of the alveolar socket damage which was due to the alveolar bone fracture (Figures 3 and 4).

Oral hygiene instructions were given, and the patient was discharged to the care of his parents. The parents were asked to keep the teeth as clean as possible, and a chlorohexidine mouthwash was given for rinsing. Amoxicillin with clavulanic acid (375 mg t.i.d.) and acetaminophen was prescribed as discharge medicine. Patient was advised to take soft diet for 10-14 days.

After 10 days, satisfactory postoperative healing was there and the sutures were removed. The patient was followed for 2, 4, and 6 weeks. The healed maxillary and mandibular arches can be appreciated in Figures 1(d) and 2(b). After 4 weeks, the splint was removed as per the Guidelines of International Association of Dental Traumatology (Revised in June 2020) [11] and American Associations of Endodontists [12]. Maxillary and mandibular arch alginate (Plastalgin, Septodont Healthcare India Pvt. Ltd. Raigad, Maharashtra, India) impressions were taken after 6 weeks of soft tissue healing to fabricate an acrylic prosthesis (Figures 1(c)–1(f)). Teeth numbers 31 and 42 were asymptomatic clinically as well as radiographically with intact lamina dura. The patient was reevaluated for the removable prosthesis in recall visits, and the patient was well adapted to the appliance with no complaints regarding mastication and speech. The patient was advised to report periodically for further adjustments in the prosthesis in case of permanent tooth eruption and for radiographic evaluation.

3. Discussion`

Traumatic dental injury is not a result of a disease but can be a consequence of many factors that will get accumulated through entire life if not treated properly [13]. Emotional preparation of the child is required prior to the dental treatment. Trauma can increase patient's apprehension towards the treatment. However, extensive trauma to dentoavleolar part requires immediate intervention and treatment for the stability of child's physical and emotional integrity [14]. It also prepares the child and the family for an expensive and extensive restorative future [2]. This case report involved extensive lesions of extraoral soft tissue over lip and chin area, teeth, and alveolar bone which are rarely seen in dental practice as most of the dental avulsions affect only a single tooth [14–16]. The most common teeth involved in the dental trauma were maxillary incisors as compared to mandibular incisors because any blow to the mandibular teeth was dissipated due to nonrigid connection of the mandible to the base of cranium [13].

According to the studies in the literature, boys had suffered more traumatic injuries than girls which could be attributed to the behavioural factors as boys tend to be more energetic and inclined towards outdoor activities and contact sports [5]. Severe damage was occurred to the left half of the maxilla following loss of multiple permanent teeth and fracture of the alveolar bone. The permanent maxillary anterior teeth and premolars could not be reimplanted because of the damage to the alveolar bone [2]. The deciduous tooth was also not reimplanted because of its proximity to permanent tooth germ, and it can cause significant alteration to the succedaneous tooth [17]. It may result in worst consequences like dilacerations, enamel hypoplasia, imapctions, or deviation from the normal path of eruption. Some studies have also reported radicular cyst associated with the replanted

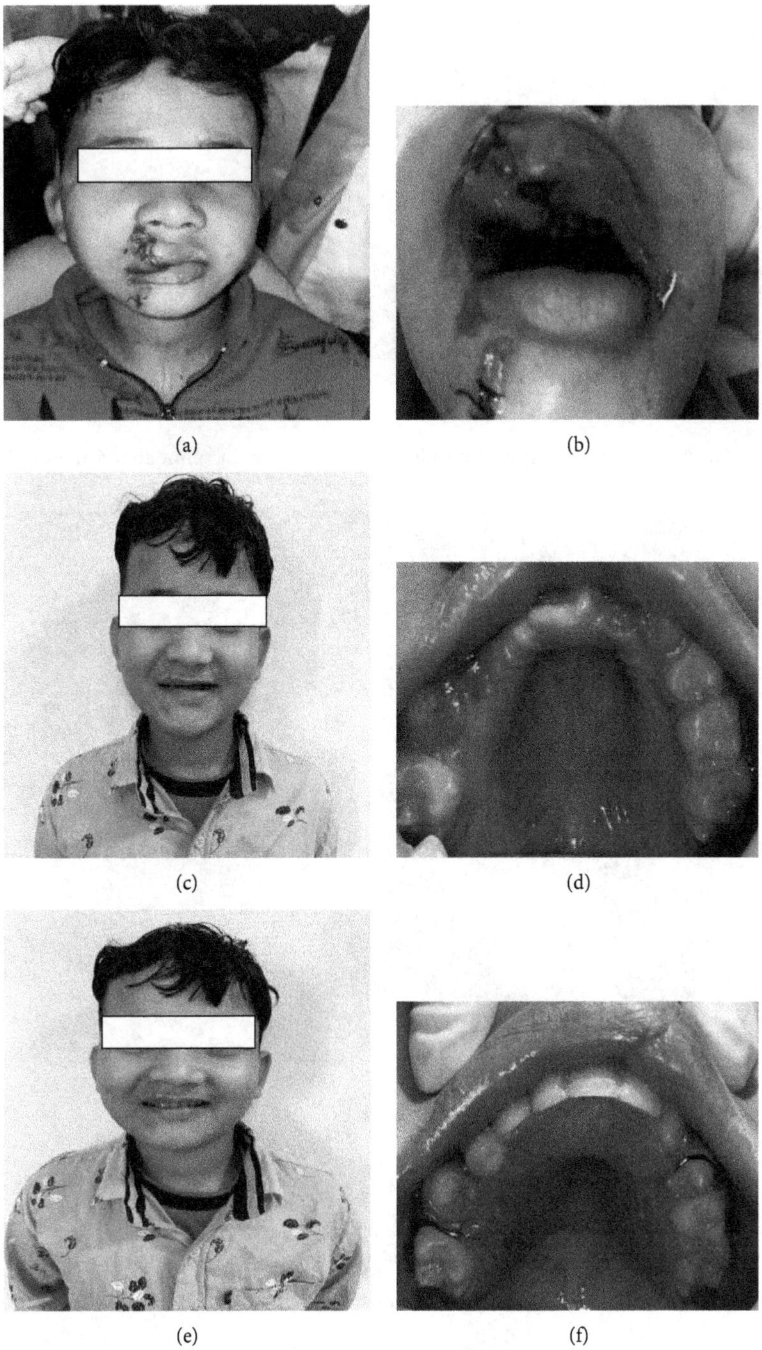

Figure 1: (a–f) Preoperative and postoperative (installation of removable prosthesis in the maxillary arch) photographs of the pat.

primary tooth [18]. Also, it should be noted that the dry storage time beyond 60 minutes had a strong relationship with replacement resorption [19]. Poor prognosis of the treatment done can develop because of periodontal ligament death, pulp necrosis which leads to ankylosis, internal resorption, replacement resorption, and eventually the loss of tooth [19]. The main reason for loss of replanted teeth is resorption. The risk of early resorption is increased in teeth which are having additional damage or contamination or which are kept in dry extraoral conditions for more than 15 min. The teeth, whose periodontal ligaments have dried, destroyed, and removed from the root surface, result in replacement resorption and get fused with the alveolar bone [20].

After healing of the alveolar tissue, maxillary prosthesis was given for restoration of aesthetics and phonetics of the young child [2, 14] (Figures 1(d)–1(f)). The mandibular teeth were splinted with wire composite splint [1–3, 21]. This nonrigid splint was removed after 4 weeks [19, 21] as "splinting for 4 weeks was shown to influence the healing pattern" [19]. The dental trauma healing mainly depends upon firstly on repositioning and splinting and secondly, the infection prevention. Antibiotic prophylaxis was mainly used for controlling

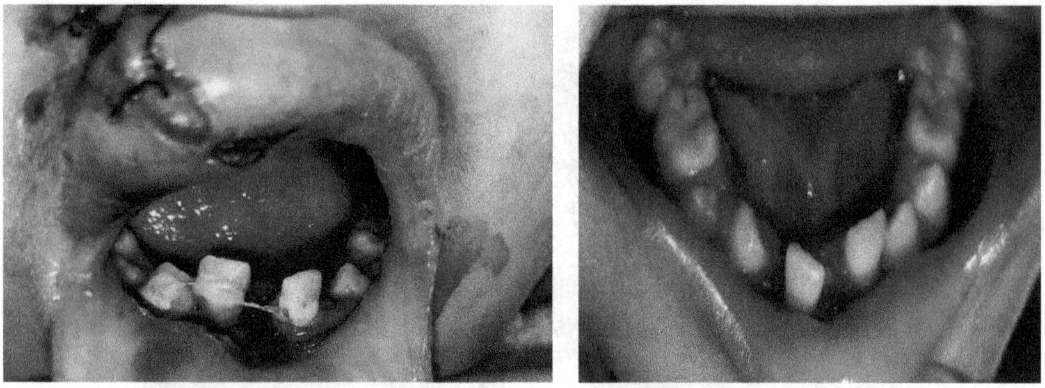

(a) (b)

Figure 2: (a) Composite wire splint and (b) removal of splint after 4 weeks.

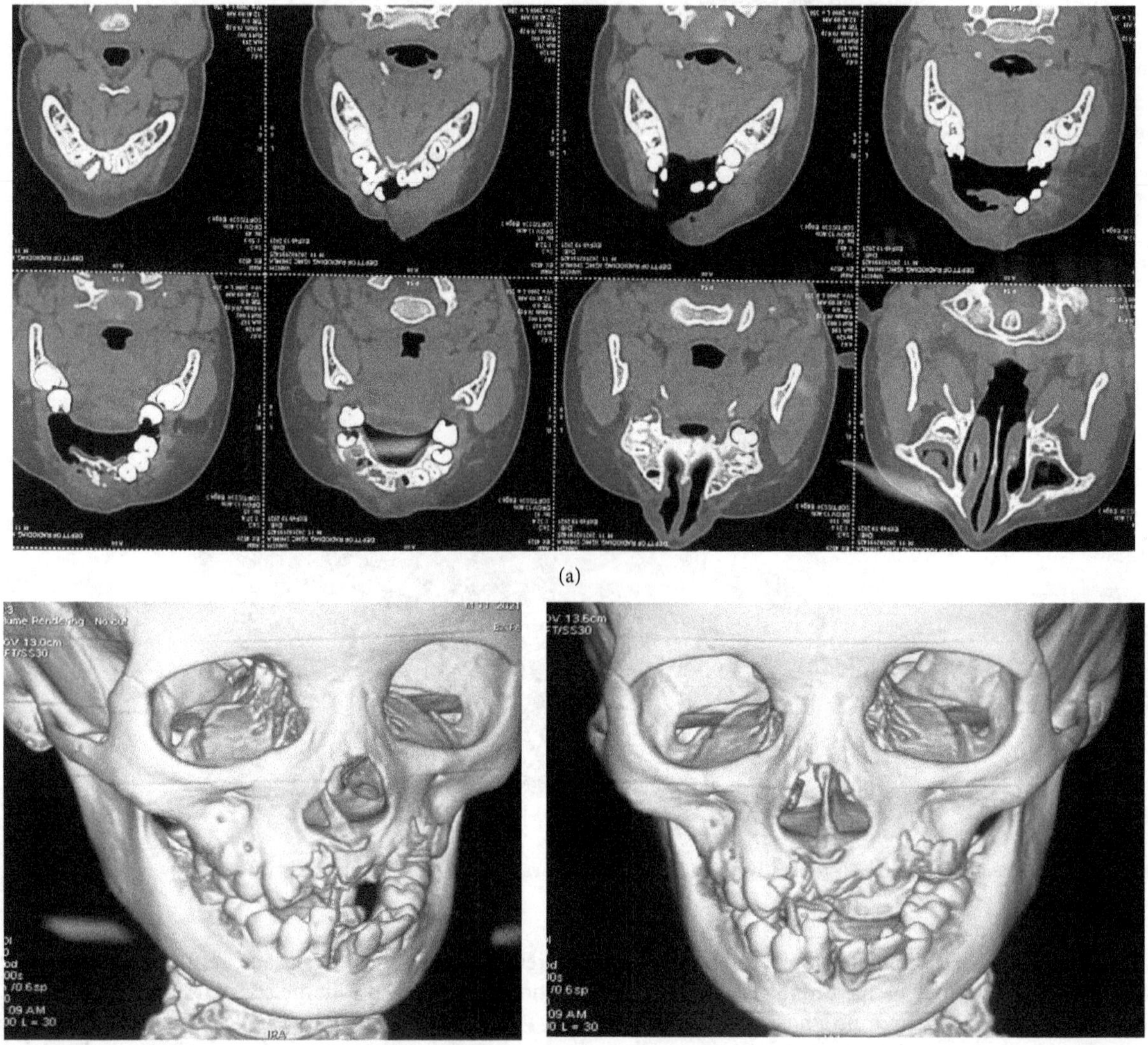

(a)

(b) (c)

Figure 3: (a–c) Computed tomography (CT) scan showing multiple avulsions along with alveolar bone fracture.

soft tissue infections; however, its role to influence the wound healing has not been found in traumatic dental injuries. In clinical studies, application of splints in some cases can add extra damage to the periodontal and pulpal tissue [22].

There are many consequences after early loss of permanent teeth, and the indication of a prosthetic rehabilitation with miniscrew-assisted provisional restorations in aesthetic zone may be an alternative for an effective treatment. This

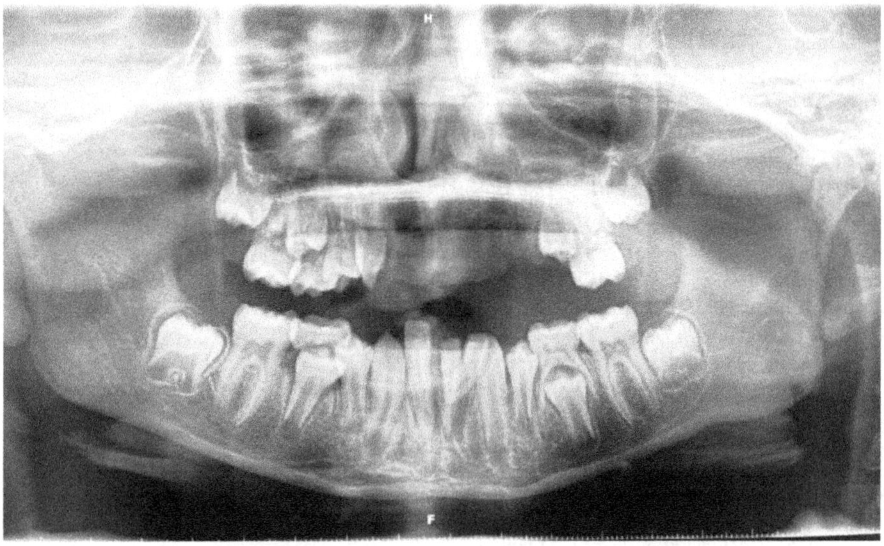

FIGURE 4: Radiograph showing multiple avulsions of the teeth.

technique can also be used in growing patients as miniscrews have been demonstrated to have excellent mechanical properties and can support the patient until adult age, when conventional implants can be placed [23, 24]. Along with restoring aesthetics, it will also help in avoiding any alterations in phonetic and masticatory functions. However, it prepares the child psychologically to accept and collaborate with the proposed treatment in order to be socially reintegrated [14].

Within the limitation of the present case report, it was a matter of trying what was believed to be the best approach for this patient. However, reviewing the literature, it is apparent that the approach to deal with these aspects of trauma needs constant update, which is based on our clinical decisions.

4. Summary

To summarize, knowledge and ability of the professional are put to test while handling a pediatric traumatic emergency. Acute dental treatment is an important aspect following dental traumatic injuries. Awareness regarding tooth storage media and preventive education programs should be instituted at the level of parents (including pregnant mothers), school teachers, and common people so that they can contribute to better prognosis of traumatized tooth. Another important aspect is to improve knowledge among general dentists regarding aetiology, diagnosis, treatment, and complications of trauma.

References

[1] H. Sobczak-Zagalska and K. Emerich, "Best splinting methods in case of dental injury- a literature review," *The Journal of Clinical Pediatric Dentistry*, vol. 44, no. 2, pp. 71–78, 2020.

[2] M. M. Sheroan and M. W. Roberts, "Management of a complex dentoalveolar trauma with multiple avulsions: a case report," *Dental Traumatology*, vol. 20, no. 4, pp. 222–225, 2004.

[3] J. E. Rutar, "Paediatric dentistry avulsion: case reports," *Australian Dental Journal*, vol. 42, no. 6, pp. 361–366, 1997.

[4] K. M. Sangeetha, P. Surendra, N. M. Roshan, V. V. S. Reddy, R. G. Chaur, and S. B. Srinivasa, "Management of dentoalveolar fracture with multiple avulsions: a case report with three years follow-up," *International Journal of Case Reports and Images*, vol. 5, no. 12, pp. 835–838, 2014.

[5] P. Juneja, S. Kulkarni, and S. Raje, "Prevalence of Traumatic Dental Injuries and their relation with predisposing factors among 8-15 years old school children of Indore city, India," *Medicine and Pharmacy Reports*, vol. 91, no. 3, pp. 328–335, 2018.

[6] E. B. Bastone, T. J. Freer, and J. R. McNamara, "Epidemiology of dental trauma: a review of the literature," *Australian Dental Journal*, vol. 45, no. 1, pp. 2–9, 2000.

[7] A. S. Kaba and S. C. Marechaux, "A fourteen-year follow-up study of traumatic injuries to the permanent dentition," *Journal of Dentistry for Children*, vol. 56, no. 6, pp. 417–425, 1989.

[8] J. E. Onetto, M. T. Flores, and M. L. Garbarino, "Dental trauma in children and adolescents in Valparaiso, Chile," *Endodontics & Dental Traumatology*, vol. 10, no. 5, pp. 223–227, 1994.

[9] N. Altay and H. C. Gungor, "A retrospective study of dentoalveolar injuries of children in Ankara, Turkey," *Dental Traumatology*, vol. 17, no. 5, pp. 201–204, 2001.

[10] U. Glendor, "Aetiology and risk factors related to traumatic dental injuries–a review of the literature," *Dental Traumatology*, vol. 25, no. 1, pp. 19–31, 2009.

[11] C. Bourguignon, N. Cohenca, E. Lauridsen et al., "International Association of Dental Traumatology guidelines for the management of traumatic dental injuries: 1. Fractures and luxations," *Dental Traumatology*, vol. 36, no. 4, pp. 314–330, 2020.

[12] American Association of Endodontists, "Recommended guidelines of the AAE for the treatment of traumatic dental

injuries," http://www.aae.org/specialty/wp-content/uploads/sites/2/2019/02/19_TraumaGuidelines.pdf.

[13] M. C. Patel and S. G. Sujan, "The prevalence of traumatic dental injuries to permanent anterior teeth and its relation with predisposing risk factors among 8–13 years school children of Vadodara city: an epidemiological study," *Journal of the Indian Society of Pedodontics and Preventive Dentistry*, vol. 30, no. 2, pp. 151–157, 2012.

[14] M. C. M. Freitas, A. R. F. de Castilho, S. N. Marta, L. A. Francischone, C. E. Carrara, and S. de Oliveira Braga Franzolin, "Consequences and treatment after multiple avulsions of deciduous teeth - a case report," *Dental Traumatology*, vol. 24, no. 3, pp. e381–e384, 2008.

[15] M. S. N. P. Corrêa and M. T. Wanderley, *Sucesso no atendimento odontopediátrico: aspectos psicológicos*, pp. 461–473, aspectos psicológicos, Santos: São Paulo, Brazil, 2002.

[16] M. Sabas, C. Alonso, D. M. Pascual, M. A. Castillo, and G. Weisstaub, "Frecuencia de traumatismos dentarios en pediatria," *Revista de la Asociación Odontológica Argentina*, vol. 88, pp. 611–614, 2000.

[17] P. A. Martins-Júnior, F. A. D. A. S. Franco, R. V. de Barcelos, L. S. Marques, and M. L. Ramos-Jorge, "Replantation of avulsed primary teeth: a systematic review," *International Journal of Paediatric Dentistry*, vol. 24, no. 2, pp. 77–83, 2014.

[18] A. S. Al-Khayatt and L. E. Davidson, "Complications following replantation of a primary incisor: a cautionary tale," *British Dental Journal*, vol. 198, no. 11, pp. 687-688, 2005.

[19] S. B. Misra and K. J. Toumba, "A combined avulsion and root fracture/avulsion trauma with ten years review," *European Archives of Paediatric Dentistry*, vol. 9, no. 3, pp. 153–159, 2008.

[20] M. Donaldson and M. J. Kinirons, "Factors affecting the time of resorption on avulsed and replanted incisor teeth in children," *Dental Traumatology*, vol. 17, no. 5, pp. 205–209, 2001.

[21] A. E. Koyuturk and A. Kusgoz, "Multiple dentoalveolar traumatic injury: a case report (3 years follow up)," *Dental Traumatology*, vol. 24, no. 4, pp. e16–e19, 2008.

[22] J. O. Andreasen, E. Lauridsen, and F. M. Andreasen, "Contradictions in the treatment of traumatic dental injuries and ways to proceed in dental trauma research," *Dental Traumatology*, vol. 26, no. 1, pp. 16–22, 2010.

[23] D. Michelogiannakis, F. Javed, and H. Vastardis, "Mini-screw implant-supported pontics for the transitional management of missing permanent maxillary lateral incisors in children and adolescents: a review of currently available evidence," *European Archives of Paediatric Dentistry*, vol. 21, no. 3, pp. 285–293, 2020.

[24] M. F. Sfondrini, P. Gandini, R. Alcozer, P. K. Vallittu, and A. Scribante, "Failure load and stress analysis of orthodontic miniscrews with different transmucosal collar diameter," *Journal of the Mechanical Behavior of Biomedical Materials*, vol. 87, pp. 132–137, 2018.

5

Possibility of using Flexible Dentures over Iliac Bone Graft in Adolescent Patients with Ameloblastoma: A 9-Month Follow-Up Clinical Report

Ammar Belal,[1] **Bassil Monther**,[2] **and Wael Alzarif**[3]

[1]*Master's Degree, Clinical Instructor, School of Dentistry, Hama University, Removable prosthodontic Department, Hama, Syria*
[2]*Professor, Doctorate, School of Dentistry, Hama University, Removable prosthodontic Department, Hama, Syria*
[3]*Oral and Maxillofacial Surgery, Syrian Board of Medical Specialties, Head of Oral and Maxillofacial Surgery, National Hospital of Hama, Hama, Syria*

Correspondence should be addressed to Ammar Belal; dr.ammar.belal@gmail.com

Academic Editor: Giuseppe Colella

Introduction. The use of bone grafts is a common procedure after excision and reconstruction of the mandible, although it is rare in children and adolescents due to incomplete growth, which means a long transition period until reaching an appropriate age for implants or more predictable outcomes. *Case Report.* This article describes a 9-month follow-up of the use of a flexible denture above a bone graft taken from the anterior iliac crest for adolescent patients with resected mandible due to ameloblastoma. Taking into account prosthetic considerations, radiography, and clinical observation, no complications were seen with the graft. *Conclusion.* It is safe to use a flexible denture as a prosthetic over an iliac bone graft block during the healing period.

1. Introduction

Ameloblastoma is a rare tumor, but it affects all ages, especially between the second and fifth decades, and equally, in both sexes, its incidence in the lower jaw is 80% compared to the upper jaw. Although it is a benign tumor, it has a pandemic effect because it grows without symptoms and tends to be recurrent in 90% of conservative approach (enucleation, marsupialization, or curettage) [1–4]. Therefore, to get the best results, 1 to 2 cm of healthy bone around the tumor must be excised, whatever its type (multicystic, peripheral, and unicystic tumors) [5–7]. This excision may lead to a dramatic collapse of the patient's swallowing, pronunciation, chewing, and aesthetic functions, and the loss of anatomical structures will make the procedures of prosthetics difficult, especially in cases of the lower jaw, in addition to the deviation of the remaining segment toward the defect side which may lead to the loss of occlusal contacts on the defect side and a shift in the posterior functional contacts on the normal side [8, 9]. Therefore, expeditiously rehabilitation after marginal or segmental mandibulectomy is preferred [10, 11]. There are many techniques for the management of mandibular continuity defects such as nonvascularized bone graft, iliac crest free flap, and vascularized osseous free graft [12]. Whatever the donor site is (the fibula, scapula, rib, and the iliac crest) [13], it is desirable to preserve the bone graft until full healing to make the final prosthetic whatever its types including implant-supported fixed prostheses [14], or removable dentures whether supported by implants or not [15, 16], but until then, the bone graft must be protected in addition to helping the patient during this stage to restore the masticatory, aesthetic, and verbal function, as well as improving his psychological state through the interim prosthesis, which is mostly a removable denture. Although interim care is not indicated for mandibular defects, most cases and discussions usually talk about maxillary ones; unless, they have to wait for the surgical site to heal and if it is dimensionally stable [17, 18]. Many studies describe the factors influencing the success or failure of bone grafts especially those related to surgery or postsurgery procedures such as type of defect and scope of excision, bone graft infection, extrusion, malocclusion, facial nerve involvement, or deformation of lower face [19, 20], while factors related to the prosthetics are studied extensively in terms of its effect on alveolar bone resorption in conventional cases, such as its type, design, method of impressions, or occlusal scheme [21–25]. Prosthodontics considerations in cases of mandibular resection were mentioned in articles and references that also mentioned about acrylic and hybrid prosthetics due to their ability to be modified with an interim or resin lining material; they also talked about their design such as not extending the base widely as normal dentures, reducing the occlusal surface, and the use of existing teeth for additional retention in metal or acrylic dentures [18, 26–28]; however, it is rare to find an article about using the flexible dentures maybe because the controversy about it is not over yet; anyway, it is still a viable option (polyamide, polyester, acrylic resin, polycarbonate, and polypropylene); in addition to having many useful advantages and indications, interim dentures or spare dentures for patients with metal allergy or for whom esthetics must be given top priority [29]. The purpose of this clinical report is to describe the possibility of using interim flexible acrylic dentures over iliac bone graft for a considerable period in cases of mandibular resection in adolescent patients with ameloblastoma.

2. Clinical Report

A 12-year-old male patient reported to the Department of Oral and Maxillofacial Surgery at the National Hospital of Hama with visible swelling; intraorally, there was a noticeable expansion of the mandible body in the posterior section. After the radiographic examination, the presence of multicystic ameloblastoma was suspected (Figure 1), which was confirmed by histological examination. On the CBCT scan, the tumor was extending from tooth 34 to tooth 38 with part of the ramus. According to Ord et al. [30], the treatment of ameloblastoma would be complicated because of continued growth and a higher percentage of cancellous bone which increased bone turnover and high periosteal reactivity, so the treatment should be in the same way used with adults; therefore, a partial resection of the mandible from the tooth 33 until the ramus was done while keeping the condyle (Figure 2).

A titanium reconstruction plate was adapted and contoured to the mandible body to reinforce and help stabilize a block graft, but we waited 8 months before applying the bone graft to ensure that there was no recurrence of excision, and due to the lack of technology required to operate a microsurgical reconstruction beside, the patient was unable to travel to another place where these experiences are available, so a nonvascularized bone graft was taken from the anterior iliac crest, and because the patient's bone is spongy and fragile, we waited a whole year, and after that, we confirm the success of the graft and the stability of its dimensions. During this period, a transpalatal arch was applied to prevent rotation of upper molars and maintain the arch width (Figures 3 and 4). The second stage of treatment involved a removable partial denture until the patient reaches an appropriate age to place implants and fixed prosthetic where the additional bone graft may be applied before placing the implants.

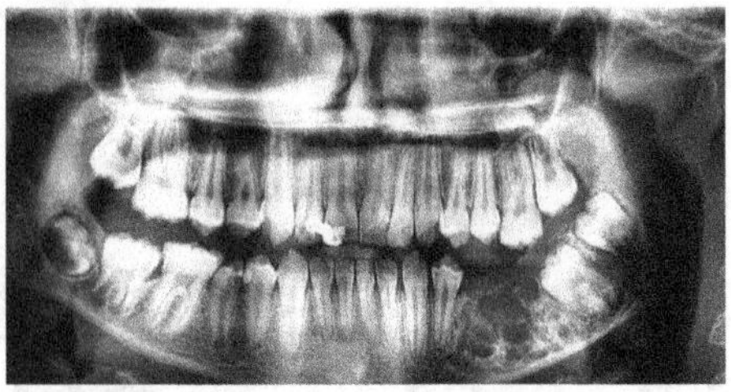

Figure 1: Preoperative panoramic radiograph.

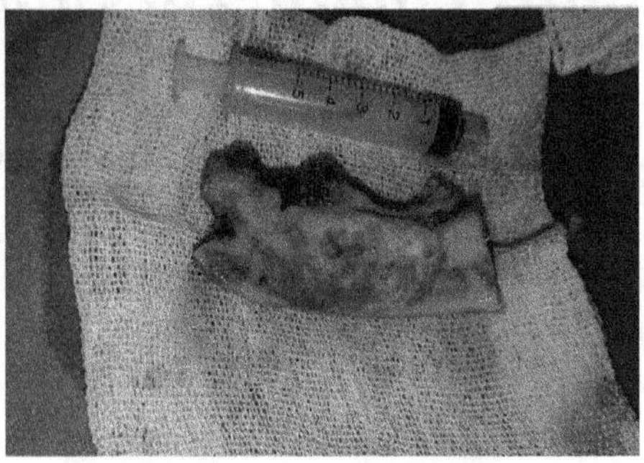

Figure 2: Excised bone.

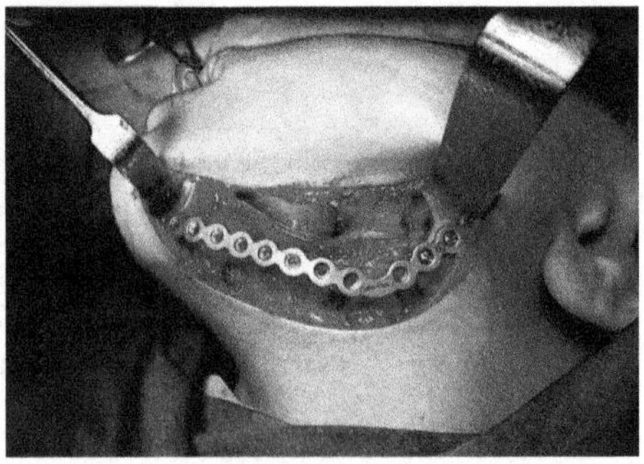

Figure 3: The titanium reconstruction plate.

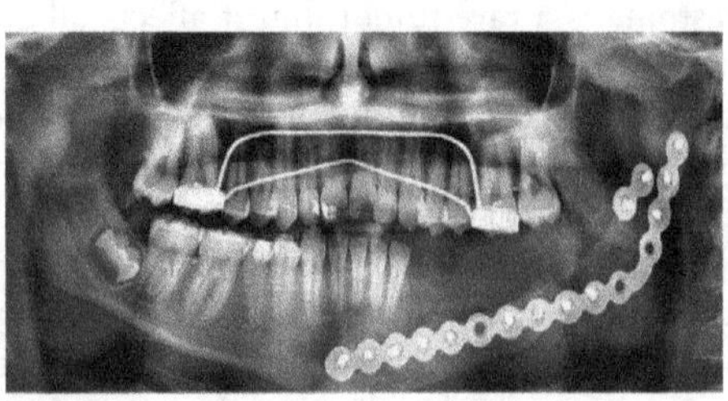

Figure 4: Postoperative view with the graft.

Intraoral examination showed an obvious volume of soft tissue in the iliac graft region which had healed well (Figure 5), and all options were discussed with the patient's parents regarding their economic situation or expectations who refused to perform another surgical procedure to remove the flabby soft tissue, so the prosthodontic plan was designed to fabricate a flexible partial denture.

As usual, the procedures began with making a primary impression using irreversible hydrocolloid material. The custom tray was made by autopolymerizing acrylic resin (Simplex Hi, Kemdent, UK) and checked in the patient mouth. To fill the missed area of the resected mandible in the tray, impression compound sticks (Kerr, Italy) were used to support the final impression material and to make the border molding; then, the functional impression was made with irreversible hydrocolloid material (Zetaplus, Zhermak, Italy) and poured with the pink gypsum type IV (Shera, Italy) (Figure 6).

The occlusal relationship was registered using a register plate made with autopolymerizing acrylic resin and modeling wax (Tenatex, Kemdent, UK) to make the rim that holds the medium (Chemi Sil Bite, Hyvincare, Korea), taking into account the situation of the mandible and its deviation, and because this stage is considered critical, the relationship was manually directed until reaching the most stable position, taking advantage of the remaining teeth on the natural side, and then was confirmed during the clinical trial.

The denture was processed with flexible acrylic resin (Valplast, Tianjin Iris, China) and delivered to the patient after adjustment procedures and assessment of both speech and mastication (Figures 7 and 8); after that, the artificial teeth were prepared according to class I of black and restored with an amalgam filling to create a natural look for a young man of this age.

A digital panoramic radiograph was made with a silicone bite on the biting block of the radiographic device to ensure that the patient bites the same situation after the end of the observation period which was 9 months (Figure 9).

3. Discussion

The initial plan chosen for this patient was a flexible partial denture that will be used for a considerable period. All options for the type of the removable partial denture have been taken into account, starting with the cast metal one. But it is not considered a logical option due to the incomplete growth of young patient besides its high price, especially with the possibility of making a new denture after a while, in addition to the difficulty of controlling the lever effect around the rest with the presence of flabby tissue which may cause damage to the bone graft or natural teeth, as leaving the patient without a denture in this age is also illogical because of the need to restore the mastication and cosmesis in addition to the possibility of food trapping and possible infections of the surgical area due to the difficulty cleaning or impaired neuromuscular function [17]. The second option was a heat polymerizing resin denture as an interim prosthetic due to its cheap price and lining capacity, but the presence of the large volume of flabby tissue and the difficulty of obtaining sufficient stability or the possibility of damage to adjacent teeth and the health of supporting soft tissues [17], especially above the graft area, make the flexible denture a more acceptable choice for several reasons:

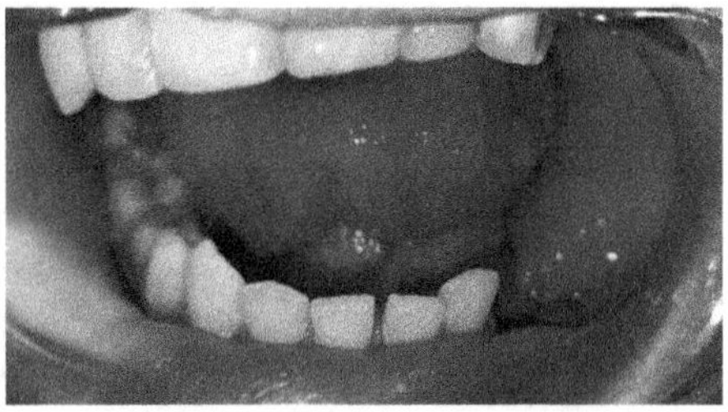

Figure 5: Intraoral view.

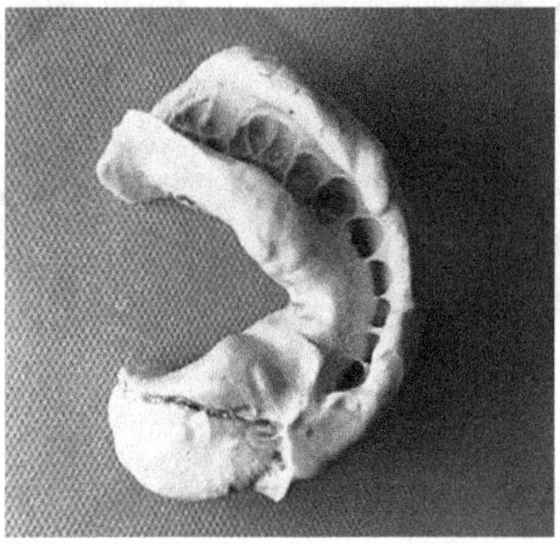

Figure 6: Final impression.

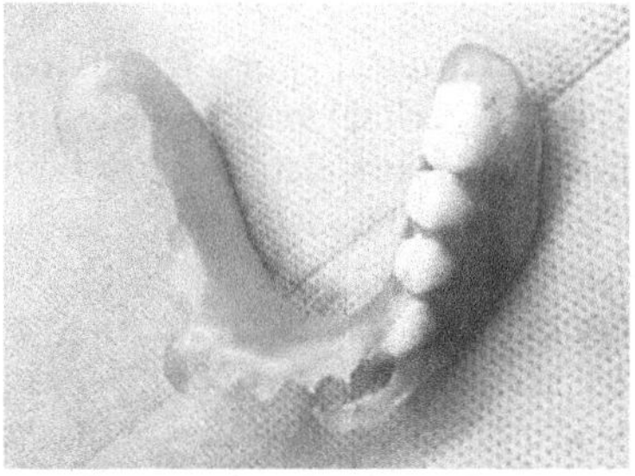

Figure 7: The flexible denture.

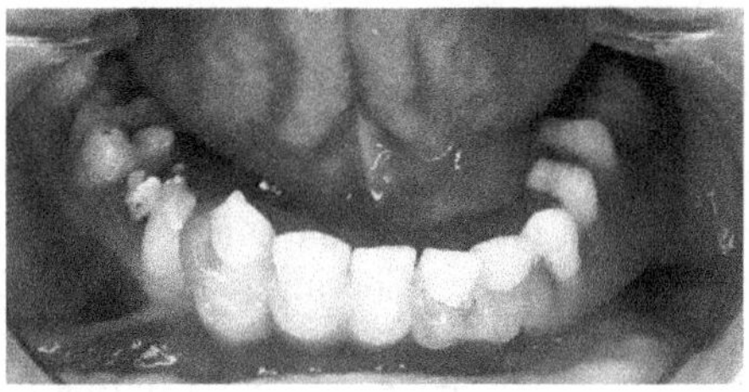

Figure 8: Flexible dentures inside the mouth.

(i) Its flexibility allows obtaining additional stability and retention by increasing the flange extension under hard or soft tissue undercuts, in addition to extending the clasp of more teeth [24, 29]

(ii) Softer surface compared with acrylic resin means that patients feel better when wearing it and there appears to be no problem with the fit [24, 29]

(iii) Thermoplastic resins have hygienic advantages due to their low water absorption and solubility [24]

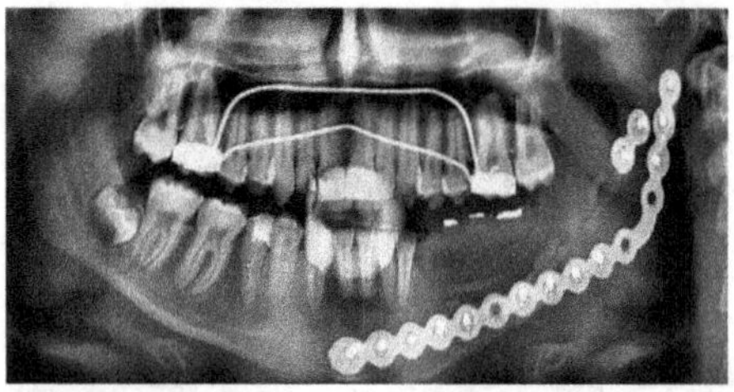

Figure 9: A radiographic image after denture delivery.

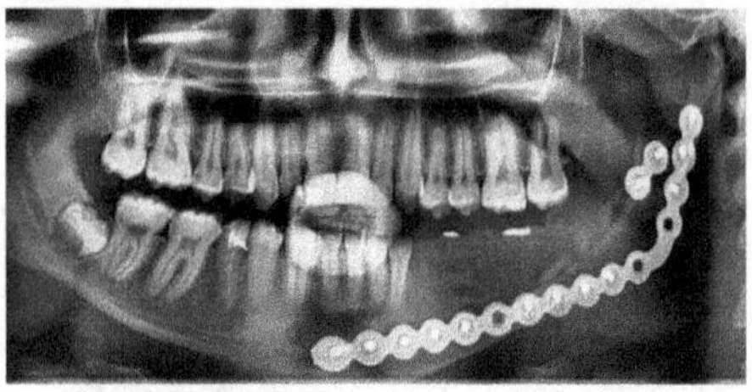

Figure 10: After 9 months.

(iv) Aesthetically, it is better than acrylic resin [24]

Taking into account some of its disadvantages, such as difficulty to repair or poor resistance to scratching [24], the patient was alerted to the need for oral hygiene and regular reviews.

To reduce the functional efforts transferred to the graft by reducing the total occlusal load applied in the supporting tissue, the lingualized articulation at the premolars was adopted but anatomic one at the first molar. For more effective chewing but with the deletion of the second molar [17, 24], panoramic imaging is an accepted procedure for observing vertical changes in the bone [31], which after nine months showed no bone resorption or has not exceeded bone remodeling (Figure 10); besides, the intraoral examination showed healthy tissue with no wasting or any infection.

4. Conclusions

Within the limits of this case and the duration of observation of a bone graft taken from the anterior iliac crest under a flexible partial denture, adhering to prosthetic considerations, it can be said that it is safe to use a flexible denture as a prosthetic over iliac bone graft block during the healing period [32].

References

[1] M. Oomens and I. van der Waal, "Epidemiology of ameloblastomas of the jaws; a report from the Netherlands," *Medicina Oral Patología Oral y Cirugia Bucal*, vol. 19, no. 6, pp. e581–e583, 2014.

[2] R. Netto, W. Cortezzi, T. Nassif, M. Calasans-Maia, and R. S. Louro, "Rehabilitation with dental implants in microvascular iliac graft after solid ameloblastoma Resection," *Implant Dentistry*, vol. 22, no. 6, pp. 561–565, 2013.

[3] S. Anil Kumar, N. K. Sahoo, and H. S. Sandhu, "Vascularised fibula osteocutaneous flap for mandibular reconstruction and multiple implant retained fixed prosthetic rehabilitation of a patient with mandibular ameloblastoma," *Medical Journal Armed Forces India*, vol. 71, pp. S534–S537, 2015.

[4] C. Moreno-Soriano, A. Estrugo-Devesa, P. Castañeda-Vega, E. Jané-Salas, and J. López-López, "Postsurgical prosthetic rehabilitation after mandibular ameloblastoma resection: a 7-year follow-up case report," *Case Reports in Dentistry*, vol. 2021, Article ID 5593973, 5 pages, 2021.

[5] H.-J. Yoon, S.-P. Hong, J.-I. Lee, S.-S. Lee, and S.-D. Hong, "Ameloblastic carcinoma: an analysis of 6 cases with review of the literature," *Oral Surgery, Oral Medicine, Oral Pathology, Oral Radiology, and Endodontology*, vol. 108, no. 6, pp. 904–913, 2009.

[6] M. A. Pogrel and D. M. Montes, "Is there a role for enucleation in the management of ameloblastoma?," *International Journal of Oral and Maxillofacial Surgery*, vol. 38, no. 8, pp. 807–812, 2009.

[7] H. P. Philipsen and P. A. Reichart, "Classification of odontogenic tumors and allied lesions," in *Odontogenic tumors and allied lesions*, pp. 21–23, Quintessence Pub. Co. Ltd, 2004.

[8] J. Beumer, "Maxillofacial Rehabilitation Prosthodontic and Surgical Considerations," *Ishigaki Euroamerica*, pp. 143-144, 1996.

[9] T. D. Taylor, "Clinical Maxillofacial Prosthetics," *Assessment*, vol. 20, pp. 155–188, 2000.

[10] I. Petrovic, Z. U. Ahmed, J. M. Huryn et al., "Oral rehabilitation for patients with marginal and segmental mandibulectomy: a retrospective review of 111 mandibular resection prostheses," *The Journal of Prosthetic Dentistry*, vol. 122, no. 1, pp. 82–87, 2019.

[11] R. M. Lustosa, D. d. V. Macedo, L. C. V. Iwaki et al., "Continuity resection of the mandible after ameloblastoma - feasibility of oral rehabilitation with rhBMP-2 associated to bovine xenograft followed by implant installation," *Journal of Cranio-Maxillofacial Surgery*, vol. 43, no. 8, pp. 1553–1560, 2015.

[12] R. P. Fernandes and J. G. Yetzer, "Reconstruction of acquired oromandibular defects," *Oral and Maxillofacial Surgery Clinics of North America*, vol. 25, no. 2, pp. 241–249, 2013.

[13] R. P. Mehta and D. G. Deschler, "Mandibular reconstruction in 2004: an analysis of different techniques," *Current Opinion in Otolaryngology & Head and Neck Surgery*, vol. 12, no. 4, pp. 288–293, 2004.

[14] U. Cakan, N. Anil, and Y. Aslan, "Prosthetic rehabilitation of a mandibular gunshot defect with an implant- supported fixed partial denture: A clinical report," *The Journal of Prosthetic Dentistry*, vol. 95, no. 4, pp. 274–279, 2006.

[15] B. Gökçen-Röhlig, B. Atalay, E. Baca, D. Işik, and U. Meriç, "Prosthetic rehabilitation of a patient with a mandibular defect caused by a gunshot wound," *Journal of Craniofacial Surgery*, vol. 20, no. 5, pp. 1614–1617, 2009.

[16] R. de Freitas, O. B. Kaizer, M. M. Hamata, D. R. B. de Resende, and R. de Oliveira Fortes Kaizer, "Prosthetic rehabilitation of a bone defect with a teeth-implant supported, removable partial denture," *Implant Dentistry*, vol. 15, no. 3, pp. 241–247, 2006.

[17] A. B. Carr, *McCracken's Removable Partial Prosthodontics-E-Book*, Elsevier Health Sciences, 2016.

[18] J. Beumer III, M. T. Marunick, and S. J. Esposito, "Maxillofacial rehabilitation: prosthodontic and surgical management

of cancer-related, acquired, and congenital defects of the head and neck," *Quintessence Pub*, vol. 172, 2011.

[19] S.-H. Chen, H.-C. Tai, T.-J. Cheng et al., "Reconstruction for mandibular implant failure," *Issues in Flap Surgery*, vol. 103, 2018.

[20] M. A. Pogrel, S. Podlesh, J. P. Anthony, and J. Alexander, "A comparison of vascularized and nonvascularized bone grafts for reconstruction of mandibular continuity defects," *Journal of Oral and Maxillofacial Surgery*, vol. 55, no. 11, pp. 1200–1206, 1997.

[21] D. D. S. Ammar Belal and D. D. S. Hussain Al-Eisa, "Effect of the functional impression on the alveolar resorption beneath the flexible acrylic resin bases for the partial removable dentures patients of class I of Kennedy," *International Journal of Medical and Health Research.*, vol. 5, no. 10, pp. 100–106, 2019.

[22] A. Aljammal, "In-vivo and in-vitro comparative study between removable partial dentures fabricated," in p. 106, Damascus University, 2013.

[23] H. Alisa, "A comparative study between movable denture bases prepared by different methods and their effect on oral mucosa," in p. 50, Damascus University, 2007.

[24] O. Şakar, Ed., *Removable Partial Dentures: A Practitioners' Manual*, Springer, 2015.

[25] F. Jnaid, "Evaluation of three methods for management of stress distribution of mandibular distal extension removable partial dentures-Kennedy class I-(in vivo and in-vitro study)," in pp. 69-98–157,158, Damascus University, 2015.

[26] R. Cantor and T. A. Curtis, "Prosthetic management of edentulous mandibulectomy patients. Part I. Anatomic, physiologic, and psychologic considerations," *The Journal of Prosthetic Dentistry*, vol. 25, no. 4, pp. 446–457, 1971.

[27] R. Cantor and T. A. Curtis, "Prosthetic management of edentulous mandibulectomy patients. Part II. Clinical procedures," *The Journal of Prosthetic Dentistry*, vol. 25, no. 5, pp. 546–555, 1971.

[28] E. W. J. Leong, A. C. Cheng, N. Tee-Khin, and A. G. Wee, "Management of acquired mandibular defects-prosthodontic considerations," *Singapore Dental Journal*, vol. 28, no. 1, p. 22, 2005.

[29] K. Fueki, C. Ohkubo, M. Yatabe et al., "Clinical application of removable partial dentures using thermoplastic resin- Part I: Definition and indication of non-metal clasp dentures," *Journal of Prosthodontic Research*, vol. 58, no. 1, pp. 3–10, 2014.

[30] R. A. Ord, R. H. Blanchaert Jr., N. G. Nikitakis, and J. J. Sauk, "Ameloblastoma in children," *Journal of Oral and Maxillofacial Surgery*, vol. 60, no. 7, pp. 762–770, 2002.

[31] S. Acharya, V. K. Lohe, and R. R. Bhowate, "Evaluation, and comparison of alveolar bone loss of maxilla and mandible in completely edentulous patients on digital panoramic radiographs," *Journal of Oral Medicine, Oral Surgery, Oral Pathology and Oral Radiology*, vol. 2, no. 3, pp. 112–119, 2016.

[32] A. Belal, B. Monther, and W. Alzarif, "Possibility of using flexible dentures over iliac bone graft in adolescent patients with ameloblastoma: a case report," *Research Square*, 2021.

6

Unpredictable Outcomes of a Regenerative Endodontic Treatment

Zahra Mohammadi, Hadi Assadian, Behnam Bolhari, Mohammadreza Sharifian, Mehrfam Khoshkhounejad, and Nazanin Chitsaz

Department of Endodontics, School of Dentistry, Tehran University of Medical Sciences (TUMS), Iran

Correspondence should be addressed to Nazanin Chitsaz; chitsaz.nazanin11@yahoo.com

Academic Editor: Andrea Scribante

Regenerative endodontic treatment (RET) is a valuable treatment for necrotic immature teeth with many advantages such as increasing root length and thickness of root wall. The success of RETs is based on healthy stem cells, suitable scaffolds, and growth factors and takes place when bacterial contamination is well controlled. The aim of this article is to address controversy in a case with multiple success criteria. This paper reports a 9-year-old boy with a complicated crown fracture of the maxillary left central incisor about three years prior to referral with a diagnosis of intrusive luxation with spontaneous reeruption. The tooth had an underdeveloped root and a well-defined periapical radiolucent lesion around the root apex. RET was considered according to the stage of root development. Upon the three-week recall session, the clinical examination indicated that the patient was asymptomatic in the affected site. However, the patient returned two weeks later with a sinus tract pertaining to the apex of tooth #9. Therefore, debridement of the root canal space was repeated and the RET redone. On the second trial, the patient was symptom-free, but no more evidence of root maturation was observed on 18-month follow-up. The tooth was asymptomatic (without swelling, drainage, and pain) during this time, and esthetics was provided for the patient.

1. Introduction

All endodontic treatments are aimed at prevention or treatment of apical periodontitis (AP). The goal for treatment of immature permanent teeth is to restore the physiologic structures and functions of the pulp dentin complex [1]. As a substitute to conventional root canal treatment, regenerative endodontic treatment (RET), is a valuable treatment for necrotic immature teeth with many advantages such as increasing root length and thickness of root walls unlike other treatments such as apical plug or apexification with calcium hydroxide [2–4].

The success in RETs relies on the tripod of healthy stem cells, suitable scaffolds, and growth factors [5–7] and takes place when bacterial contamination is eliminated from the environment [8]. The successful regenerative endodontic procedure is measured via increased root length, thickened canal walls, and closure of the root apex and even in some cases with positive responses to pulpal sensibility tests [9]. Several published cases with immature roots indicate that the RET has the potential to encourage continued maturation of the root in terms of width and length. This procedure includes competent infection control, a suitable scaffold for fresh tissue ingrowth, and adequate coronal seal [10]. Achievement of success in RETs requires no signs and symptoms of disease such as pain, swelling, or sinus tract, as well as radiographic evidence of periapical healing with increased root length and root canal wall thickness, indicating continued root development [11]. Unhealed periapical lesions, fractures, and failures to induce periapical bleeding are the main causes associated with RET failure [12].

There are several factors which affect the outcome of RET such as apex diameter, patient age, and degree of root canal infection [13].

Histological examinations of the nature of the tissue formed in humans and animals showed a tissue similar to cementum and osteodentin [14–16] and a soft tissue similar to fibrous connective tissue containing vessels [15, 17].

The success of RETs is dependent on the patient's potential to heal the dental pulp tissues. The provision of RETs should be restricted to healthy patients who can heal and benefit from the procedure [18]. The survival of cells and regeneration of tissues is sensitive to the conditions within the intracanal environment. The materials should be biocompatible, because they can cause cell death and allow bacterial leakage [19].

There are various guidelines and studies that have defined the success of RET more precisely.

Diogenes et al. [20] describe the RET outcome in three levels: patient-based outcome (absence of swelling, drainage, pain, tooth survival and function, and tooth esthetics); clinician-based outcome (radiographic healing, radiographic root development, and positive vitality responses); and scientist-based outcome (histologic evidence of complete regeneration) are taken into account.

Staffoli et al. [18] suggested treatment success as healing of apical radiolucency within an average of 8 months and root development within 18 months after treatment and stated that absence of these radiographic features within 2 years or the presence of signs and symptoms equals treatment failure. American Association of Endodontics (AAE) [21] categorized success rates of RETs as primary, secondary, and tertiary goals, with elimination of symptoms and bone healing as primary, root maturation as secondary, and positive response to vitality testing as the tertiary goals. European Society of Endodontology (ESE) [22] describes success of regenerative endodontic procedure as lack of signs and symptoms, discoloration, and patient's acceptance and radiographic detection of new PDL along the inner wall of root canal.

Even though the primary goal of healing AP and continued root development is mostly reached in REPs, the unpredictability of the regeneration evidence from histological point of view is a shortcoming. It is completely comprehensible that achieving this goal is very demanding due to its multifactorial nature [23].

Most studies in regenerative endodontics are limited to successful cases with an increase in root length or closure of the apex [24–26], while cases that are limited to relieving the patient's symptoms have been neglected, although these treatments can be categorized as successful in the patients' view [20].

The aim of the current case report was to describe clinical RET using calcium hydroxide mixed with chlorhexidine as intracanal medicament for a patient's postoperative functional teeth without any signs of root development on 18-month follow-up.

2. Case Report

The patient was a 9-year-old boy referred by a general dentist to the School of Dentistry, Tehran University of Medical Sciences (TUMS), Tehran, Iran, in 2018. His medical history revealed a systemically healthy patient categorized as class I according to ASA health status. His dental history indicated a complicated crown fracture of the maxillary left central incisor about three years ago due to a fall. The patient was admitted to the Department of Endodontics with a prereferral diagnosis of intrusive luxation with spontaneous reeruption and complicated crown fracture by a general dentist. Extraoral examination showed no scar in the pertinent soft tissues. Upon intraoral examination, complicated crown fracture of tooth #9 was noted (Figure 1(a)). The patient's oral hygiene was good.

A pulp sensitivity test to cold stimulus using CO_2 snow spray (Luber cool, Luber, Germany) showed no response in the involved teeth. The periodontal examinations revealed normal conditions (i.e., probing < 3 mm, mobility < 1 mm, and insensitive to percussion/palpation). Periapical radiographic examination showed that tooth #9 had an open apex shorter root and thinner radicular walls in comparison with the adjacent teeth. A well-defined periapical radiolucent lesion was evident around the root apex (see Figure 2(a)). The maxillary left central incisor was diagnosed as having a necrotic pulp with asymptomatic apical periodontitis. RET was considered according to the stage of root development. The patient's parents were informed about the treatment process, and informed consent was provided. In the first session, local anesthesia was administered using 2% lidocaine with 1 : 80,000 epinephrine (Daru Pakhsh, Tehran, Iran), and the access cavity was prepared under rubber dam isolation. The working length was determined using an electronic apex locator (Root ZX, J. Morita Corp., Tokyo, Japan) and confirmed radiographically. Then, chemical disinfection was performed using 20 mL of 1.5% sodium hypochlorite (Hypo-EndoX, Morvabon, Iran) with passive ultrasonic activation using a piezoelectric ultrasonic unit (Varios 970, NSK, Japan), with the power setting at 10, for 5 min. Then, calcium hydroxide (Golchadent, Tehran, Iran) was applied into the canal in a creamy consistency, using a #15 K-file (MicroMega, Besangon, France) placed 2 mm short of the working length. Then, the access cavity was sealed with reinforced zinc-oxide eugenol cement (Zoliran, Golchadent, Iran). Upon the three-week recall session, the clinical examination indicated that the patient was asymptomatic in the affected site. Local anesthesia was administered using infiltration of 3% mepivacaine plain (Daru Pakhsh, Tehran, Iran), and the tooth was isolated with rubber dam. The remnants of the intracanal medicament were removed using passive ultrasonically activated irrigation (Varios 970, NSK, Japan) with 20 mL normal saline solution. The canal was irrigated with 20 mL of 17% EDTA solution for 5 min and then dried with sterile paper points. Blood was harvested from patient's brachial artery, and PRF was provided using a centrifuge (DUO Quattro, Process for PRF, Nice, France) at 208 g for 8 min. Bleeding was induced by a sterile manual #60 K-file (MicroMega, Besangon, France), within the canal. The intracanal PRF was placed 3 mm apical to the CEJ level. Dentin-bonding agent (Single Bond, 3M, ESPE, USA) was applied to the internal access cavity walls, and then, MTA Angelus (Angelus, Londrina, PR, Brazil) as a coronal barrier was applied using an MTA carrier. A moist cotton pellet was placed on top of the bulk of MTA, and the access cavity was sealed with reinforced zinc-oxide eugenol cement (Zoliran, Golchadent, Iran). It was scheduled to check MTA setting 1 day later, but the patient missed the appointment and returned two weeks later with a sinus tract. Upon

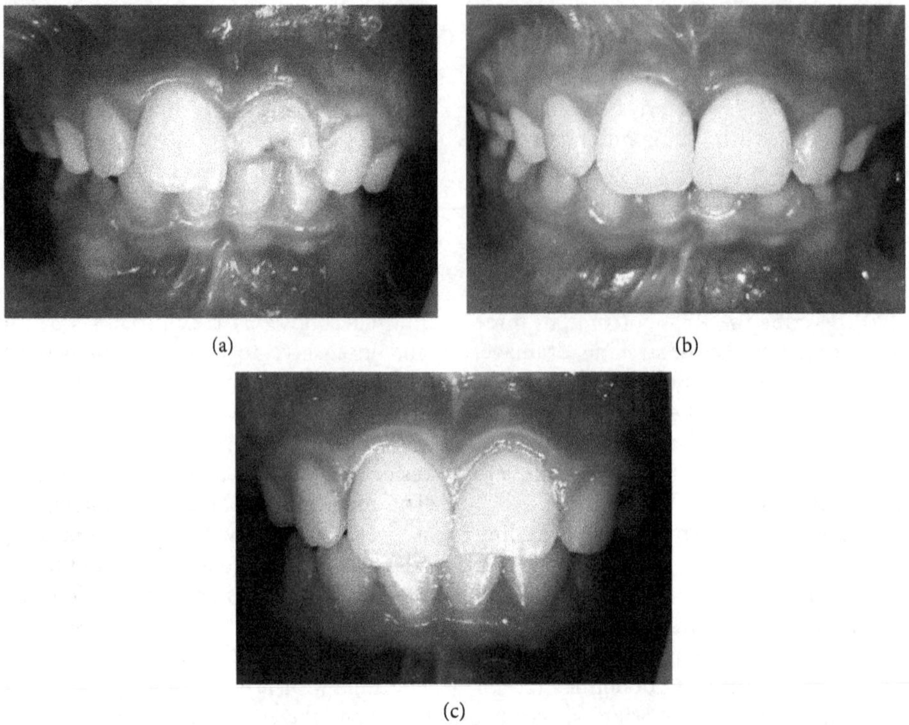

Figure 1: Intra-oral photograph of the fractured maxillary left central incisor in a 9-year-old boy (a) preoperative image, (b) 3-month recall, and (c) 18-month recall.

radiographic evaluation, the sinus tract was traced with a #30/0.02 gutta percha point and its extension to the apex of tooth #9 was confirmed (see Figure 2(b)). Due to the presence of the draining sinus tract, debridement of the root canal space was repeated after injection of 2% lidocaine anesthesia and 1 : 80,000 epinephrine (Daru Pakhsh, Tehran, Iran), using 20 mL of ultrasonically (Varios 970, NSK, Japan) activating 1.5% sodium hypochlorite solution (Hypo-EndoX, Morvabon, Iran) under rubber dam isolation. Mechanical instrumentation was carried out using light circumferential filing with a #25 Hedstrom file (Dentsply Sirona, Ballaigues, Switzerland). Then, calcium hydroxide (Golchadent, Tehran, Iran) mixed with 2% chlorhexidine solution (Morvabon, Tehran, Iran) dressing was inserted into the root canal in a creamy consistency, and the tooth was temporarily filled with reinforced zinc oxide eugenol (Zoliran, Golchadent, Iran). The draining mucosal sinus tract healed after 10 days.

Therefore, after infiltration of 3% mepivacaine without a vasoconstrictor (Daru Pakhsh, Tehran, Iran), the dressing was removed similar to previous try under rubber dam isolation. The canal was rinsed with 20 mL of 17% EDTA solution (Sigma-Aldrich, St. Louis, MO, USA). PRF was prepared, and bleeding was induced by a sterile manual file as described above. The PRF, Dentin-bonding agent (Single Bond, 3M, ESPE, USA), and coronal barrier (Retro-MTA (bioMTA, Seoul, South Korea)) was placed as pervious try, access cavity sealed with reinforced zinc-oxide eugenol (Zoliran, Golchadent, Iran). (Figure 2(c)) After 1 week, the MTA was set and the crown was restored by composite resin (FGM, Joinville, Brazil). Follow-up sessions were planned. On recall visits, the tooth was asymptomatic and had a normal condition during periodontal tests. The follow-up radiographs and photographs are shown in Figures 1 and 2.

3. Discussion

In this case report, the patient had a history of dental trauma. After more than 18 months of recall, the teeth were in normal condition during periodontal tests and were still functional. In addition, the tooth functionality and esthetics were restored but no further root development was observed.

A recent study revealed that root development potential of immature necrotic teeth is related to the vitality of Hertwig's epithelial root sheath. Therefore, there might be a correlation between dental traumatic history and root development; the longer the duration of pulp necrosis, the lower the rate of root development after RET [27].

The patient represented a history of dental traumatic injury with possibly 3 years of pulpal necrosis. There is no evidence of root canal development in an 18-month recall.

In the classic RET protocol, passive decontamination is performed with sodium hypochlorite without conventional mechanical instrumentation for prevention of periapical cellular destruction. However, more recently mechanical instrumentation is used to wipe out necrotic pulp and remove the intracanal medicament [28].

A previous review claimed that immature teeth with an extended history of pulp necrosis had an unfavorable radiographic outcome after RET [29]. The contention of this argument is that even in the presence of some residual bacteria, traditional root canal treatment can result in the healing of periapical disease, but at the same way, it may not apply to

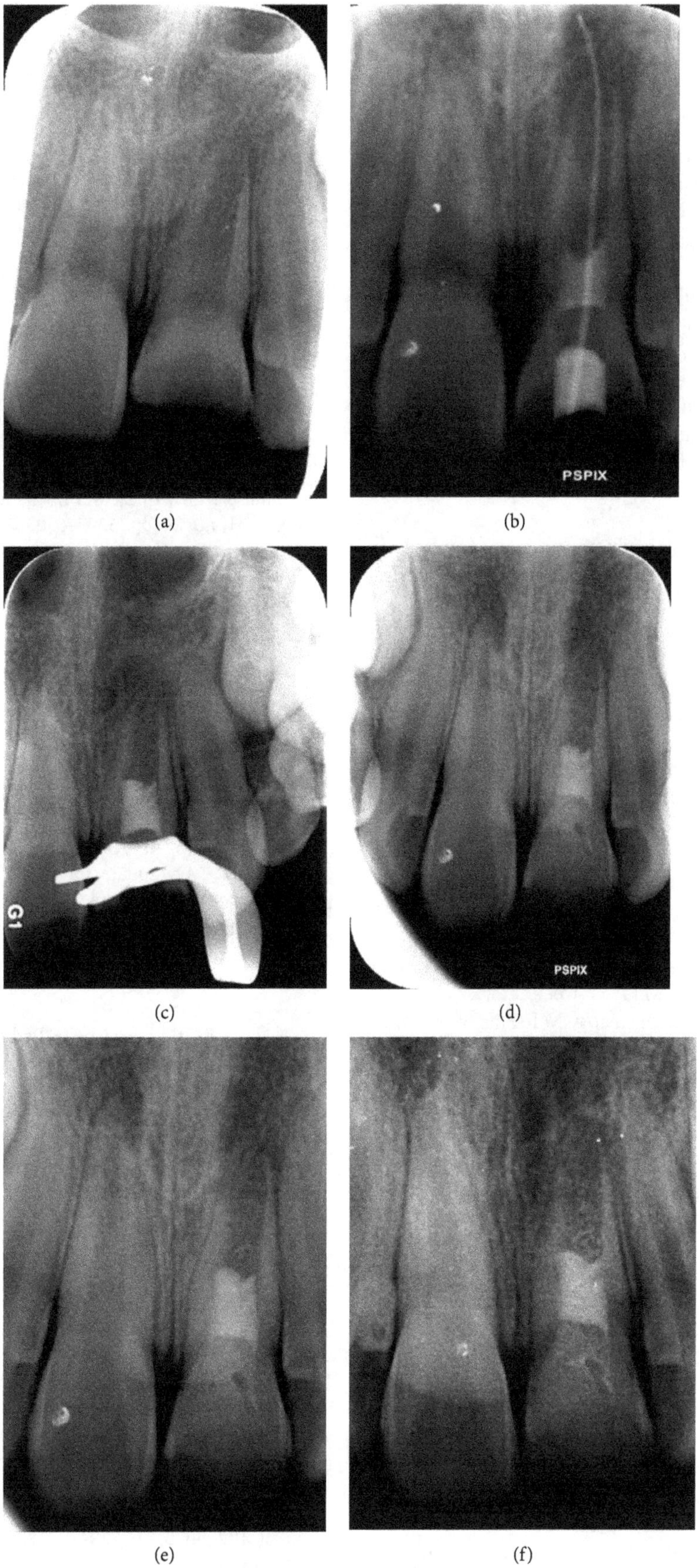

FIGURE 2: The radiographic images showing (a) the initial preoperative condition, (b) tracing the mucosal sinus tract with a gutta percha point, (c) second try, (d) 3-month recall, (e) 9-month recall, and (f) 18-month recall.

RET [19]. Residual bacteria have a critical negative effect on the outcome of RETs [8]. Eradication of bacteria from the pulp canal has an important role in successful RET because revascularization halts in the presence of infection [17].

One approach for disrupting the biofilm is gentle brushing of the root canal wall with endodontic instruments (e.g., Hedstrom files) [30]. In case of persisting symptoms, repetition of the protocol using root canal disinfection by another regimen or the same drugs for a longer period of time is recommended [18].

In this case, on a second try, in addition to gentle brushing of the root canal walls, the intracanal medicament was used once more. Hence, 2% chlorhexidine was added to improve antimicrobial efficacy of calcium hydroxide. Correspondingly, de Jesus et al. reported successful treatment results with the use of calcium hydroxide mixed with chlorhexidine as an intracanal medicament in a patient with a past history of intrusive luxation and complicated crown fracture [31].

One of the limitations of regeneration in compromised teeth is the lack of space for intracanal posts. In the present case, due to the sufficient remaining enamel surface, direct composite build-up was performed. In immature permanent teeth with necrotic pulp when the pulp space is needed for a post/core in the final restoration, the modified apexification procedure has been suggested [32]; of course, it will be difficult to remove the MTA in case of treatment failure.

MTA prevents microleakage in addition to being biocompatible and promoting regeneration of the tissue when placed in contact with the dental pulp or periradicular, but one of the major problems with MTA, beside its setting time, is the very low value and unpredictable bonding to restorative materials. Therefore, delayed restoration improves bond strength [33]. Permanent restoration of the tooth in the present case was performed with composite resin after ensuring complete setting of MTA (1 week later).

Another shortcoming with using MTA as a coronal barrier is color change possibility in the medium/long term [34].

In order to prevent discoloration, dentin bonding was applied to seal the dentin tubules, in addition to limiting MTA placement under the CEJ level.

The results of the present study have shown that root development or increase in root canal wall thickness are not the only success criteria of treatment but also the tooth functionality and esthetic for young patients to give time for bone growth should be sufficient; so if the tooth becomes symptomatic in the future, the tooth site will be suitable for alternative treatments such as dental implants.

From this point of view, this case can belong to "primary success" according to AAE [21]. However, taking the ESE guidelines into consideration, the treatment was considered as "failed" due to the lack of root length increase [22]. Therefore, AAE criteria for success in RETs seem to be more comprehensive more specifically in border line cases.

There is also a strong need to report failed or ambiguous RET cases in endodontic literature besides successful ones to have a more accurate evaluation about RET rate of success.

References

[1] K. M. Galler, R. N. D'Souza, M. Federlin et al., "Dentin conditioning codetermines cell fate in regenerative endodontics," *Journal of Endodontics*, vol. 37, no. 11, pp. 1536–1541, 2011.

[2] M. Alasqah, S. I. R. Khan, K. Alfouzan, and A. Jamleh, "Regenerative endodontic management of an immature molar using calcium hydroxide and triple antibiotic paste: a two-year follow-up," *Case reports in dentistry*, vol. 2020, Article ID 9025847, 5 pages, 2020.

[3] K. M. Hargreaves, T. Giesler, M. Henry, and Y. Wang, "Regeneration potential of the young permanent tooth: what does the future hold?," *Pediatric Dentistry*, vol. 30, no. 3, pp. 253–260, 2008.

[4] G. T.-J. Huang, "Apexification: the beginning of its end," *International Endodontic Journal*, vol. 42, no. 10, pp. 855–866, 2009.

[5] F.-M. Chen, M. Zhang, and W. Zhi-Fen, "Toward delivery of multiple growth factors in tissue engineering," *Biomaterials*, vol. 31, no. 24, pp. 6279–6308, 2010.

[6] K. M. Gathani and S. S. Raghavendra, "Scaffolds in regenerative endodontics: a review," *Dental research journal*, vol. 13, no. 5, pp. 379–386, 2016.

[7] A. A. Volponi, Y. Pang, and P. T. Sharpe, "Stem cell-based biological tooth repair and regeneration," *Trends in cell biology*, vol. 20, no. 12, pp. 715–722, 2010.

[8] M. C. M. Conde, L. A. Chisini, R. Sarkis-Onofre, H. S. Schuch, J. E. Nör, and F. F. Demarco, "A scoping review of root canal revascularization: relevant aspects for clinical success and tissue formation," *International Endodontic Journal*, vol. 50, no. 9, pp. 860–874, 2017.

[9] A. Diogenes, M. A. Henry, F. B. Teixeira, and K. M. Hargreaves, "An update on clinical regenerative endodontics," *Endodontic Topics*, vol. 28, no. 1, pp. 2–23, 2013.

[10] P. J. Palma, J. Martins, P. Diogo et al., "Does apical papilla survive and develop in apical periodontitis presence after regenerative endodontic procedures?," *Applied Sciences*, vol. 9, no. 19, p. 3942, 2019.

[11] S.-J. Chen and L.-P. Chen, "Radiographic outcome of necrotic immature teeth treated with two endodontic techniques: a retrospective analysis," *biomedical journal*, vol. 39, no. 5, pp. 366–371, 2016.

[12] J. Y. Nagata, A. J. Soares, F. J. Souza-Filho et al., "Microbial evaluation of traumatized teeth treated with triple antibiotic paste or calcium hydroxide with 2% chlorhexidine gel in pulp revascularization," *Journal of endodontics*, vol. 40, no. 6, pp. 778–783, 2014.

[13] B.-N. Lee, J.-W. Moon, H.-S. Chang, I.-N. Hwang, W. M. Oh, and Y.-C. Hwang, "A review of the regenerative endodontic treatment procedure," *Restorative dentistry & endodontics*, vol. 40, no. 3, pp. 179–187, 2015.

[14] L. A. B. da Silva, P. Nelson-Filho, R. A. B. da Silva et al., "Revascularization and periapical repair after endodontic treatment using apical negative pressure irrigation versus conventional irrigation plus triantibiotic intracanal dressing in dogs' teeth with apical periodontitis," *Oral Surgery, Oral Medicine, Oral Pathology, Oral Radiology, and Endodontology*, vol. 109, no. 5, pp. 779–787, 2010.

[15] G. Martin, D. Ricucci, J. L. Gibbs, and L. M. Lin, "Histological

findings of revascularized/revitalized immature permanent molar with apical periodontitis using platelet-rich plasma," *Journal of Endodontics*, vol. 39, no. 1, pp. 138–144, 2013.

[16] X. Wang, B. Thibodeau, M. Trope, L. M. Lin, and G. T.-J. Huang, "Histologic characterization of regenerated tissues in canal space after the revitalization/revascularization procedure of immature dog teeth with apical periodontitis," *Journal of endodontics*, vol. 36, no. 1, pp. 56–63, 2010.

[17] E. Shimizu, D. Ricucci, J. Albert et al., "Clinical, radiographic, and histological observation of a human immature permanent tooth with chronic apical abscess after revitalization treatment," *Journal of endodontics*, vol. 39, no. 8, pp. 1078–1083, 2013.

[18] S. Staffoli, G. Plotino, B. Nunez Torrijos et al., "Regenerative endodontic procedures using contemporary endodontic materials," *Materials*, vol. 12, no. 6, p. 908, 2019.

[19] M. C. Valera, M. T. P. Albuquerque, M. C. Yamasaki, F. N. S. Vassallo, D. A. e. S. A. da Silva, and J. Y. Nagata, "Fracture resistance of weakened bovine teeth after long-term use of calcium hydroxide," *Dental Traumatology*, vol. 31, no. 5, pp. 385–389, 2015.

[20] A. Diogenes, N. B. Ruparel, Y. Shiloah, and K. M. Hargreaves, "Regenerative endodontics: a way forward," *The Journal of the American Dental Association*, vol. 147, no. 5, pp. 372–380, 2016.

[21] American Association of Endodontists, "AAE clinical considerations for a regenerative procedure," 2016.

[22] K. M. Galler, G. Krastl, S. Simon et al., "European Society of Endodontology position statement: revitalization procedures," *International endodontic journal*, vol. 49, no. 8, pp. 717–723, 2016.

[23] P. J. Palma, J. C. Ramos, J. B. Martins et al., "Histologic evaluation of regenerative endodontic procedures with the use of chitosan scaffolds in immature dog teeth with apical periodontitis," *Journal of Endodontics*, vol. 43, no. 8, pp. 1279–1287, 2017.

[24] O. Austah, R. Joon, W. M. Fath et al., "Comprehensive characterization of 2 immature teeth treated with regenerative endodontic procedures," *Journal of Endodontics*, vol. 44, no. 12, pp. 1802–1811, 2018.

[25] A. Nosrat, A. Seifi, and S. Asgary, "Regenerative endodontic treatment (revascularization) for necrotic immature permanent molars: a review and report of two cases with a new biomaterial," *Journal of Endodontics*, vol. 37, no. 4, pp. 562–567, 2011.

[26] Z. C. Cehreli, B. Isbitiren, S. Sara, and G. Erbas, "Regenerative endodontic treatment (revascularization) of immature necrotic molars medicated with calcium hydroxide: a case series," *Journal of Endodontics*, vol. 37, no. 9, pp. 1327–1330, 2011.

[27] M. H. Chen, K. L. Chen, C. A. Chen, F. Tayebaty, P. A. Rosenberg, and L. M. Lin, "Responses of immature permanent teeth with infected necrotic pulp tissue and apical periodontitis/abscess to revascularization procedures," *International Endodontic Journal*, vol. 45, no. 3, pp. 294–305, 2012.

[28] T. W. Lovelace, M. A. Henry, K. M. Hargreaves, and A. Diogenes, "Evaluation of the delivery of mesenchymal stem cells into the root canal space of necrotic immature teeth after clinical regenerative endodontic procedure," *Journal of Endodontics*, vol. 37, no. 2, pp. 133–138, 2011.

[29] A. Nosrat, N. Homayounfar, and K. Oloomi, "Drawbacks and unfavorable outcomes of regenerative endodontic treatments of necrotic immature teeth: a literature review and report of a case," *Journal of Endodontics*, vol. 38, no. 10, pp. 1428–1434, 2012.

[30] I. Rotstein and J. I. Ingle, *ngle's endodontics*, vol. 945, PMPH USA, Raleigh, 7th ed edition, 2019.

[31] A. d. J. Soares, F. F. Lins, J. Y. Nagata et al., "Pulp revascularization after root canal decontamination with calcium hydroxide and 2% chlorhexidine gel," *Journal of endodontics*, vol. 39, no. 3, pp. 417–420, 2013.

[32] K. Songtrakul, T. Azarpajouh, M. Malek, A. Sigurdsson, B. Kahler, and L. M. Lin, "Modified apexification procedure for immature permanent teeth with a necrotic pulp/apical periodontitis: a case series," *Journal of Endodontics*, vol. 46, no. 1, pp. 116–123, 2020.

[33] P. J. Palma, J. A. Marques, R. I. Falacho, A. Vinagre, J. Santos, and J. Ramos, "Does delayed restoration improve shear bond strength of different restorative protocols to calcium silicate-based cements?," *Materials*, vol. 11, no. 11, p. 2216, 2018.

[34] P. J. Palma, J. A. Marques, J. Santos et al., "Tooth discoloration after regenerative endodontic procedures with calcium silicate-based cements—an ex vivo study," *Applied Sciences*, vol. 10, no. 17, p. 5793, 2020.

7

Pediatric Dental Management of an Uncommon Case of Mucopolysaccharidosis Type IV A (Morquio A Syndrome): A Case Report of a Three-Year Follow-Up

Andrea Gómez-González, Miguel Ángel Rosales-Berber, Paola De Ávila-Rojas, Amaury Pozos-Guillén, and Arturo Garrocho-Rangel

Pediatric Dentistry Postgraduate Program, Faculty of Dentistry, San Luis Potosi University, SLP, San Luis Potosi, Mexico

Correspondence should be addressed to Arturo Garrocho-Rangel; agarrocho@hotmail.com

Academic Editor: Muawia A. Qudeimat

Mucopolysaccharidosis type IV A or Morquio syndrome is an uncommon inherited metabolic condition caused by the deficient intralysosomal storage of glycosaminoglycans. Diagnosis is typically based on clinical examination, skeletal radiographs, and histochemical tests in blood cells or fibroblasts. It is characterized by evident skeletal deformities, poor joint mobility, severe growth deficit, occlusal anomalies, and enamel defects. The aim of the present clinical case report is to describe the general oral management provided to a 6-year-old female patient and its corresponding evolution for more than three years.

1. Introduction

Mucopolysaccharidoses (MPS) constitute a group of rare inherited lysosomal storage diseases produced by deficiencies in the metabolism and degradation of special enzymes called glycosaminoglycans (GAGs). These disorders are skeletal dysplasias, in which GAGs are accumulated within lysosomes of skeletal, diverse connective tissues, and teeth, resulting in progressive and permanent skeletal deformities, poor joint mobility, severe growth deficit, coarse facial features, and enlarged organs [1, 2]. MPS are clinically characterized by short stature, mental retardation, multiple dysostoses, cardiovascular/digestive anomalies, ocular impairments, and skin thickening. Early detected mild forms of MPS have a good prognosis and relatively normal life; however, most severe cases exhibit an average survival age of 10 years [3].

The MPS prevalence around the world varies between 1.9 and 4.5 cases per 100,000 live births, depending on the geographic region. MPS have different identified forms, ranging from MPS-I to MPS-VII, according to the clinical/radiographic and biochemical characteristics, the degree of severity, and the involved deficient GAGs [4, 5]. Specifically, the MPS type IV A or Morquio A syndrome (MAS) consists in the intralysosomal accumulation of two GAGs, keratan sulfate, and chondroitin-6-sulfate, interfering with the chondrocyte function in cartilage, bone, and ligaments; this accumulation is due to mutations in the gene encoding of the enzyme N-acetylgalactosamine-6-sulfate sulfatase (GALNS) [6]. MAS is typically featured by the presence of the notorious short neck and trunk, prominent forehead, cervical spinal deformities with cord and medullary compression, general osteoporosis, lungs/heart dysfunction, *pectus carinatum* (malformation of the chest characterized by a protrusion of the sternum and ribs), muscle weakness, kyphoscoliosis, flat feet and knock-knees (or *genua valga*, a condition in which the legs curve inward and the feet are apart when the knees are touching), and frequent falls associated to an abnormal gait [7]. Unlike other MPS, affected children usually exhibit normal intelligence [8]. The most common orofacial anomalies are a short nose and broad mouth; unerupted, malposition, and spaced permanent teeth; abnormally thin and porous enamel and loss of dental structure; anterior open bite associated to macroglossia; and flattened condyle [3, 4, 8–10]. The diagnosis of MAS is carried out through raised

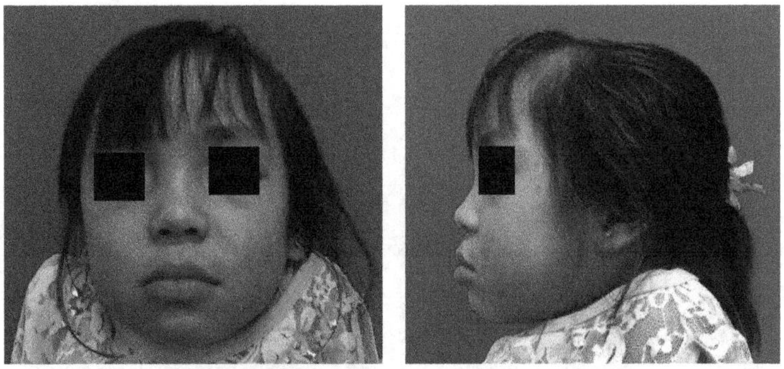

Figure 1: Initial extraoral views (August 2016).

urinary levels of keratan sulfate, GALNS activity testing, skin biopsy, leucocyte and fibroblast cultures, genetic analysis, and distinctive radiographic features [8, 11]. General management usually consists of the substitution of abnormal GAGs through enzyme replacement therapies; for more severe cases, the hematopoietic stem cell transplantation is sometimes used [10].

The aim of the present case report is to describe the most representative systemic and orofacial characteristics, diagnostic procedures, and dental management provided to a female pediatric patient aged 6 years and 6 months suffering from Morquio A syndrome. The patient has been followed up closely for more than two years.

2. Case Report

In August 2016, a six-year-six-month-old female was referred to the Pediatric Dentistry Postgraduate Program Clinic for routine oral examination and possible treatment. The general and craniofacial features were suggestive of a rare syndrome, with retarded growth according to her chronological age, strange walking, and normal speech. The parents (father 26 and mother 29 years old, both healthy) reported that the patient was diagnosed with a nonsevere form of Morquio syndrome four years ago, confirmed by a significant increase in keratan sulfate in urine and a marked deficiency of galactosamine-6-sulfate activity in leucocyte cultures. No additional diagnostic tests (e.g., genetic analyses) for the condition were undertaken because the condition was diagnosed previously, and they represented a strong monetary outlay for the parents. At that time, the parents were recommended by the medical team to initiate treatment with enzyme replacement; however, the child had not received any type of therapy since the diagnosis by their own decision. The family history did not reveal any other relevant information. According to an exhaustive nutrition/diet questioning through the clinical history, her carbohydrate daily consumption (food and drinks) was considered low.

The clinical body examination manifested evident short stature and neck, slight scaphocephaly, bony deformities, protruded chest, stubby hands, kyphosis, and rotated legs. No neurological abnormalities were detected. The most important craniofacial features were brachycephaly, convex/-biprotusive profile, flat nasal bridge, closed nasolabial angle, apparent large mouth, and broad lips (Figure 1). Intraoral findings included a partially complete mixed dentition with several deep caries or cavities in all primary molars, ovoid arcades, anterior crossbite, mild open bite, macroglossia, and tongue thrusting; soft tissues were normal, but generalized moderate gingivitis was present; there also was high labial frenum (Figure 2). Parents reported occasional oral abnormal habits such as onychophagia, thumb sucking, and mouth breathing. Both temporomandibular joints were diagnosed as normal, according to a clinical examination involving manual palpation of the masticatory muscles; mouth opening, closing, and lateral movements, or deviations of the mandible; and lateral and dorsal extra-auricular auscultation with the aid of a stethoscope for the determination of abnormal joint sounds. Oral hygiene was considered poor. The patient exhibited significant anxiety and difficulties in maintaining an adequate supine posture on the dental chair.

An adequate restorative/endodontic/orthodontic treatment plan was designed and presented to the parents. They agreed and signed an informed consent form. Initially, the patient was behaviorally managed employing persistently different noninvasive psychological techniques (e.g., conditioning, gradual desensitization, "tell-show-do," and positive reinforcement), dental prophylaxis, and fluoride varnish applications; subsequently, a fair-to-good cooperation level was achieved. The restorative treatment consisted of the placement of preformed metallic crowns on all primary molars. Pulpotomies were performed in the right and left maxillary first and second primary molars, left mandibular first primary molar, and right mandibular second primary molar; and pulpectomies were performed in the left mandibular second primary molar and right mandibular first primary molar, under local anesthesia (lidocaine plus epinephrine) and rubber dam isolation. Pit and fissure sealants were also applied on the four permanent first molars (October 2016) (Figure 3). Additionally, a preventive program was initiated and supervised. Anterior teeth exhibited some small enamel chalky irregularities (Figure 4).

Then, the orthodontic clinical and cephalometric diagnosis (Figures 5(a) and 5(b)) was carried out, determining the presence of a pseudo-class III malocclusion. A Hyrax appliance was placed for four months (June 2017) (Figure 6). In October 2017, Hawley and Schwartz removable orthodontic appliances were placed, and in November 2017, a laser labial

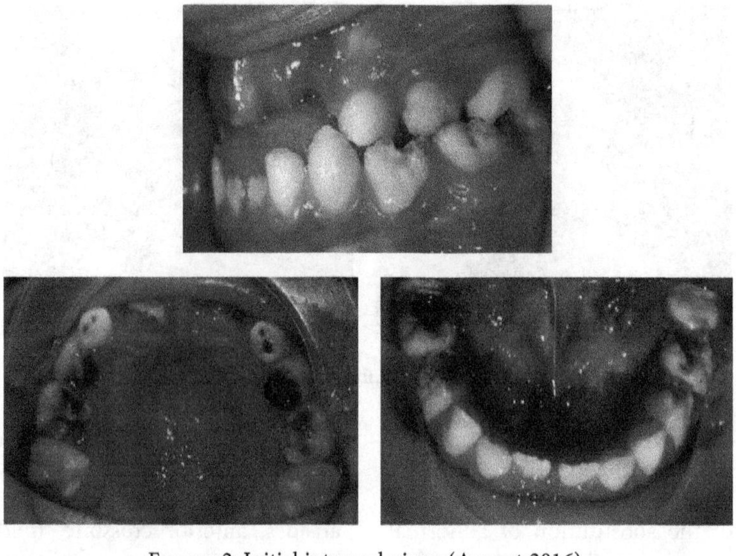

Figure 2: Initial intraoral views (August 2016).

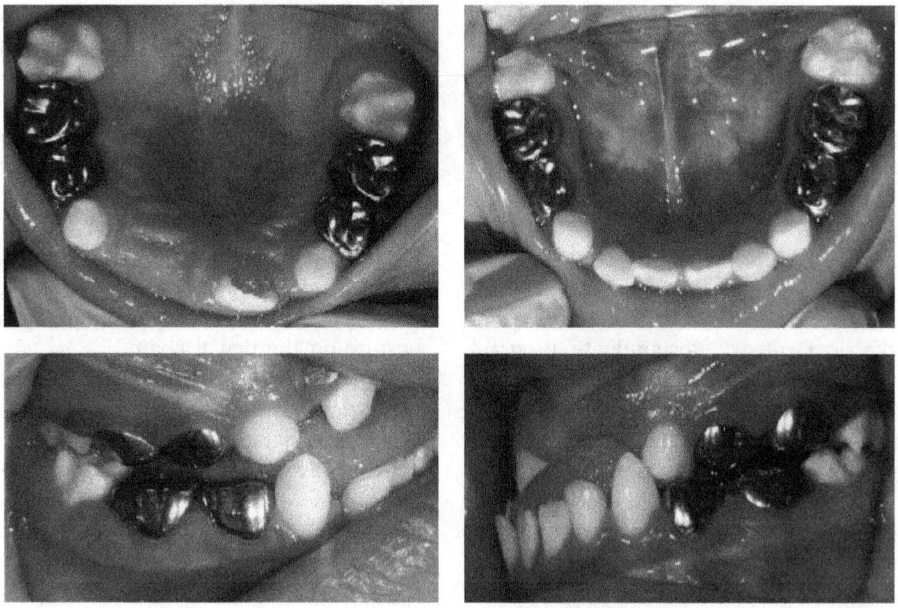

Figure 3: Oral rehabilitation treatment images (October 2016).

frenulectomy was carried out. Nine months later, the Hawley appliance was substituted by a fixed Nance button with "Z" springs over the upper incisors for treating the anterior crossbite (Figure 7).

Unexpectedly, two months later, a gingival lesion appeared above the right upper central incisor, diagnosed presumptively as a "localized juvenile spongiotic gingival hyperplasia (LJSGH)" (Figure 8(a)); after discussing with the oral surgeon, it was decided only to observe the lesion, without any kind of treatment. It healed spontaneously during the next 10 months approximately (Figure 8(b)).

In July 2019, the occlusal problems have been almost resolved (Figure 9). The last appointment was in September 2019 for clinical and radiographic control (Figure 10). In this orthodontic stage, the cooperation and participation levels of the child and her parents were considered excellent. The patient will be closely followed in order to assess the evolution of the potential class III malocclusion.

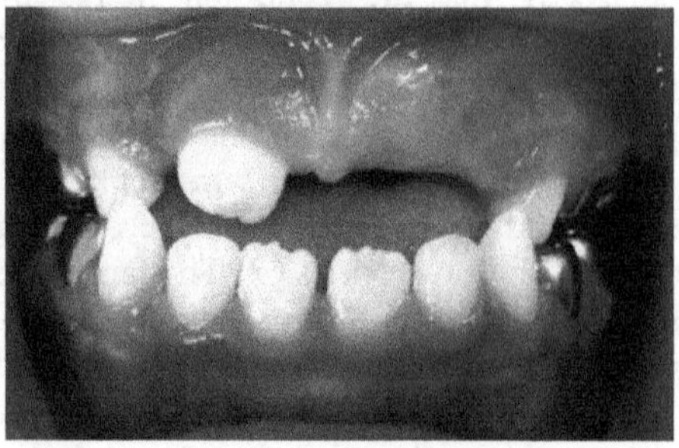

Figure 4: Postrehabilitation treatment (anterior view) (October 2016).

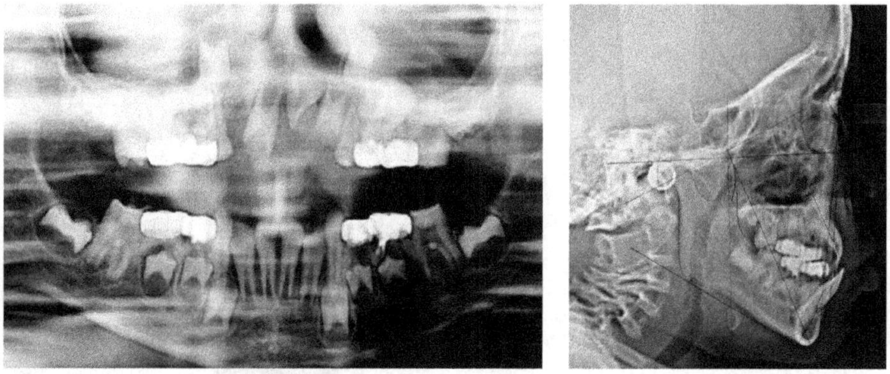

(a) (b)

FIGURE 5: (a) Radiographic view and (b) Ricketts cephalometric analysis (June 2017).

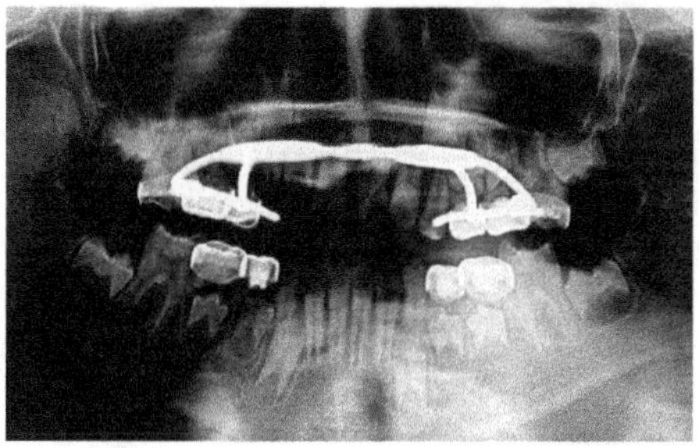

FIGURE 6: Hyrax appliance (June 2017).

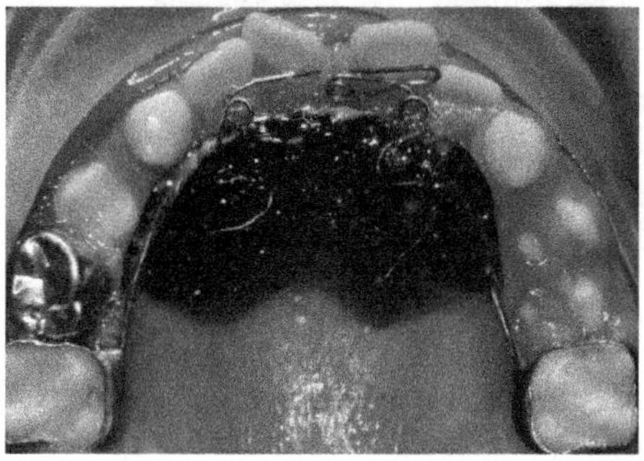

FIGURE 7: Fixed orthodontic appliance with Z springs (July 2018).

3. Discussion

According to the American Academy of Pediatric Dentistry guidelines, one of the most important purposes of this dental area is to provide "both primary and comprehensive preventive and therapeutic oral health care to individuals with Special Health Care Needs (SHCNs)," as an integral part of the pediatric dentistry practice. In this same context, the term SHCNs refers to those children with "any physical, developmental, cognitive, or emotional impairment or limiting condition that requires medical management, healthcare intervention, and/or the use of specialized services or programs" [12]. Mucopolysaccharidosis IV A or MAS is not an exception.

MAS is an uncommon autosomal recessive condition with multisystemic and progressive involvement. The syndrome has two variants: A and B. Type B is caused by a deficiency of β-galactosidase, and unlike type A, it usually lacks enamel hypoplasia [10]. Also, the latter finding suggests that GALNS is more determinant for enamel hypoplasia in patients with MAS, who are deficient in the enzyme. In this same regard, these authors theorize that GALNS deficiency may be the result of the abnormal accumulation of chondroitin-6-sulfate within the lysosomes of ameloblasts in the early secretory stage, in the course of odontogenesis [10]. It has been also suggested that during the first phases of amelogenesis, GAGs (mainly keratan sulfate) act as a matrix for a normal attachment between enamel and dentin through the production of amelogenin at the amelodentinal junction. In addition, Al-Jawad et al. [1] demonstrated that, in patients with MAS, deficient keratin sulfate in the dentine tubules disrupts the proper integration of enamel and dentin of primary and permanent teeth and causes an irregular hydroxyapatite crystal orientation and geometry throughout the enamel layer. As a consequence, in MAS-affected children, the occurrence of failures in enamel acid etching is frequent, affecting the adequate bonding of adhesive restorations. These histopathological findings have been as well associated with dental impactions and formation of dentigerous cysts [10]. In addition to the occurrence of enamel hypoplasia, there are other differences between mucopolysaccharidosis IV types A and B. It has been mentioned that patients with type B usually exhibit skeletal dysplasia of the long bones and extremities, with a more normal stature regarding type A; other authors have described the symptoms of type B as being mild (less severe) relative to those observed in patients with MAS [13].

On the other hand, reports along the recent history have mentioned the different oral, dental, and radiographic features in patients suffering from MAS [3, 8, 9, 14–18]. These manifestations are consistent between the studies and are helpful for performing a differential oral diagnosis with other similar disorders, for example, hypoplastic forms of amelogenesis imperfecta (AI), in which dental characteristics notoriously resemble those observed in MAS patients; however, AI lacks skeletal problems [4]. Regarding caries susceptibility, there are contradictory reports in the literature; some authors mention an increased risk for caries development while others establish that the risk is lower [8].

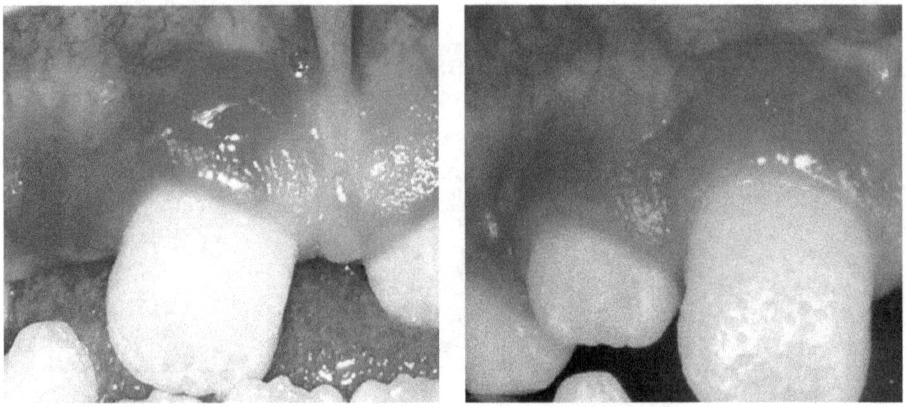

(a) (b)

Figure 8: (a) Spongiotic localized juvenile hyperplasia localized above the upper right central permanent incisor (October 2017). (b) The same lesion disappeared without any type of treatment (July 2018).

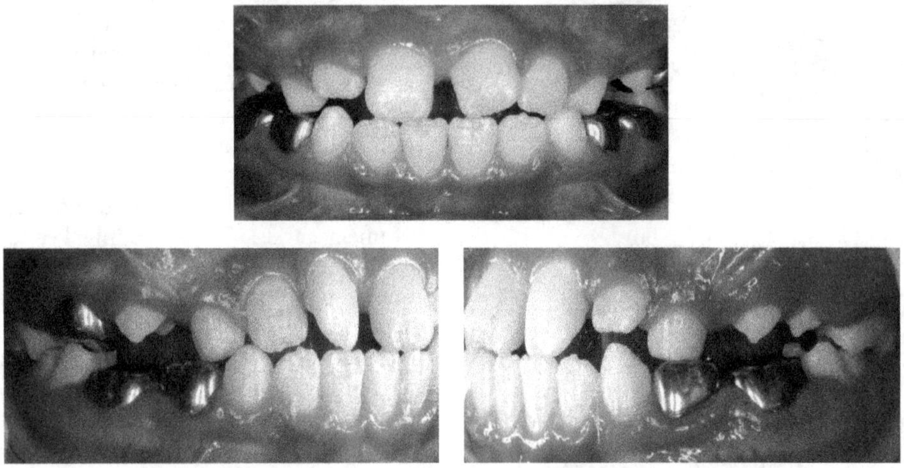

Figure 9: Recent intraoral views (July 2019).

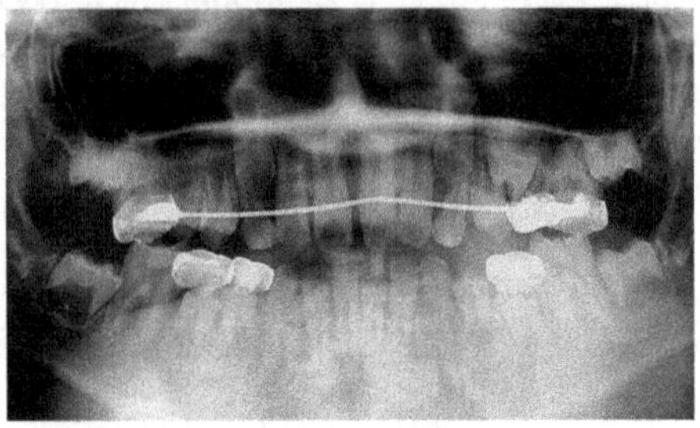

Figure 10: Radiographic control, Nance appliance (September 2019).

One relevant intraoral sign seen in the present patient was the occurrence of LJSGH during the orthodontic treatment. This is an unusual and painless type of self-limiting gingival inflammatory hyperplasia with female predilection. The lesion is characterized by a micropapillary or granular surface, with a bright red overgrowth on the attached gingiva, which may bleed easily during tooth brushing [19–21]. LJSGH may be clinically confounded with other similar conditions, such as simple inflamed gingiva, puberty gingivitis, pyogenic granuloma, inflammatory gingival hyperplasia, foreign body gingivitis, and linear gingival erythema, among others; demographic and clinical features are sufficient characteristics for an adequate diagnosis [21, 22]. According to Darling and coworkers [23], only persistent lesions should be surgically excised and sent to hystopatological analysis. Lack of response to periodontal therapy or topical corticoid therapy provides additional evidence for the diagnosis of LJSGH [21].

4. Conclusions

Pediatric dentistry practitioners must know all relevant bodily, craniofacial, and dental characteristics proper of MAS for early detection and to provide adequate oral management. As mentioned, this disease is frequently confounded with other similar dental conditions, such as AI in its hypoplastic form. Therefore, the pediatric dentist should be part of a multidisciplinary health team in order to perform a precise and opportune diagnosis. Then, it will be possible to offer some advice to the parents regarding the medical management and, of course, on the preventive, endodontic, restorative, and orthodontic procedures for improving the patient's general and oral health and, as consequence, her/his quality of life.

Consent

The patient's parents signed a prior informed consent form, approving the publication of the present case report and emphasizing the absolute confidentiality of the patient's personal identification.

Acknowledgments

This work was supported partially by the PFCE 2019 grant.

References

[1] M. Al-Jawad, O. Addison, M. A. Khan, A. James, and C. J. Hendriksz, "Disruption of enamel crystal formation quantified by synchrotron microdiffraction," *Journal of Dentistry*, vol. 40, no. 12, pp. 1074–1080, 2012.

[2] E. M. Ribeiro, C. S. R. Fonteles, A. B. Freitas, K. S. D. S. Alves, A. J. Monteiro, and C. A. B. Da Silva, "A clinical multicenter study of orofacial features in 26 Brazilian patients with different types of mucopolysaccharidosis," *The Cleft Palate Craniofacial Journal*, vol. 52, no. 3, pp. 352–358, 2015.

[3] D. J. de Santana Sarmento, S. H. G. de Carvalho, S. L. S. Melo et al., "Mucopolysaccharidosis: radiographic findings in a series of 16 cases," *Oral Surgery, Oral Medicine, Oral Pathology and Oral Radiology*, vol. 120, no. 6, pp. e240–e246, 2015.

[4] P. Rekka, P. V. Rathna, S. Jagadeesh, and S. Seshadri, "Mucopolysaccharidoses type IV A (Morquio syndrome): a case series of three siblings," *Journal of the Indian Society of Pedodontics and Preventive Dentistry*, vol. 30, no. 1, pp. 66–69, 2012.

[5] R. S. Lachman, B. K. Burton, L. A. Clarke et al., "Mucopolysaccharidosis IVA (Morquio A syndrome) and VI (Maroteaux-Lamy syndrome): under-recognized and challenging to diagnose," *Skeletal Radiology*, vol. 43, no. 3, pp. 359–369, 2014.

[6] S. Tomatsu, A. M. Montaño, H. Oikawa et al., "Mucopolysaccharidosis type IVA (Morquio A disease): clinical review and current treatment," *Current Pharmaceutical Biotechnology*, vol. 12, no. 6, pp. 931–945, 2011.

[7] S. Tomatsu, C. J. Alméciga-Díaz, H. Barbosa et al., "Therapies of mucopolysaccharidosis IVA (Morquio A syndrome)," *Expert Opinion on Orphan Drugs*, vol. 1, no. 10, pp. 805–818, 2013.

[8] D. Barker and R. R. Welbury, "Dental findings in Morquio syndrome (mucopolysaccharidoses type IVa)," *ASDC Journal of Dentistry for Children*, vol. 67, no. 6, pp. 431–3, 407, 2000.

[9] M. J. Kinirons and J. Nelson, "Dental findings in mucopolysaccharidosis type IV A (Morquio's disease type A)," *Oral Surgery, Oral Medicine, and Oral Pathology*, vol. 70, no. 2, pp. 176–179, 1990.

[10] R. Q. de Almeida-Barros, P. F. V. de Medeiros, M. Q. de Almeida Azevedo et al., "Evaluation of oral manifestations of patients with mucopolysaccharidosis IV and VI: clinical and imaging study," *Clinical Oral Investigations*, vol. 22, no. 1, pp. 201–208, 2018.

[11] T. C. Wood, K. Harvey, M. Beck et al., "Diagnosing mucopolysaccharidosis IVA," *Journal of Inherited Metabolic Disease*, vol. 36, no. 2, pp. 293–307, 2013.

[12] American Academy of Pediatric Dentistry, "Guideline of management of dental patients with special health care needs," *Pediatric Dentistry*, vol. 4, no. 6, pp. 237–242, 2018.

[13] C. J. Hendriksz, P. Harmatz, M. Beck et al., "Review of clinical presentation and diagnosis of mucopolysaccharidosis IVA," *Molecular Genetics and Metabolism*, vol. 110, no. 1-2, pp. 54–64, 2013.

[14] S. M. Garn and V. O. Hurme, "Dental defects in three siblings affected with Morquio's disease," *British Dental Journal*, vol. 93, no. 3, pp. 210–212, 1952.

[15] L. O. Langer Jr and L. S. Carey, "The roentgenographic features of the KS mucopolysaccharidosis of Morquio (MORQUIO-BRAILSFORD'S disease)," *The American Journal of Roentgenology, Radium Therapy, and Nuclear Medicine*, vol. 97, no. 1, pp. 1–20, 1966.

[16] D. G. Gardner, "The dental manifestations of the Morquio syndrome (mucopolysaccharidosis type IV). A diagnostic aid," *American Journal of Diseases of Children*, vol. 129, no. 12, pp. 1445–1448, 1975.

[17] L. S. Levin, R. J. Jorgenson, and C. F. Salinas, "Oral findings in the Morquio syndrome (mucopolysaccharidosis IV)," *Oral Surgery, Oral Medicine, and Oral Pathology*, vol. 39, no. 3, pp. 390–395, 1975.

[18] J. Nelson and M. Kinirons, "Clinical findings in 12 patients with MPS IV A (Morquio's disease). Further evidence for heterogeneity. Part II: dental findings," *Clinical Genetics*, vol. 33, no. 2, pp. 121–125, 1988.

[19] J. Y. F. Chang, H. P. Kessler, and J. M. Wright, "Localized juvenile spongiotic gingival hyperplasia," *Oral Surgery, Oral Medicine, Oral Pathology, Oral Radiology, and Endodontology*, vol. 106, no. 3, pp. 411–418, 2008.

[20] E. M. Kalogirou, K. Chatzidimitriou, K. I. Tosios, E. P. Piperi, and A. Sklavounou, "Localized juvenile spongiotic gingival hyperplasia: report of two cases," *Journal of Clinical Pediatric Dentistry*, vol. 41, no. 3, pp. 228–231, 2017.

[21] D. T. Fernandes, J. M. Wright, S. M. P. Lopes, A. R. Santos-Silva, P. A. Vargas, and M. A. Lopes, "Localized juvenile spongiotic gingival hyperplasia: a report of 4 cases and literature review," *Clinical Advances in Periodontics*, vol. 8, no. 1, pp. 1–14, 2017.

[22] L. W. Solomon, W. R. Trahan, and J. E. Snow, "Localized juvenile spongiotic gingival hyperplasia: a report of 3 cases," *Pediatric Dentistry*, vol. 35, no. 4, pp. 360–363, 2013.

[23] M. R. Darling, T. D. Daley, A. Wilson, and G. P. Wysocki, "Juvenile spongiotic gingivitis," *Journal of Periodontology*, vol. 78, no. 7, pp. 1235–1240, 2007.

8

Clinical Evaluation of Solitary Median Maxillary Central Incisor Syndrome

Malaz M. Mustafa, M. Zakirulla, Ibrahim AlShahrani, Rafi A. Togoo, Zuhair M. Alkahtani, and Tasneem S. Ain

Department of Pediatric Dentistry & Orthodontic Sciences, College of Dentistry, King Khalid University, Abha, Saudi Arabia

Correspondence should be addressed to M. Zakirulla; tamer@kku.edu.sa

Academic Editor: Alberto C. B. Delbem

Solitary median maxillary central incisor (SMMCI) is a rare dental anomaly. It is estimated to occur in 1 : 50,000 live births. The SMMCI tooth differs from the normal central incisor in that the crown form is symmetric and it develops and erupts precisely in the midline of the maxillary dental arch in both primary and permanent dentitions. The presence of SMMCI with hemifacial microsomia (HFM) is a very rare clinical condition. We report a case of SMMCI in a female of African ethnic origin, who presented with SMMCI in permanent dentition with mild nasal stenosis. An early diagnosis of SMMCI is important, since it may be a sign for other severe congenital or developmental abnormalities. Therefore, systematic follow-up and close monitoring of the growth and development of SMMCI patients are crucial.

1. Introduction

A solitary median maxillary central incisor (SMMCI) is a rare malformation associated with defects of midline structures, including the craniofacial bones, nasal airways (choanal atresia and nasal pyriform aperture stenosis), and developing brain (holoprosencephaly [HPE]), along with an increased risk of pituitary malformation and malfunction [1]. A large number of midline developmental defects, such as hypotelorism (closely spaced eyes) and microcephaly (small head circumference), have been reported in patients with SMMCI [2]. Sex predominance in SMMCI is a debatable issue, with some studies stating a female predominance, while others not stating any sex predilection [3, 4]. The etiology of SMMCI is unknown, but it may be related to a disruption in the development of the maxilla, which occurs during gestation at approximately 35 to 38 days, with abnormal formation of tooth germs and alveolar bone. The most common clinical characteristic of this malformation in the oral cavity is the presence of a single central incisor in the midline of the maxilla in both the dentitions [5].

The name originally given to this syndrome by Hall et al. [1] was "solitary median maxillary central incisor, short stature, choanal atresia/midnasal stenosis syndrome." It has now been customarily shortened to "solitary median maxillary central incisor syndrome" or SMMCI syndrome.

A family history of SMMCI or of holoprosencephaly, slow learning or intellectual disability, congenital nasal obstruction, microcephaly, epilepsy, very short stature, or other midline defects are seen in 25% of the cases [2, 6, 7]. Furthermore, studies have confirmed the suggestion that congenital nasal pyriform aperture stenosis (CNPAS) probably represents a manifestation of HPE [8]. SMMCI is detected in approximately 60% of CNPAS cases. The purpose of this paper was to report a case of a patient with a SMMCI.

2. Case Report

A 12-year-old female of African ethnic origin was reported to the pediatric dental clinic of King Khalid University, College of Dentistry. She was the third child among her five siblings, with no history of hereditary diseases reported by the

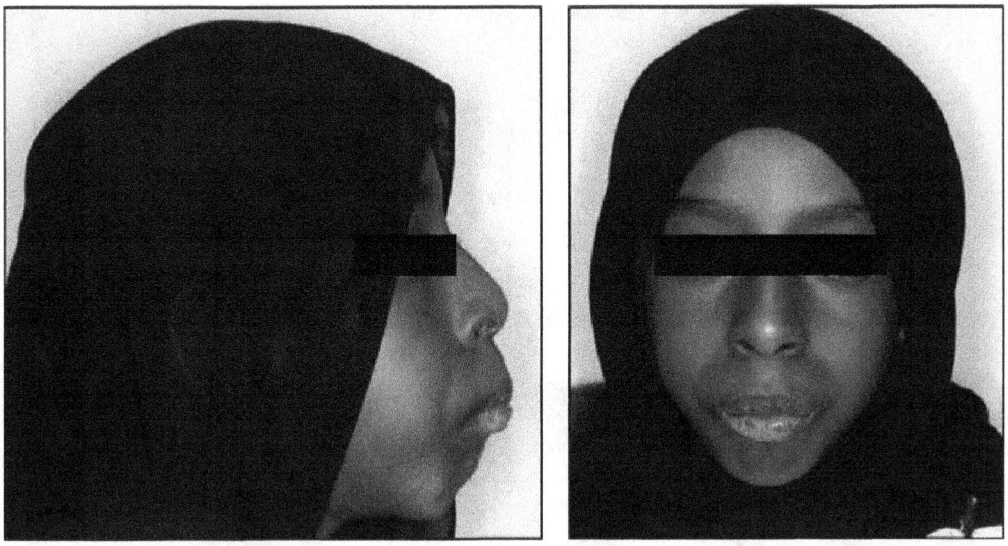

(a) (b)

FIGURE 1: Extraoral photograph of the patient showing (a) convex lateral facial profile and (b) frontal facial view where prominent nasal bone, narrow nose, indistinctive philtrum, and incompetent lips can be seen.

accompanying mother. The birth history of the patient was uneventful and was born as a full-term neonate of average birth weight by spontaneous normal delivery to healthy, nonconsanguineous parents. However, soon after birth, she suffered breathing difficulties and respiratory distress that necessitated her hospital admission for 37 days under observation. A diagnosis of mild nasal stenosis was made that did not require any intervention or treatment. The patient was then discharged, but there was no follow-up due to the patient's failure to appear for follow-up visits.

On extraoral examination, the patient had a noticeable convex facial profile, poorly distinctive philtrum of the upper lip, prominent nasal bone, narrow nose, and obviously incompetent lips (Figure 1). Intraorally, the maxillary labial frenum was entirely absent, and the palate was narrow, high arched, and V-shaped with a prominent midpalatal suture (Figure 2(a)). The dentition was in the mixed dentition stage, with Angle's quarter cusp class II molar occlusal relation on the right side, while the left side indicated a full cusp class II relation. An extreme horizontal overbite (>7 mm) was noted. Rampant caries was evident with retained root stumps of primary molars. On the left side, the maxillary and mandibular teeth exhibited heavy plaque and calculus accumulation as compared to the right, indicating a right-side chewing dominance. No abnormality was detected with respect to the oral mucosa and gingival tissues, except for a small sinus tract related to the remaining root stumps of the maxillary right first primary molar (Figures 2(b)–2(d)).

An SMMCI was present precisely at the midline, and the patient's mother reported its presence in the primary dentition as well. It exhibited mirror image symmetry between its right and left sides, which mimicked the anatomic contour of the distal surface of a normal maxillary central incisor (Figure 3). The patient was referred for orthodontic evaluation and assessment. A true lateral view (lateral cephalogram) of the patient revealed a class II skeletal pattern with a downward and backward mandibular rotation. Both Anterior Nasal Spine (ANS) and Sella Nasion-Mandibular Plane (SNMP) angles showed a huge disparity from normal values, which reflected a highly prominent premaxilla (Figure 4(a)). The child was later referred to a pediatrician for the assessment of her overall physical status and for further investigation. The patient was categorized as underweight as her body mass index (BMI) at the time of consultation was 13.4, which put her below the fifth percentile in the growth chart. No abnormalities were detected in the child's intelligence quotient level, brain structure, or growth hormone levels. However, nasal stenosis was observed on frontal cone beam computed tomography (Figure 4(b)).

The treatment plan for the current case consisted of two main phases: a preparatory phase of comprehensive oral rehabilitation of dental diseases, including extraction of all residual roots of primary molars and restoration of carious permanent teeth, followed by a corrective phase that would involve complex orthodontic treatment.

3. Discussion

SMMCI is a rare developmental anomaly that may occur as an isolated dental disorder or may be a part of a syndrome accompanied by a range of midline field defects [9]. The SMMCI syndrome is a complex syndrome comprising various defects, mainly midline defects of development that result from unknown factor(s) operating in utero around the 35th to 38th day from conception [1]. Although the etiology is unknown, it is believed to have a genetic background involving a mutation in gene Sonic Hedgehog (SHH) in chromosome 7q36.1 [10]. SMMCI has been reported to occur due to the fusion of two deciduous tooth germs and the permanent maxillary central incisors [11]. The single central incisor erupts exactly in the midaxial region and differs in morphology from the normal central incisors in that

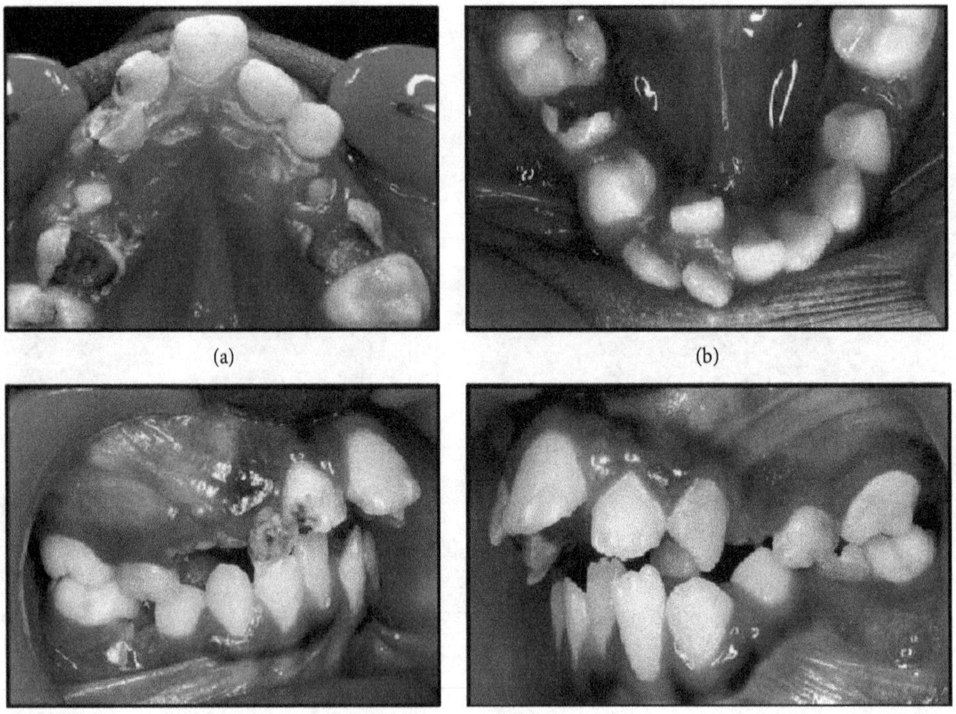

(a) (b) (c) (d)

Figure 2: Intraoral photographs are showing (a) upper jaw with characteristic prominent median palatal suture, (b) lower jaw with lingually erupting #42 indicating crowding; (c) right side view is showing sinus tract related to #54; and (2d) left side view showing heavy calculus accumulation.

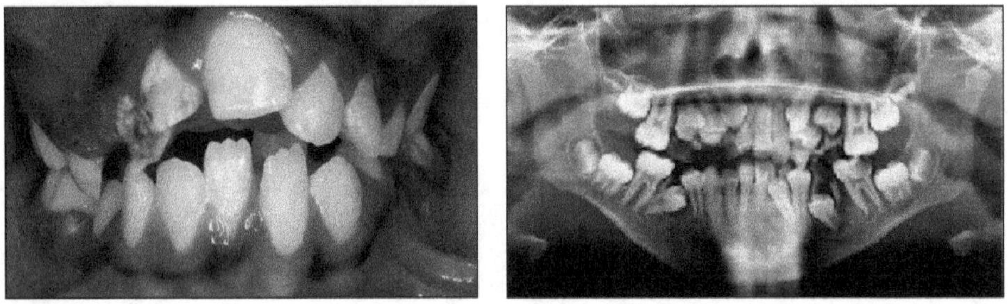

(a) (b)

Figure 3: Images show (a) an intraoral image showing the frontal view of SMMCI and (b) orthopantomography (OPG) showing SMMCI.

it exhibits a symmetrical dental crown (as seen in the present case report where an SMMCI was located precisely in the midline) with identical right and left surfaces, unlike a normal central incisor [2, 12].

The condition of SMMCI can be recognized prior to the eruption of the deciduous single incisor. Diagnosis can be made prenatally with ultrasound or genetic testing; however, it is more commonly confirmed at birth. The child may present a notched upper lip, along with the absence of a labial frenulum and a narrow nose. Preterm birth and low birth weight are also seen in 37% of the cases [1]. In the present case, the patient was a full-term neonate with average birth weight, as reported by her mother.

In the literature, more than 70 systemic abnormalities have been described in SMMCI patients without a defined syndrome [13, 14]. SMMCI may occur as an isolated trade or along with various other midline developmental defects including "congenital heart disease" [15]; "short stature" [14–18]; "congenital nasal pyriform aperture stenosis" [19, 20]; "pituitary insufficiency" [17, 18]; "microcephaly" [15]; "midnasal stenosis" [16]; "scoliosis" [15]; choanal atresia; cleft lip and cleft palate; less commonly microcephaly, hypopituitarism, hypotelorism, convergent strabismus, esophageal and duodenal atresia, cervical hemivertebrae, cervical dermoid, hypothyroidism, scoliosis, absent kidney, micropenis, and ambiguous genitalia. 50% of the reported cases exhibited short stature [14, 16]. On the other hand, numerous identified syndromes have been reported in SMMCI patients, including ectodermal dysplasia [21], Duane retraction syndrome [22], velocardiofacial syndrome, CHARGE syndrome, vacterl associations, and HPE. Systemic conditions were found in 50% of cases including 20% asthma and allergies; multiple hemangiomas; alopecia with parchment skin; ptosis; ocular coloboma; congenital talipes

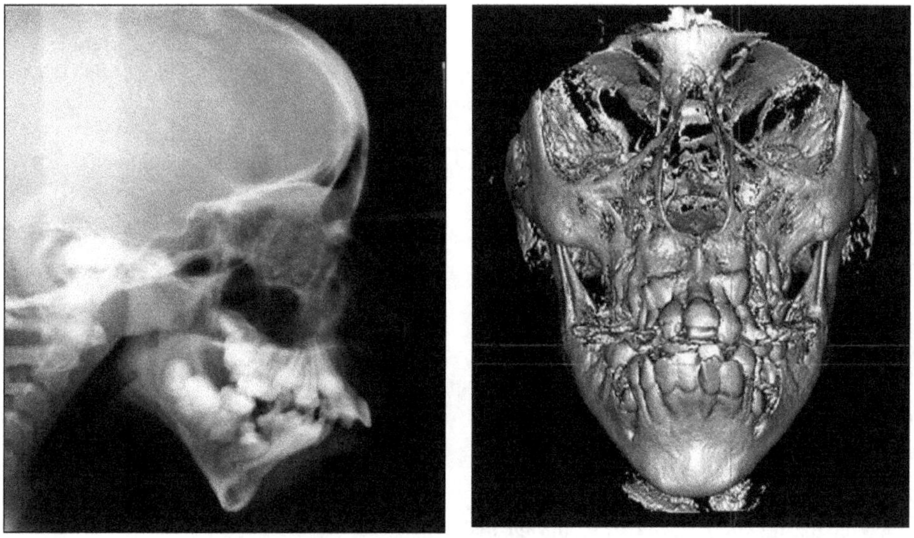

(a) (b)

FIGURE 4: Images shows (a) lateral cephalogram and (b) cone beam computed tomography (CBCT) frontal view showing SMMCI.

equinovarus; oligodontia; and absent thumb [16]. Less common manifestations comprise diabetic pregnancies (14%), preterm labor, and low birth weight (37%) [1].

In our case report, the patient was diagnosed with mild nasal stenosis since birth. Congenital nasal malformation associated with SMMCI (midnasal stenosis, choanal atresia, or congenital narrowing of nasal pyriform aperture). The patient's mother reported that the patient suffered severe respiratory distress soon after birth for which she was hospitalized for approximately 37 days. Previous studies have reported that respiratory problems are quite frequent among SMMCI cases due to nasal stenosis, which makes it difficult for newborn babies to breathe through the nostrils. The presence of an SMMCI tooth can be an indicator of associated anomalies, particularly of the serious anomaly of holoprosencephaly [23].

On extraoral examination, the patient presented a noticeable convex facial profile, poorly distinctive philtrum of the upper lip, prominent nasal bone, narrow nose, and obvious incompetent lips. Previous cases have been reported wherein SMMCI was associated with features such as pseudo-notched or arch-shaped upper lip appearance with an indistinct philtrum, which is believed to be due to the prominent maxillary alveolus over the developing primary SMMCI tooth. Other features include nonexistence of the labial frenulum, with a narrow nose, a V-shaped palate, and narrow ridge along the midpalatal suture.

In several studies conducted earlier, SMMCI syndrome has been associated with a short stature and growth hormone deficiency [7, 11, 24]. The patient in this report was found to be underweight as per her BMI. Dental experts are familiar with the fundamentals of SMMCI syndrome and can help detect serious associated abnormalities such as HPE. Thus, they can suggest proper referral or treatment to the affected patients. Bolan et al. rightly mention that dentists are usually the first health professionals to face patients with SMMCI, which makes it obligatory for them to know and understand the appropriate diagnosis and treatment plan [25]. Various treatment options can be adopted for treating SMMCI cases depending upon its severity and associated problems.

Proper management of SMMCI (following diagnosis and genetic counseling) necessitates comprehensive pediatric dental care if the case presentation included SMMCI and mild nasal airway narrowing exclusively without other manifestations. A facial growth pattern in both transverse and sagittal directions should be analyzed in addition to serial photographs taken as part of routine dental reviews. Intervention is not required in the primary dentition [14]. In the permanent dentition stage, orthodontic intervention will be in the form of palatal expansion to accommodate sufficient space for the SMMCI and growing maxilla. Furthermore, a space required to accommodate for a contralateral artificial central incisor can be provided by either distalization of the first permanent molars or, otherwise, extraction of premolars. Artificial replacement of the contralateral missing central incisor can be in the form of a spoon denture, bridge, or single tooth implant at an older age (17-18 years old) [1]. Some cases might require extraction of the SMMCI followed by mesialization and reshaping of the laterals, canines, and premolars [12]. In case of associated syndromes, a more complex treatment requiring interdisciplinary care might be necessary [14].

4. Conclusion

A multidisciplinary approach is essential for the management of affected individuals and their families. Early diagnosis of SMMCI is important, as it may be a sign of other severe congenital or developmental abnormalities. Therefore, systematic follow-up and close monitoring of the growth and development of SMMCI patients are crucial. Referral to a pediatrician for further investigation is important. Comprehensive dental management for the patient should be tailored to suit the patient's need. Medical input needs to be supplemented by a team including a pedodontist, an orthodontist, an endodontist, and an oral surgeon, as well as a speech therapist and a psychologist.

Consent

Informed consent was obtained from all individual participants included in the study.

References

[1] R. K. Hall, "Solitary median maxillary central incisor (SMMCI) syndrome," *Orphanet Journal of Rare Diseases*, vol. 1, no. 1, p. 12, 2006.

[2] L. Nanni, J. E. Ming, Y. du et al., "*SHH* mutation is associated with solitary median maxillary central incisor: a study of 13 patients and review of the literature," *American Journal of Medical Genetics*, vol. 102, no. 1, pp. 1–10, 2001.

[3] E. Machado, P. Machado, B. Grehs, and R. A. Grehs, "Síndrome do incisivo central superior solitário: relato de caso," *Dental Press Journal of Orthodontics*, vol. 15, no. 4, pp. 55–61, 2010.

[4] S. Nuvvula, N. Gokhale, V. Yamini, and G. Shilpa, "Concomitant solitary median maxillary central incisor and fused right mandibular incisor in primary dentition," *Contemporary Clinical Dentistry*, vol. 3, no. 6, pp. 203–205, 2012.

[5] A. T. Lim, K. L. Hung, T. H. Chen, and H. T. Liao, "Solitary median maxillary central incisor syndrome with midnasal stenosis: case report," *Fu-Jen Journal of Medicine*, vol. 9, no. 1, pp. 37–42, 2011.

[6] S. Viana Eda, P. F. Kramer, L. Q. Closs, and G. Scalco, "Solitary median maxillary central incisor syndrome and holoprosencephaly: a case report," *Pediatric Dentistry*, vol. 32, no. 5, pp. 424–427, 2010.

[7] H. Hattori, T. Okuno, T. Momoi et al., "Single central maxillary incisor and holoprosencephaly," *American Journal of Medical Genetics*, vol. 28, no. 2, pp. 483–487, 1987.

[8] M. Devambez, A. Delattre, and P. Fayoux, "Congenital nasal pyriform aperture stenosis: diagnosis and management," *The Cleft Palate-Craniofacial Journal*, vol. 46, no. 3, pp. 262–267, 2009.

[9] N. Johnson, R. Windrim, K. Chong, S. Viero, M. Thompson, and S. Blaser, "Prenatal diagnosis of solitary median maxillary central incisor syndrome by magnetic resonance imaging," *Ultrasound in Obstetrics & Gynecology*, vol. 32, no. 1, pp. 120–122, 2008.

[10] A. Utreja, S. N. Zahid, and R. Gupta, "Solitary median maxillary central incisor in association with hemifacial microsomia: a rare case report and review of literature," *Contemporary Clinical Dentistry*, vol. 2, no. 4, pp. 385–389, 2011.

[11] O. Ilhan, Y. Pekcevik, S. Akbay et al., "Solitary median maxillary central incisor, holoprosencephaly and congenital nasal pyriform aperture stenosis in a premature infant: case report," *Archivos Argentinos de Pediatría*, vol. 116, no. 1, pp. 130–134, 2018.

[12] K. B. Becktor, L. Sverrild, C. Pallisgaard, J. Burhøj, and I. Kjaer, "Eruption of the central incisor, the intermaxillary suture, and maxillary growth in patients with a single median maxillary central incisor," *Acta Odontologica Scandinavica*, vol. 59, no. 6, pp. 361–366, 2001.

[13] S. Y. Cho and B. K. Drummond, "Solitary median maxillary central incisor and normal stature: a report of three cases," *International Journal of Paediatric Dentistry*, vol. 16, no. 2, pp. 128–134, 2006.

[14] A. E. Sekerci, F. I. Uçar, H. Gümüş, M. Aydınbelge, and Y. Sisman, "Solitary median maxillary central incisor: a report of 2 cases," *Pediatric Dentistry*, vol. 34, no. 2, pp. 150–155, 2012.

[15] E. D. Fulstow, "The congenital absence of an upper central incisor," *British Dental Journal*, vol. 124, pp. 186–188, 1968.

[16] R. K. Hall, A. Bankier, M. J. Aldred, K. Kan, J. O. Lucas, and A. G. B. Perks, "Solitary median maxillary central incisor, short stature, choanal atresia/midnasal stenosis (SMMCI) syndrome," *Oral Surgery, Oral Medicine, Oral Pathology, Oral Radiology, and Endodontics*, vol. 84, no. 6, pp. 651–662, 1997.

[17] E. B. Rappaport, R. A. Ulstrom, and R. J. Gorlin, "Monosuperocentroincisivodontic dwarfism," *Birth Defects Original Article Series*, vol. 12, pp. 243–245, 1976.

[18] M. Vanelli, S. Bernasconi, and P. Balestrazzi, "Solirary maxillary central incisor with growth hormone deficiency," *Archives Françaises de Pédiatrie*, vol. 37, pp. 321-322, 1980.

[19] S. A. Royal, G. L. Hedlund, and B. J. Wiatrak, "Single central maxillary incisor with nasal pyriform aperture stenosis: CT diagnosis prior to tooth eruption," *Pediatric Radiology*, vol. 29, no. 5, pp. 357–359, 1999.

[20] K. Blackmore and D. M. Wynne, "A case of solitary median maxillary central incisor (SMMCI) syndrome with bilateral pyriform aperture stenosis and choanal atresia," *International Journal of Pediatric Otorhinolaryngology*, vol. 74, no. 8, pp. 967–969, 2010.

[21] I. Buntinx and M. Barairser, "A single maxillary incisor as a manifestation of an ectodermal dysplasia," *Journal of Medical Genetics*, vol. 26, no. 10, pp. 648–651, 1989.

[22] F. Parentin and P. Perissutti, "Solitary median maxillary central incisor, Duane retraction syndrome, growth hormone deficiency and duplicated thumb phalanx: a case report," *Clinical Dysmorphology*, vol. 12, no. 2, pp. 141-142, 2003.

[23] S. Yang, P. Orta II, E. M. Renk, and J. C. Inman, "Congenital nasal pyriform aperture stenosis in association with solitary median maxillary central incisor: unique radiologic features," *Radiology Case Reports*, vol. 11, no. 3, pp. 178–181, 2016.

[24] N. N. Lygidakis, K. Chatzidimitriou, N. Petrou, and N. A. Lygidakis, "Solitary median maxillary central incisor syndrome (SMMCI) with congenital nasal puriform aperture stenosis: literature review and case report with comprehensive dental treatment and 14 years follow-up," *European Archives of Paediatric Dentistry*, vol. 14, no. 6, pp. 417–423, 2013.

[25] M. Bolan, C. D.'. A. Derech, M. Côrrea, G. L. U. Ribeiro, and I. C. S. Almeida, "Palatal expansion in a patient with solitary median maxillary central incisor syndrome," *American Journal of Orthodontics and Dentofacial Orthopedics*, vol. 138, no. 4, pp. 493–497, 2010.

9

Gingival Bleeding in a Child with Fanconi Anemia: A Case Report and Literature Review

Dorsaf Touil, Rahma Bouhouch, Raoua Belkacem Chebil, Lamia Oualha, and Nabiha Douki

University of Monastir, Dental Faculty of Monastir, Research Laboratory LR12ES11, Tunisia

Correspondence should be addressed to Dorsaf Touil; touil.oueslati.dorsaf@gmail.com

Academic Editor: Leandro Napier de Souza

Fanconi anemia (FA) is a rare autosomal recessive disorder characterized by multiple congenital abnormalities, bone marrow failure, and higher susceptibility to malignancies, especially to head and neck carcinomas. Only few reports about the oral manifestations of FA are available. The main reported oral conditions associated with FA are microdontia and advanced periodontitis. The aim of this paper was to report a case of a 10-year-old patient with FA presenting severe spontaneous gingival bleeding, as well as to discuss the role of the dentist in the management and treatment of this condition.

1. Introduction

Fanconi anemia (FA) is a genetic disorder occurring in 1-2 per 100000 births [1]. In 90% of the cases, it is caused by a mutation in 3 genes: FNCA, FANCC, and FANCA. All the genes implicated in the development of FA DNA are involved in the crosslink repair pathway. Thus, patients with FA exhibit impaired capacity to repair the DNA crosslinks [2].

Clinically, FA is often characterized by multiple congenital abnormalities, progressive bone marrow failure, and an increased risk of developing squamous cell carcinomas, particularly head and neck squamous cell cancer, at a young age [3]. The clinical course of FA begins in the first decade of life, during which patients exhibit congenital abnormalities, hematological disturbances, or both [4]. Their physical abnormalities may include a short stature, abnormal skin pigmentation, thumb and radial anomalies, structural renal defects, microcephaly, and delayed development that are recognizable at birth and/or during early childhood [5].

There are only few reports with regard to the oral manifestations of FA. The main described oral conditions associated with FA are microdontia, missing teeth, and advanced periodontitis [6].

Patients with severe periodontitis may present gingival bleeding, tooth mobility, and halitosis. These manifestations are often related to the host defense impairment seen in these subjects, which increases their susceptibility to periodontal infection, and to the poor oral hygiene [6, 7].

The thrombocytopenia exacerbates the gingival bleeding and complicates its management, especially in young patients who are affected not only by the disease but also by the heavy treatment that often requires long hospitalization periods, which dramatically reduces their access to oral hygiene [8].

The aim of this paper was to report a case of a 10-year-old patient with FA presenting severe spontaneous gingival bleeding, as well as to discuss the role of the dentist in the management and the treatment of this condition.

2. Case Report

Written informed consent of the patient's father was obtained prior to this paper's publication.

A 10-year-old male patient (Figure 1) was referred by his hematologist to the Department of Oral Medicine at the University Hospital Sahloul, Tunisia, for spontaneous severe gingival bleeding during the last two days before consultation.

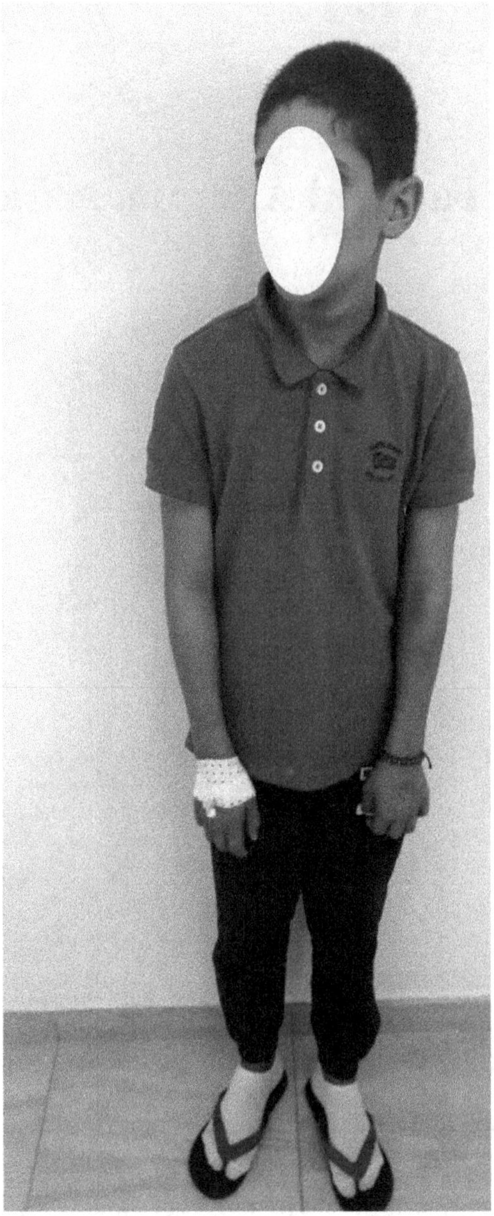

FIGURE 1: Physical examination of the patient showing a short stature.

The patient was diagnosed with FA at the age of five. The patient's family history was significant as he was the second child of a consanguineous marriage. His parents and sibling were healthy. The patient was operated for bifid thumbs at the age of 2 years (Figure 2) and for cryptorchidism at the age of seven.

The child's physical examination revealed a short stature (Figure 1). He had a pale skin as well as skin pigmentations in the form of "café au lait" spots that were noticeable on his face and arms.

The intraoral examination revealed petechial hemorrhages with oozing blood from the gingiva which was more evident in the lower anterior region with a blood collection in the lower vestibule.

His total blood count showed hemoglobin (Hb) = 6.2 g/dL, platelet (PLT) = 6000/μL, and white blood cell (WBC) = 1170/mm^3.

Given the patient's agitation, the pancytopenia, and the severe bleeding, no dental therapeutics were possible.

Our therapeutic approach consisted in the application of a sterile compress soaked in tranexamic acid (Exacyl 1 mL/10 L) in local compression for 5 minutes in each bleeding area. A prescription of tranexamic acid, four times a day, as a passive mouthwash was recommended. The patient was asked to avoid hot foods and drinks.

The patient was hospitalized to keep him under supervision and to correct his blood count. Given the FA-related severe thrombocytopenia, a platelet concentrate was necessary to raise the platelet count above 50000/μL. The patient was therefore given a single unit of leuko-depleted and irradiated apheresis platelet.

We received the patient two days later—during his hospital setting—for dental scaling. His blood count revealed Hb = 8.2 g/L, PLT = 51000/mm^3, and WBC = 1170/mm^3.

The oral examination showed poor oral hygiene and discolored teeth. However, the gingival bleeding was scarce (Figures 3(a) and 3(b)).

Sixty minutes before the dental scaling, the patient received 1.5 g ampicillin per os to reduce the risk of postoperative infection. We started by rinsing the patient's mouth for 2 minutes with 0.2% chlorhexidine solution; after that, manual supragingival scaling was performed under local anesthesia. The gingival bleeding was controlled by local compression using gauze saturated with tranexamic acid.

At the end of the treatment session, the patient and his parents received succinct instructions with regard to the importance of maintaining good oral hygiene, as well as the regular monitoring of his mouth.

The patient's parents were informed of the risks of developing malignancies, and they were asked to perform a regular mouth inspection to their child to detect any possible suspicious lesion. Follow-up sessions were scheduled.

3. Discussion

Fanconi anemia is a rare autosomal recessive syndrome caused by mutations in one of at least 19 genes. The proteins encoded by these genes act together to protect the genomic integrity [1].

FA belongs to a group of hereditary disorders clinically characterized by bone marrow failure, congenital malformations, and susceptibility to cancer [4].

The early symptoms of FA include multiple anomalies, such as skin pigmentation in the form of "café au lait" spots, short stature, thumb and genital anomalies, microcephaly, and cognitive impairment [9].

However, some patients with FA may not have any physical anomalies or skin lesions [10]. In the International Fanconi Anemia Registry (IFAR), a third of patients with FA were reported as not having any congenital malformations [11]. In our case, the patient was operated for both bifid thumb and cryptorchidism.

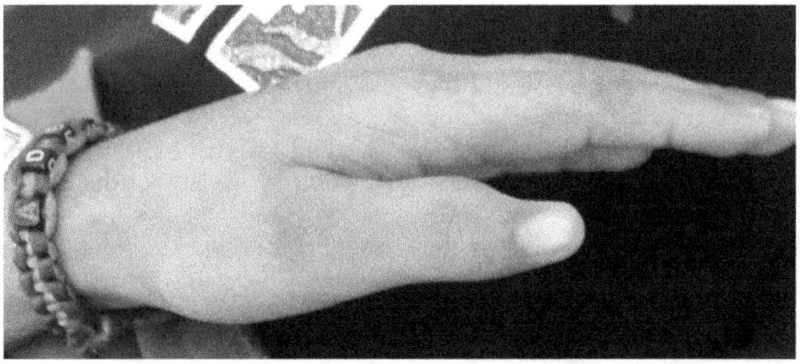

Figure 2: Operated bifid thumb.

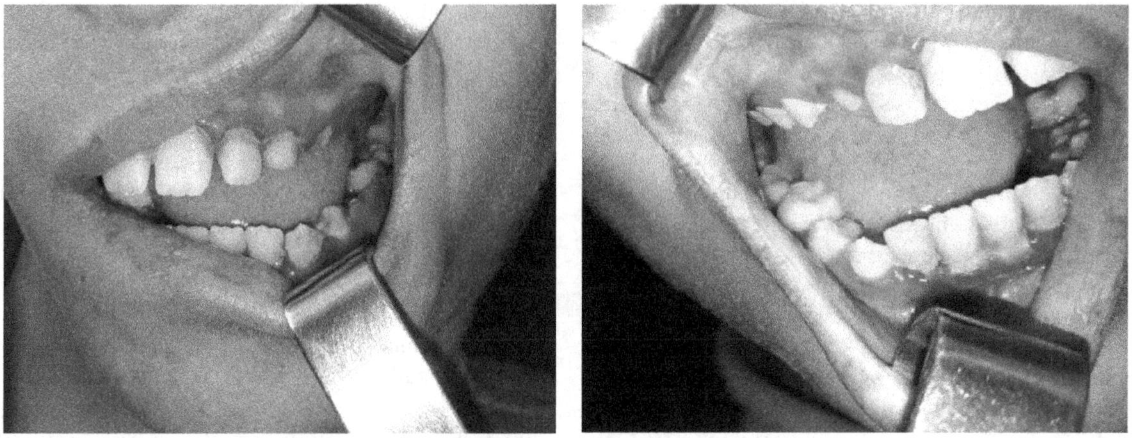

(a) (b)

Figure 3: Oral examination showing poor oral hygiene and discolored teeth.

Due to its highly variable phenotype, diagnosis may be difficult in some patients. For this reason, tests such as chromosome breakage analysis and comet assays are often performed to reach a definitive diagnosis [4].

The most frequent hematological complications of FA are pancytopenia, anemia, thrombocytopenia, and leukopenia. Because of these complications, patients affected by FA may develop severe bleeding as well as recurrent infections [12]. At the time of consultation, our patient had pancytopenia, especially a severe thrombocytopenia, which may explain the severity of the gingival bleeding.

The oral manifestations are frequently mentioned in the clinical descriptions of FA, but their prevalence has not been well documented [6]. As reported in the literature, the main oral findings associated with FA are gingivitis (41.5%) and severe periodontitis (22.3%) [7]. The high predisposition of patients with FA to periodontal disease may be due to anemia and leukopenia [13]. Moreover, the medications applied during the immunosuppressive treatment, such as corticosteroids, may further reduce the immunological defense, thus leading to a higher risk for periodontal disease [7]. It is worth mentioning that the poor oral hygiene remains a major cause of periodontal disease. Our patient had very poor oral hygiene and was not motivated to take care of his dentition. The long hospitalization periods were found to be the reason behind his demotivation and negligence.

Oral petechial hemorrhages and spontaneous gingival bleeding are common in patients with FA and are related to the very low platelet counts [14]. In previous case reports, oral traumatic and petechial hemorrhage lesions were seen in 30% of the patients and they were associated with decreased platelet level [6].

In another study, gingival bleeding was noted in 16% of patients with aplastic anemia [14].

Aphthous lesions were also reported in the literature. Some authors associated recurrent aphthous ulcers with the hematological condition, particularly anemia and neutropenia [14].

Dental anomalies such as agenesis, supernumerary teeth, microdontia, rotation, transposition, delayed eruption, and discolored teeth have been identified [9]. Oyaizu et al. reported a case of a patient with FA having macroglossia and generalized microdontia [12]. In the study of de Araujo et al., 9.1% of the patients showed anomalies in teeth on panoramic radiographs [6]. In the case we report, the patient had a complete dental formula but all his teeth were discolored.

Few studies have cited the prevalence of dental caries in the FA population. Caries were found to be associated with poor oral hygiene and accumulation of plaque but not with the systemic condition [9]. A preventive dental treatment plan should be implemented for all FA patients. It should include motivation to strict oral hygiene, conservative treatment of decayed teeth, and sealing of pits and fissures of the occlusal surfaces.

A close cooperation between the hematologist and the dentist is necessary to prevent excessive hemorrhage during dental procedures, especially when performing invasive ones, such as dental extractions, subgingival scaling, block anesthesia, or oral surgery. The platelet count should then be raised to at least 50000 μL [12, 15]. Thus, the dental treatment for these patients should be pursued in a hospital setting to ensure an appropriate follow-up of any acute complications that may arise [14]. Our patient was hospitalized to be kept under close supervision. He was given a single unit of leuko-depleted and irradiated apheresis platelets to raise his blood count. His platelet count was raised to 51000/mm^3, which was imperative to perform dental scaling without any excessive bleeding.

Moreover, dentists must use local hemostatic measures following the dental extraction in these patients as well as sutures and topic agents, such as oxycellulose, gelatine, fibrin glue, and cyanoacrylate [16, 17]. An antifibrinolytic treatment using tranexamic acid (TA) is also recommended to prevent postoperative bleeding. Various reports have described the successful local use of TA for the reduction of the oral bleeding [18]. In the case we report, a successful control of the gingival bleeding was obtained using compressive gauze saturated with TA.

Patients with FA must receive antibiotics if the absolute neutrophil count is less than 500/μL. There is no consensus on antibiotic prophylaxis for a neutrophil count greater than 500/mm^3. Antibiotic prophylaxis, typically with amoxicillin or clindamycin, should be given one hour before invasive dental procedures and should be continued until mucosal healing to prevent serious complications [19]. Dentists should also consider prescribing an antiseptic mouthwash prior to the dental management. The use of chlorhexidine mouth rinse, 30 min before the dental procedure, may be effective in reducing the risk of postoperative infection, as it has been shown to be effective in reducing plaque and gingival inflammation [12]. As antibioprophylaxis, our patient received 1.5 g ampicillin per os, 60 min before the procedure. We also used a chlorhexidine mouthwash few minutes before the gingival scaling. Our patient did not have any local or systemic complications.

The propensity to develop cancer is well documented in patients with FA. This condition is associated with a 30- to 80-fold increased risk of developing solid tumors [20] which is thought to be related to the chromosomal instability [1, 3].

The squamous cell carcinomas of the head and neck (HNSCC) represent the most frequent solid tumors. Patients with FA have up to 500-fold increased risk of developing such tumors compared to the general population [2], and these tumors are commonly located in the oral cavity [21]. Moreover, the International Fanconi Anemia Registry study observed a 20% higher risk of SCC in FA patients aged over 40 years. The median age of HNSCC diagnosis was 32 years compared to a median age of 63 in the general population [1]. On the other hand, HNSCC in the FA population have a poor prognosis and are known for their aggressive growth capacity and propensity to metastasize [5, 22].

Tobacco smoking and alcohol consumption, which are common risk factors for HNSCC in the general population, do not seem to be significant risk factors in FA patients [1, 17]. However, some authors have suggested that HPV is a leading risk factor for SCC of the head and neck in this population where 84% of the SCC contained quantifiable HPV DNA [1, 3].

Patients who underwent bone marrow transplantation have a greater incidence of malignancy development [3]. A recent study reported a 4.4-fold higher risk for SCC in FA patients who received transplants [23]. According to the authors, chronic GVHD seem to be a strong risk factor for SCC. In addition, it is suggested that in these patients, the disease onset also occurs approximately 10 years earlier [3].

Because of the high risk of developing oral cancer, an early screening together with a careful examination of the mucosal tissues is very important. Specialists recommend their patients to have an oral examination at 3- to 6-month intervals [24]. These sessions should include instruction in maintaining excellent oral hygiene. Self-examination of the mouth is recommended as a secondary preventive measure [25]. Even if our patient did not have any suspicious oral lesions, his parents were informed of the higher risk of developing carcinomas and were therefore taught how to perform meticulous examination to their child's oral cavity.

To conclude, dealing with the severe gingival bleeding of our young patient required the correction of his blood count and the use of an antifibrinolytic agent in local compression and a mouthwash. All these measures were necessary before starting the local treatment which consisted in a supragingival scaling that was aimed at reducing the local inflammation. These measures were efficient for a successful control of the severe gingival bleeding.

Still, no consensus is available with regard to the dental treatment modalities of patients with Fanconi anemia.

References

[1] D. I. Kutler, K. R. Patel, A. D. Auerbach et al., "Natural history and management of Fanconi anemia patients with head and neck cancer: a 10-year follow-up," *The Laryngoscope*, vol. 126, no. 4, pp. 870–879, 2016.

[2] T. H. Beckham, J. Leeman, C. Jillian Tsai et al., "Treatment modalities and outcomes of Fanconi anemia patients with head and neck squamous cell carcinoma: series of 9 cases and review of the literature," *Head & Neck*, vol. 41, no. 5, pp. 1418–1426, 2019.

[3] S. Goncalves, J. Montgomery-Cranny, K. D. Hunter, A. Yousefpour, L. Durham, and A. M. Hegarty, "Oral squamous cell carcinoma in patients with Fanconi anemia: a case series," *Journal of Case Reports and Images in Dentistry*, vol. 2, pp. 42–46, 2016.

[4] W. Deng, M. Zhao, Y. Liu, L. Cao, and M. Yang, "Fanconi anemia in twins with neutropenia: a case report," *Oncology Letters*, vol. 16, no. 4, pp. 5325–5330, 2018.

[5] D. I. Kutler, A. D. Auerbach, J. Satagopan et al., "High incidence of head and neck squamous cell carcinoma in patients with Fanconi anemia," *Archives of Otolaryngology – Head & Neck Surgery*, vol. 129, no. 1, pp. 106–112, 2003.

[6] M. R. de Araujo, M. de Oliveira Ribas, A. C. G. A. Koubik, T. Mattioli, and A. A. S. de Lima, "Fanconi's anemia: clinical and radiographic oral manifestations," *Oral Diseases*, vol. 13, no. 3, pp. 291–295, 2007.

[7] S. G. M. Falci, P. Corrêa-Faria, J. Tataounoff, C. R. R. dos Santos, and L. S. Marques, "Fanconi's anemia in dentistry: a case report and brief literature review," *Revista Odonto Ciência (Online)*, vol. 26, no. 3, pp. 272–276, 2011.

[8] H. Nowzari, M. G. Jorgensen, T. T. Ta, A. Contreras, and J. Slots, "Aggressive periodontitis associated with Fanconi's anemia. A case report," *Journal of Periodontology*, vol. 72, no. 11, pp. 1601–1606, 2001.

[9] M. Goswami, U. Bhushan, and M. Goswami, "Dental perspective of rare disease of Fanconi anemia: case report with review," *Clinical Medicine Insights: Case Reports*, vol. 9, p. CCRep.S37931, 2016.

[10] P. F. Giampietro, P. C. Verlander, J. G. Davis, and A. D. Auerbach, "Diagnosis of Fanconi anemia in patients without congenital malformations: an international Fanconi Anemia Registry Study," *American Journal of Medical Genetics*, vol. 68, no. 1, pp. 58–61, 1997.

[11] A. D. Auerbach, "Fanconi anemia and its diagnosis," *Mutation Research/Fundamental and Molecular Mechanisms of Mutagenesis*, vol. 668, no. 1-2, pp. 4–10, 2009.

[12] K. Oyaizu, F. Mineshiba, J. Mineshiba et al., "Periodontal treatment in severe aplastic anemia," *Journal of Periodontology*, vol. 76, no. 7, pp. 1211–1216, 2005.

[13] A. Açikgöz, F. O. Ozden, T. Fisgin et al., "Oral and dental findings in Fanconi's anemia," *Pediatric hematology and oncology*, vol. 22, no. 6, pp. 531–539, 2005.

[14] M. T. Brennan, V. Sankar, L. Baccaglini et al., "Oral manifestations in patients with aplastic anemia," *Oral Surgery, Oral Medicine, Oral Pathology, Oral Radiology, and Endodontology*, vol. 92, no. 5, pp. 503–508, 2001.

[15] A. Rai, "Aplastic anemia presenting as bleeding of gingiva: case report and dental considerations," *The Saudi journal for dental research*, vol. 7, no. 1, pp. 69–72, 2016.

[16] F. Otan, G. Açikgöz, U. Sakallioglu, and B. Ozkan, "Recurrent aphthous ulcers in Fanconi's anaemia: a case report," *International Journal of Paediatric Dentistry*, vol. 14, no. 3, pp. 214–217, 2004.

[17] L. Montebugnoli, D. B. Gissi, C. Marchetti, and M. P. Foschini, "Multiple squamous cell carcinomas of the oral cavity in a young patient with graft-versus-host disease following allogenic bone marrow transplantation," *International Journal of Oral and Maxillofacial Surgery*, vol. 40, no. 5, pp. 556–558, 2011.

[18] A. Peisker, G. F. Raschke, A. Guentsch, K. Roshanghias, and S. Schultze-Mosgau, "Management of dental extraction in a female patient with Fanconi anemia," *Journal of dentistry (Tehran, Iran)*, vol. 11, no. 5, pp. 613–619, 2014.

[19] French agency for health and health products safety, "Prescription of antibiotics in odontology and stomatology," *Agence Française de Sécurité Sanitaire des Produits de Santé .prescription des antibiotiques en odontologie et stomatologie, 2001*, 2001.

[20] Y. Hosoya, A. Lefor, Y. Hirashima et al., "Successful treatment of esophageal squamous cell carcinoma in a patient with Fanconi anemia," *Japanese Journal of Clinical Oncology*, vol. 40, no. 8, pp. 805–810, 2010.

[21] C. P. Furquim, A. Pivovar, J. M. Amenábar, C. Bonfim, and C. C. Torres-Pereira, "Oral cancer in Fanconi anemia: Review of 121 cases," *Critical Reviews in Oncology/Hematology*, vol. 125, pp. 35–40, 2018.

[22] J. Wu, Q. Mu, V. Thiviyanathan, A. Annapragada, and N. Vigneswaran, "Cancer stem cells are enriched in Fanconi anemia head and neck squamous cell carcinomas," *International Journal of Oncology*, vol. 45, no. 6, pp. 2365–2372, 2014.

[23] H. Reinhard, I. Peters, S. Gottschling, W. Ebell, and N. Graf, "Squamous cell carcinoma of the tongue in a 13-year-old girl with Fanconi anemia," *Journal of Pediatric Hematology/Oncology*, vol. 29, no. 7, pp. 488–491, 2007.

[24] A. Pivovar, C. P. Furquim, C. Bonfim, and C. C. Torres-Pereira, "Mouth examination performance by children's parents and by adolescents in Fanconi anemia," *Pediatric Blood & Cancer*, vol. 64, no. 11, article e26622, 2017.

[25] C. P. Furquim, A. Pivovar, L. G. Cavalcanti, R. F. Araújo, C. M. Sales Bonfim, and C. C. Torres-Pereira, "Mouth self-examination as a screening tool for oral cancer in a high-risk group of patients with Fanconi anemia," *Oral Surgery, Oral Medicine, Oral Pathology, Oral Radiology*, vol. 118, no. 4, pp. 440–446, 2014.

10

Restorative Treatment of Amelogenesis Imperfecta with Prefabricated Composite Veneers

Claudio Novelli,[1] Maurizio Pascadopoli,[1,2] and Andrea Scribante[1,2]

[1]*DENS Centro Medico Lombardo, Milan 20124, Italy*
[2]*Unit of Orthodontics and Pediatric Dentistry, Section of Dentistry, Department of Clinical, Surgical, Diagnostic and Pediatric Sciences, University of Pavia, 27100 Pavia, Italy*

Correspondence should be addressed to Andrea Scribante; andrea.scribante@unipv.it

Academic Editor: Konstantinos Michalakis

This case report presents the use of prefabricated composite veneers for restorative treatment of amelogenesis imperfecta (AI). This technique bridges the gap between a conventional direct technique and a conventional indirect technique and introduces an alternative semidirect restorative technique for AI patients. The aim of this case report is to describe restoration of a young girl with severe AI using prefabricated composite veneers and to discuss the benefits and limitations of this technique compared to the alternative restorative techniques.

1. Introduction

Amelogenesis imperfecta (AI) is a genetic disease caused by mutation of the genes involved in the presecretory, secretory, and maturation stages of enamel formation [1–4]. The mutation can affect both the primary and permanent dentitions and can be passed on from parents to children or develop in individuals with no family history [5, 6]. Depending on the gene involved and the timing when the disruption occurs, AI produces a wide range of enamel alterations ranging from superficial discoloration to complete enamel agenesia. Based on the phenotype of the enamel alteration, AI is classified as type I hypoplastic, type II hypomatured, type III hypocalcified, and type IV hypomatured-hypoplastic. When not only the enamel phenotype but also the inheritance pattern is considered, fifteen AI subtypes are classified. These fifteen subtypes are currently the most widely accepted AI classification system (Table 1) [7–9].

Although AI is primarily an enamel disease, not enamel-related disorders are frequently reported such as pulpal calcifications, delayed tooth eruption, congenital missing teeth, root resorption, open bite, negative overjet, and altered vertical jaw relationship [10–13]. On account of the diverse clinical manifestations, the successful treatment of AI patients requires a multidisciplinary team including a pediatric dentist, a restorative dentist, a prosthodontist, an orthodontist, and a maxillofacial surgeon [14]. Treatment always starts with restoration of the involved dentition, and minimally invasive restoration with direct composite is highly recommended due to the young age of many AI patients. However, a direct composite does not perform well in AI patients and clinical studies reveal limited longevity and high failure rate especially in AI type II and type III where the enamel qualitative alterations produce suboptimal etching pattern and impaired bond strength [15–17]. Enamel deproteinization with NaOCl was suggested to improve bond strength in type II AI patients with hypocalcified enamel and increased protein content [18, 19]. However, very limited in vivo studies are available to support the technique and the results of such studies are not always conclusive [20].

In a recent retrospective clinical study of 326 composite restorations in AI patients, the failure rate was 2.5 times higher than the control group with debonding, fracture, and secondary decay being the most frequent reasons for failure. The longevity of the composite restorations was shorter, and their quality was poorer in patients with hypomineralised/hypomaturated AI than in patients with hypoplastic AI [21]. Because

TABLE 1: Witkop classification of amelogenesis imperfecta 1989 [7].

Type	I	Hypoplastic
	IA	Hypoplastic, pitted autosomal dominant
	IB	Hypoplastic, local autosomal dominant
	IC	Hypoplastic, local autosomal recessive
	ID	Hypoplastic, smooth autosomal dominant
	IE	Hypoplastic, smooth X-linked dominant
	IF	Hypoplastic, rough autosomal dominant
	IG	Enamel agenesis, autosomal recessive
Type	II	Hypomaturation
	IIA	Hypomaturation, pigmented autosomal recessive
	IIB	Hypomaturation, X-linked recessive
	IIC	Snow-capped teeth, X-linked
	IID	Snow-capped teeth, autosomal dominant
Type	III	Hypocalcified
	IIIA	Autosomal dominant
	IIIB	Autosomal recessive
Type	IV	Hypomaturation-hypoplastic with taurodontism
	IVA	Hypomaturation-hypoplastic with taurodontism, autosomal dominant
	IVB	Hypoplastic-hypomaturation with taurodontism, autosomal recessive

of these limitations, ceramic crowns are often recommended as an alternative to direct composite especially for treatment of severe AI and multisurfaced lesions. Ceramic crowns provide excellent esthetic and function in AI patients with a longevity similar to unaffected patients and no correlation between clinical performance and type of enamel alteration [21–23]. In a split mouth study on the long-term outcome of 227 crowns in AI patients, Lundgren et al. reported a survival rate of 99.6% after 5 years with no significant difference between crowns fabricated with Procera (veneered zirconia ceramic) and IPS e.max (lithium disilicate ceramic) [24]. However, ceramic crowns involve a significant sacrifice of tooth structure and a high risk of pulp exposure in young patients with prominent pulp horns. Ceramic crowns in young patients also involve high risk of esthetic failure due to exposed margins of the restoration following craniofacial growth and soft tissue maturation [25–27].

Unfortunately, many AI patients fall in the young age group where ceramic crowns are not indicated and direct composite restorations do not perform well. When neither indirect ceramics nor direct composite seem to be the right answer for the AI patient, this paper presents an alternative restorative technique with prefabricated composite veneers. This technique bridges the gap between the conventional direct composite and the indirect ceramic techniques [28] and is indicated for the treatment of young AI patients because it provides an esthetic and functional restoration in a single appointment with minimal sacrifice of the tooth structure.

The aim of this case report is to describe the restorative treatment of a young patient with severe AI using prefabricated composite veneers and to discuss the benefits and limitations of this technique compared to the alternative restorative techniques.

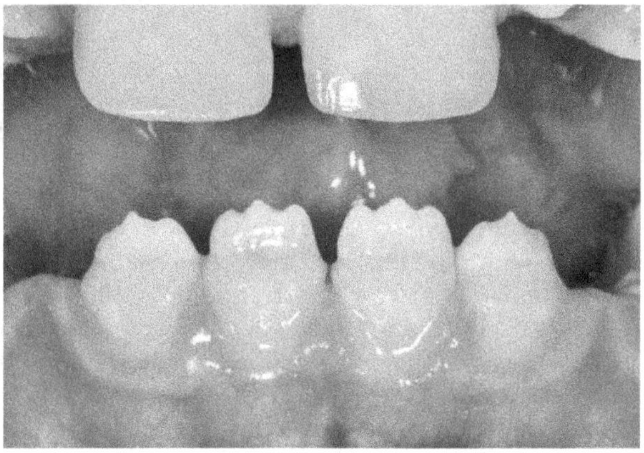

FIGURE 1: Preoperative view of the lower incisors affected by AI type 1.

2. Case Report

The patient was a 9-year-old girl with a family history of AI. At the time of the visit, the patient was in a stage of mixed dentition but all the primary teeth had been extracted by her primary dental care provider due to multiple secondary decays. The permanent first molars and the upper central incisors

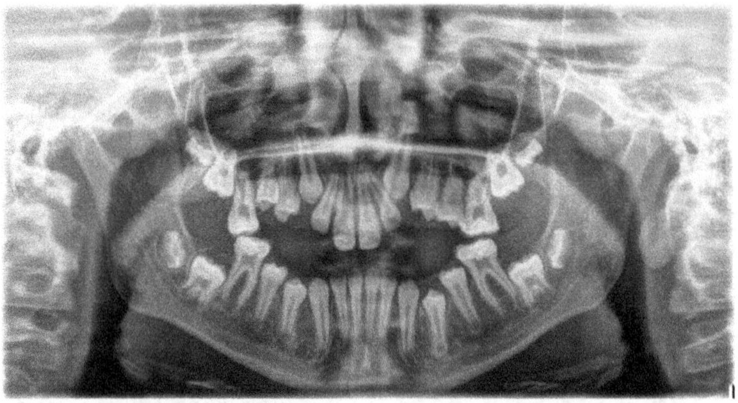

FIGURE 2: Preoperative panoramic radiographic view.

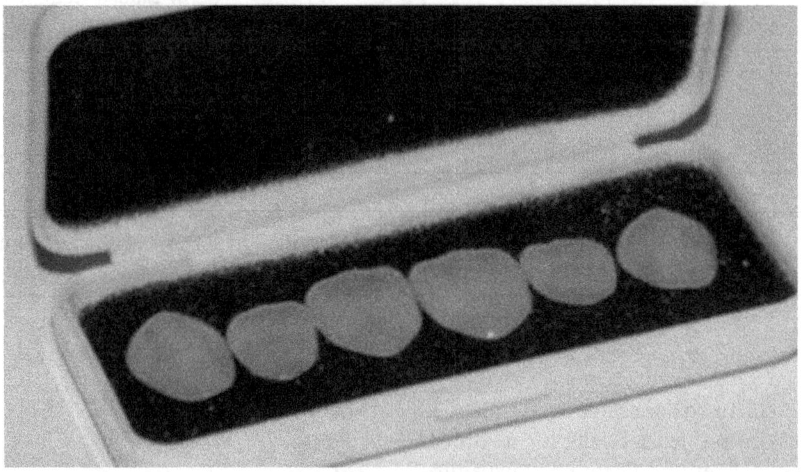

FIGURE 3: Edelweiss prefabricated composite veneers.

were less severely involved and successfully restored with direct composite.

The patient was referred for treatment of the lower incisors very sensitive upon thermal stress and unsightly due to abnormal shape, size, and color. The appearance of the lower incisors made the girl uncomfortable with her smile, and she reported bullying at school because of her teeth.

Intraoral clinical examination of the lower incisors revealed missing enamel in the incisal half and reduced enamel thickness in the cervical half of the teeth (Figure 1). Radiographic examination showed normal enamel radiopacity and normal contrast with the underlying dentin (Figure 2).

Based on the clinical and radiological examinations, a diagnosis was made of AI type I according to the Witkop classification [7]. Type l is the most common form of AI caused by a mutation in the enamelin gene ENAM 4q215 transmitted by autosomal dominant inheritance. This mutation introduces a disruption in the presecretory and secretory stages of amelogenesis resulting in a layer of hypoplastic enamel with normal mineralization but reduced thickness [28–30].

The treatment options for restoration of the lower incisors were discussed with the patient and her parents, and a final decision was made to restore the teeth with prefabricated composite veneers.

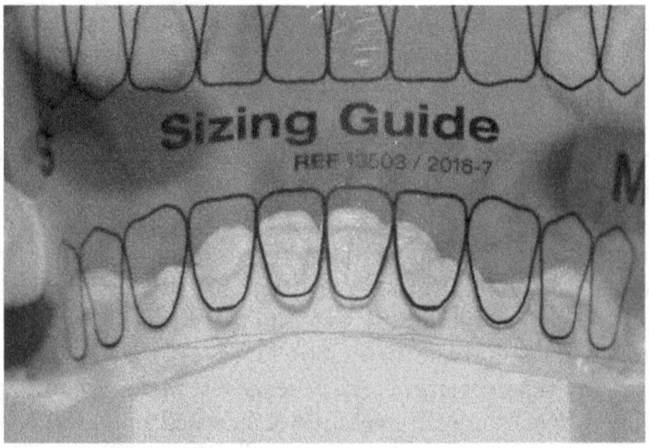

FIGURE 4: Edelweiss Veneer size selection using the Edelweiss sizing guide.

Once the treatment plan with prefabricated composite veneers was approved, the clinical procedure started with veneer size selection.

The prefabricated composite veneers for the patient in this report (Edelweiss Veneers, Edelweiss Dentistry, Wolfurt, Austria) (Figure 3) are available in four sizes (XS, S, M, and L) based on average tooth dimensions in the human population.

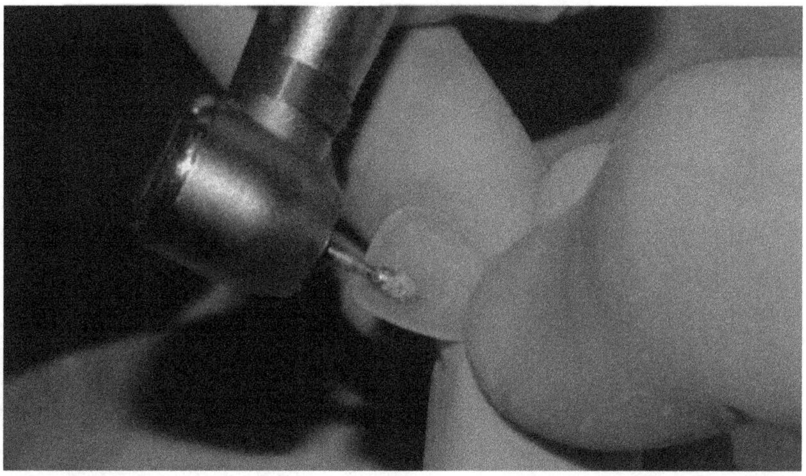

FIGURE 5: Internal adjustments to reduce the thickness of the veneer.

A custom sizing guide is included in the system to select the veneer that best fits the patient (Figure 4).

If none of the available sizes fits the patient's teeth, the width and length of Edelweiss Veneers can be altered to accommodate specific dimensional requirements. For the patient in this report, Edelweiss Veneer size M was selected, and no width or length alteration was required. However, the thickness of the veneer was reduced with a football shape diamond bur (8379, Komet USA, Rock Hill, SC, USA) to allow a more conservative tooth preparation (Figures 5 and 6). Using the same football shape diamond bur, the cervical margin of the veneer was finished to a knife-edge configuration for maximum tissue preservation in the gingival area where the enamel layer is thinner. Thanks to the combination of minimal thickness of the composite laminate and knife-edged configuration of the cervical margin, no tooth preparation was required and the thin hypoplastic enamel layer of the AI patient was fully preserved.

After veneer size selection, the next step was choosing the shade of the luting composite (Figure 7). Luting composite color selection is a critical step for successful restoration with Edelweiss Veneer because the laminate is fabricated with a colorless enamel shade, and the final color of the veneer is determined by the color of the luting composite. The Edelweiss Veneer System includes a high-viscosity nanohybrid composite for cementation available in several dentin and enamel shades (Edelweiss NH, Edelweiss Dentistry, Wolfurt, Austria). For the patient in this report, Edelweiss NH shade A2 was selected with the addition of an opalescent flowable composite in the incisal area (Effect Blue, Edelweiss Dentistry, Wolfurt, Austria) to increase incisal translucency and highlight the halo effect.

After size and shade selection, the intaglio of the veneer was conditioned with a proprietary resin primer (Veneer Bond, Edelweiss Dentistry, Wolfurt; Austria) applied with a microbrush and light cured 20 seconds according to the manufacturer recommendations (Figure 8). No acid-etching, no sandblasting, and no silane application are required inside Edelweiss Veneer. However, the manufacturer recommends internal conditioning with Veneer Bond to promote chemi-

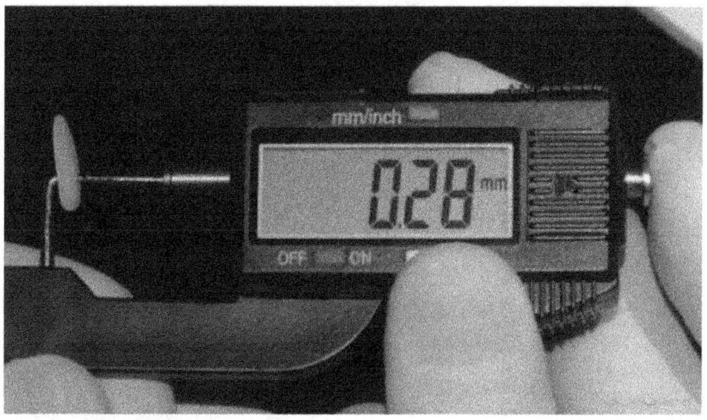

FIGURE 6: Final veneer thickness measured with a digital caliper.

cal adhesion and to increase bond strength between the highly inorganic laminate and the luting composite.

After Veneer Bond application, the veneers were ready for delivery and the working field was isolated with a rubber dam and a 212 Hu-Friedy clamp and the first lower incisor was etched with 37% H_3PO_4 (Gel Etchant, KerrHawe, Bioggio, Switzerland). Etching gel application started from enamel and after 15 seconds moved to dentin for another 15 seconds for 30 s (Figure 9) followed by water rinsing for 30 s and application of a single-step adhesive according to the manufacturer instructions (Scotchbond Universal, 3 M ESPE, Seefeld, Germany) (Figure 10).

Then, the veneer was loaded with the selected composite shade (Figure 11) and seated on the deserving tooth (Figure 12).

After gently pressing the veneer in position, the extra composite was removed with a thin spatula (CompoSculp DD 9/10, Hu-Friedy, Chicago, Ill, USA) and carefully sculpted to achieve optimal adaptation between the veneer and the tooth. Then, the veneer was light cured 20 seconds from the lingual and 20 seconds from the buccal using a high-power (1.330 mW/cm2) curing light (Demi Plus, Kerr Corporation, Brea, CA USA) (Figure 13).

Finally, the margins of the veneer were finished with composite finishing discs (Sof-Lex XT, 3M ESPE, Seefeld, Germany) (Figure 14) and interproximal finishing strips

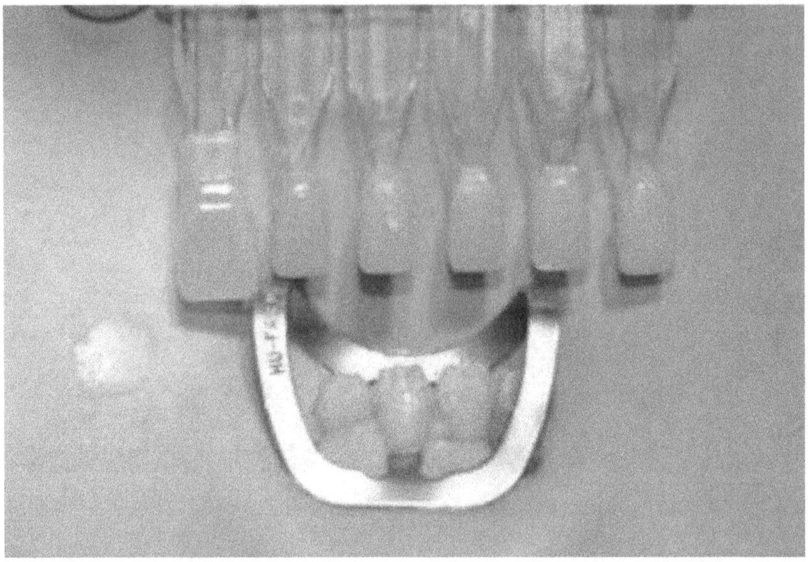

Figure 7: Shade selection of the luting composite using Edelweiss custom shade guide.

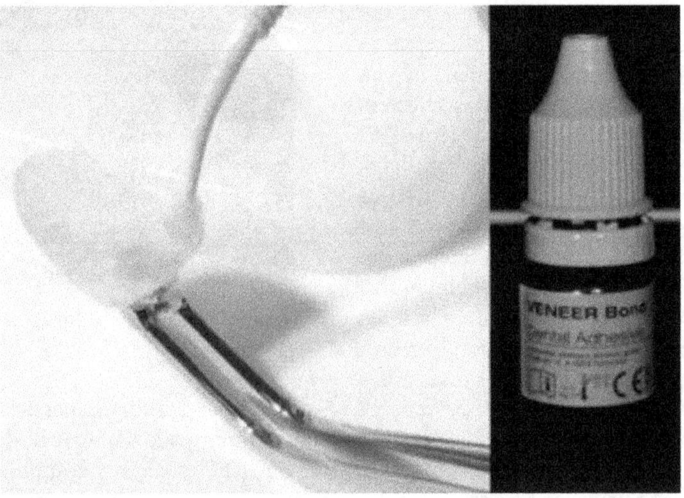

Figure 8: Veneer Bond application.

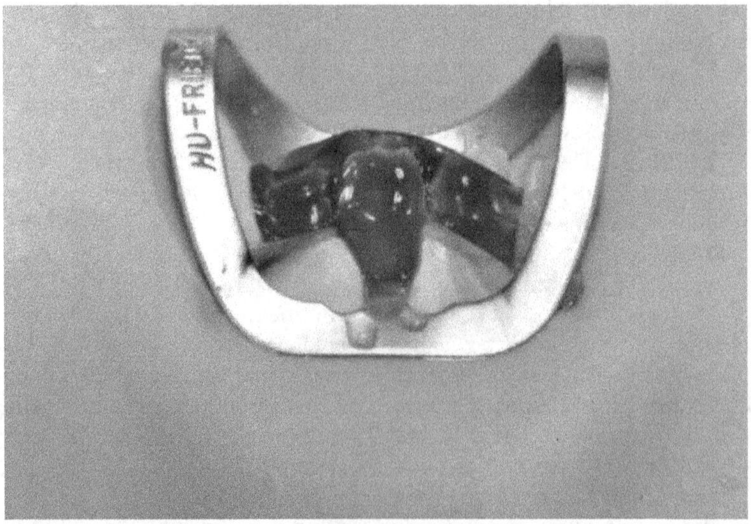

Figure 9: Tooth etching 35% H_3PO_4.

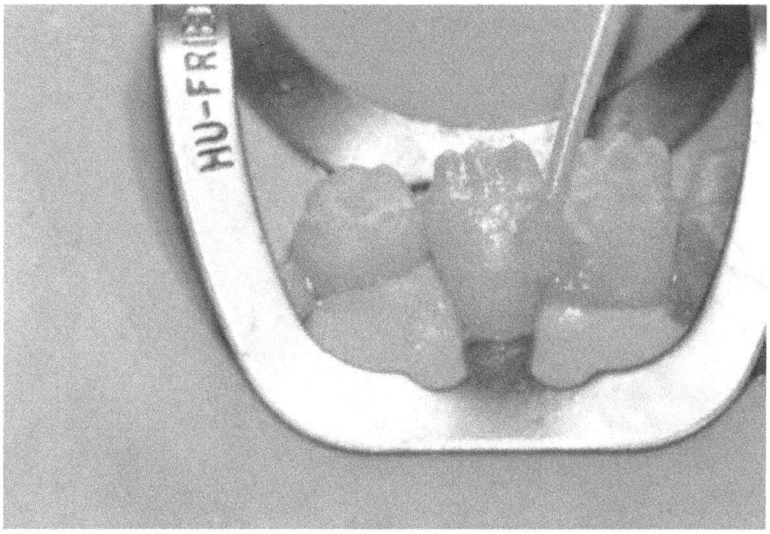

FIGURE 10: Application of single-component adhesive.

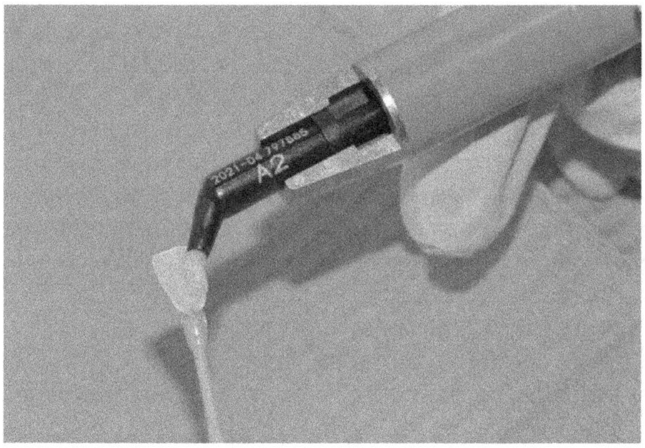

FIGURE 11: Veneer loaded with the selected composite shade.

(Sof-Lex, 3M ESPE, Seefeld, Germany) (Figure 15) followed by a diamond-impregnated silicone cup (Dia step 2, Ravelli, Milano, Italy) at 7500–10,000 rpm under water to produce the final luster.

Once the same step by step clinical procedure was completed for all the four veneers, the patient was dismissed and rescheduled for postoperative evaluation after two weeks. At the recall appointment functional evaluation (absence of fractures, marginal adaptation), biological evaluation (soft tissue response, postoperative sensitivity), and esthetic evaluation (gloss, color matching) were completed and resulted fully satisfactory (Figure 16). Radiological examination showed successful integration of the restorations (Figure 17). The patient was happy with the esthetic outcome and reported that hypersensitivity disappeared after placing the veneer.

A second recall appointment was scheduled 6 months after delivering the veneers. At the new follow-up visit, the veneers resulted fully functional with no marginal discoloration and no alteration of the original superficial luster (Figure 18). The veneers showed good soft tissue response, and the patient's oral hygiene was significantly improved as reported by the RDH who has been following the patient since the initial phase of the treatment. AI patients often experience difficulty in maintaining good oral hygiene on account of the increased tooth sensitivity that makes tooth brushing uncomfortable and the rough tooth surface that facilitates plaque accumulation. Also the impaired smile appearance with abnormal tooth shape, size, and color contributes to poor oral hygiene motivation [31–33]. Previous research demonstrates that a strong correlation exists between attractive smile appearance and positive oral health behaviors [34], and a secondary benefit of the esthetic restoration of the young AI patient presented in this report was the positive impact on the patient's strive to maintain optimal oral health.

3. Discussion

The currently available literature recommends using either direct or indirect techniques for restoration of AI patients and indicates the age of the patient as well as the extension of the enamel lesions as the main decisional criteria [31]. However, other factors should be included in the decision-making process such as the degree of esthetic alteration and the patient's esthetic expectation. AI is often associated with alterations of tooth color, size, and shape that compromise the natural appearance of the smile and have a negative impact on the oral health-related quality of life of the patient [32, 34]. AI patients frequently report being teased about their dental appearance and develop higher levels of social avoidance and psychological distress compared to the unaffected population [35, 36]. This effect is age-dependent, and young AI patients show more psychological disturbance than adult AI patients [37–39]. Hence, esthetic restoration is critical for the successful treatment of young AI patients where the smile should be restored to natural and healthy appearance despite the challenges associated with the young age. A major challenge is the limited compliance on the dental chair that impairs optimal implementation of conventional

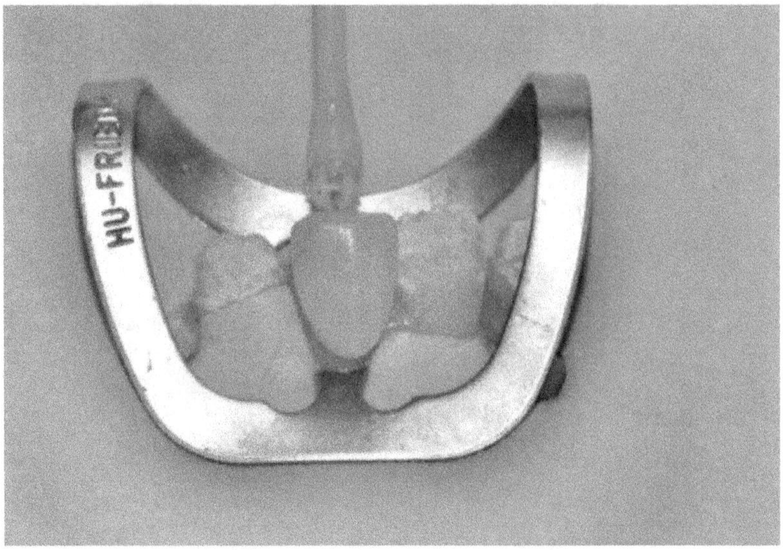

FIGURE 12: Veneer seated on the deserving tooth.

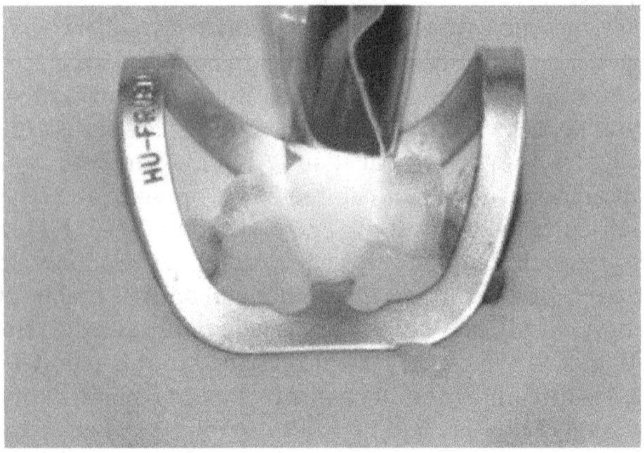

FIGURE 13: Veneer light cured on the tooth.

restorative techniques involving multiple clinical steps and extended chair time. A benefit of the prefabricated composite veneer technique is the simplified clinical procedure that produces a restoration with ideal shape, accurate anatomy, and glossy surface in a single appointment with a limited number of clinical steps and reduced chair time. In the case presented in this report, the clinical procedure was further expedited by preparing the veneers in advance on the study model (select size, adjust thickness, etc.) thereby reducing the actual chair time for each veneer to approximately 10 minutes, a time frame that every young patient can easily cope with.

Another benefit of the prefabricated composite veneer technique is the reduced thickness of the laminate that allows minimally invasive tooth preparation and maximum enamel preservation. Maximum enamel preservation is mandatory for AI type I patients where the thickness of the hypoplastic enamel layer is reduced and conventional tooth preparation easily leads to dentin exposure. Even if the initial preparation is intraenamel, after one or two cycles of veneer replacement, the thin enamel layer is likely to be lost thus limiting the option of a new veneer and leading to more invasive full coverage restoration and additional tissue loss. A secondary benefit of the reduced thickness of the prefabricated composite veneer is the optimal contact lens effect and invisible margin in the gingival area where the laminate tapers to zero. The invisible margin is a critical factor for successful restorative treatment in young patients because it reduces the risk of esthetic failure due to margin exposure following craniofacial growth and soft tissue maturation. A small margin exposure is unlikely to be an issue because the margin of the prefabricated composite veneer is not visible while a larger margin exposure can be conveniently repaired intraorally with the addition of direct composite. Intraoral composite repair increases the longevity of the prefabricated composite veneer because it allows minimally invasive intervention as opposed to replacement of the restoration with many biological and financial benefits for the patient [40–44].

The successful esthetic outcome, the simplified clinical procedure, the minimally invasive tooth preparation, the convenient intraoral repair, and the possible bonding of orthodontic brackets for orthodontic treatment to be carried out in the future were the main benefits of the prefabricated composite veneer technique for the AI patient presented in this report. Nonetheless, the technique showed some limitations such as the higher cost compared to the conventional direct composite technique. Even if the extra cost of the prefabricated composite veneer is partially compensated by the shorter chair time, the treatment fee for the patient is higher especially when multiple veneers are needed. Another limitation is the limited data available regarding the performance of prefabricated composite veneers compared to the alternative anterior restorations (i.e., direct composite and indirect ceramics). In laboratory studies, prefabricated composite veneers perform better than direct composite veneers because the extraoral curing process under controlled temperature, light, and pressure produces a significant improvement in color stability, superficial roughness, and microhardness [45–47]. The Edelweiss Veneers used for the patient in this report are expected to perform even better because the addition of high pressure (100 Pa) and high temperature (300°C) to the curing process

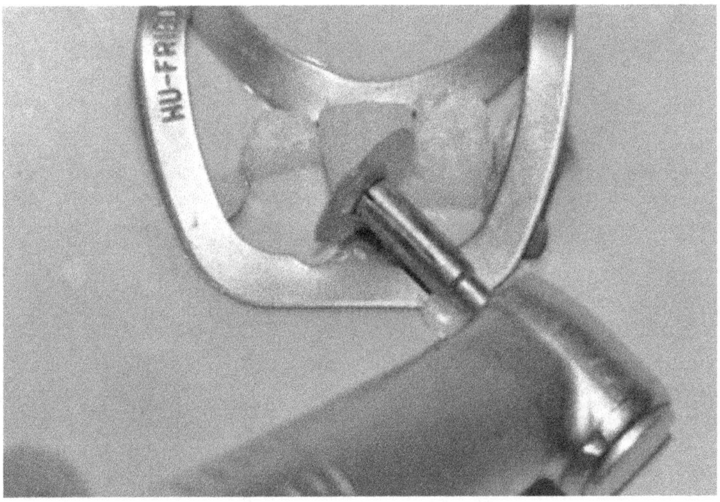

FIGURE 14: Finishing the margins with composite finishing discs.

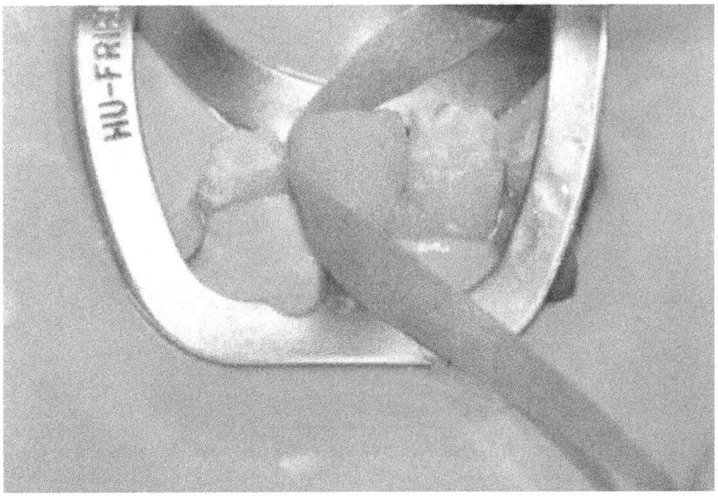

FIGURE 15: Interproximal finishing with composite paper finishing strip.

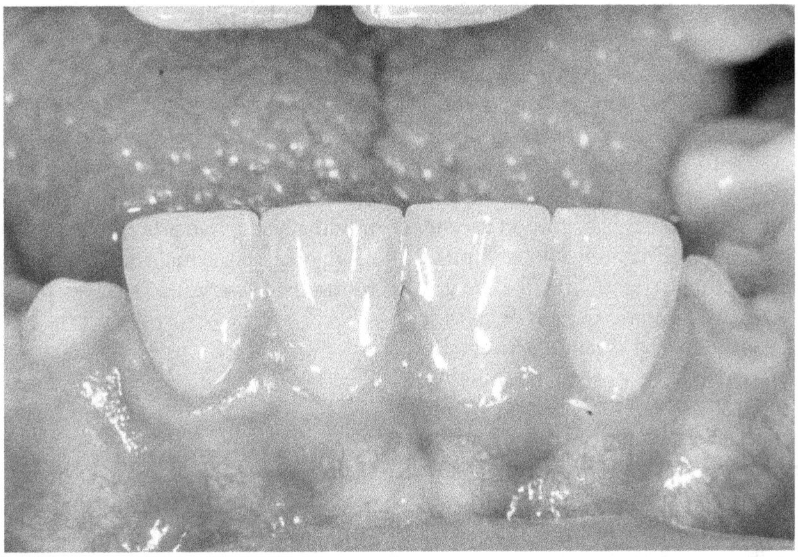

FIGURE 16: 2 weeks postoperative view of Edelweiss Veneers [31–41].

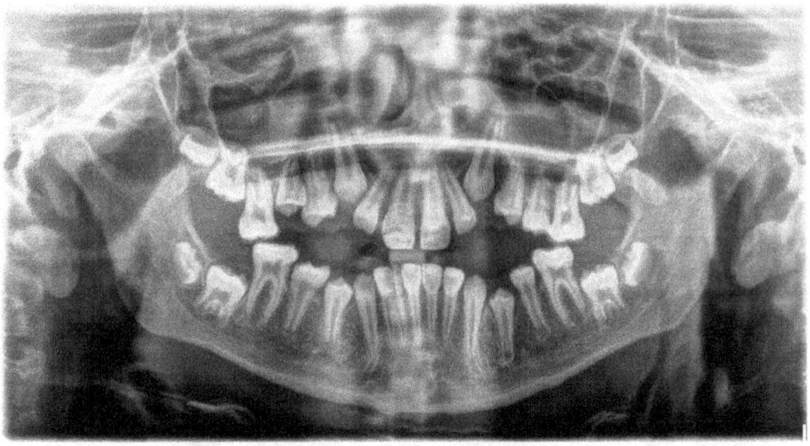

FIGURE 17: Postoperative panoramic radiographic view.

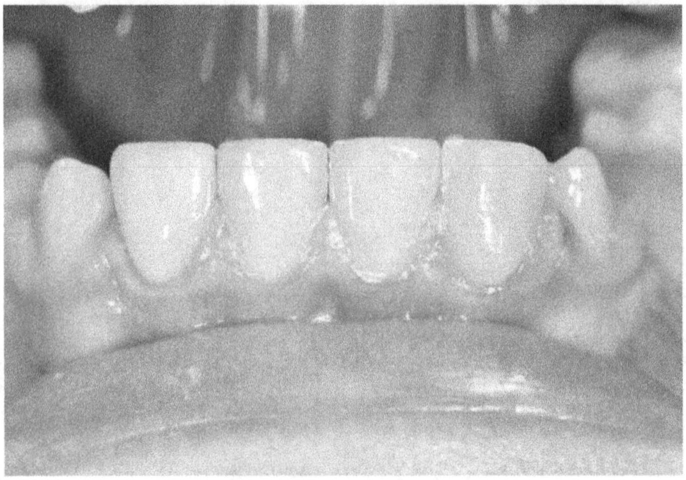

FIGURE 18: 6 months postoperative view of Edelweiss Veneers [31–41].

further improves mechanical and physical properties of the composite laminate [48]. However, no clinical studies have been published yet and it is not known how the clinical performance and longevity of prefabricated composite veneers compare within direct ceramics that are considered the gold standard for anterior restoration. It is possible that indirect ceramics provide better clinical performance and durability on account of ceramic superior mechanical properties and resistance to aging. However, indirect ceramics have limited application for restoration of young AI patients (like the girl presented in this report) because ceramic crowns involve a high risk of pulp exposure [49–51] and ceramic veneers are likely to be negatively affected by the enamel quantitative and qualitative alterations [52, 53]. When the indirect ceramic restorations are not indicated, prefabricated composite veneers provide an alternative technique for an esthetic and functional restoration of young AI patients that allows to produce a restoration with proper shape, accurate anatomy, and glossy surface with minimally invasive tooth preparation.

4. Conclusions

The treatment of severely compromised teeth in young patients suffering from amelogenesis imperfecta can be a challenge for the dental clinician, considering the kind of the disorder and the commonly known low compliance of children. The use of prefabricated veneers can be a valid approach because of the minimally invasive procedures involved and the higher esthetic result obtained, actually introducing an alternative "semidirect" restorative technique.

Acknowledgments

The authors would like to thank the manufacturer for providing the materials tested in the present case report.

References

[1] C. E. L. Smith, J. A. Poulter, A. Antanaviciute et al., "Amelogenesis imperfecta; genes, proteins, and pathways," *Frontiers in Physiology*, vol. 8, p. 435, 2017.

[2] K. Gadhia, S. McDonald, N. Arkutu, and K. Malik, "Amelogenesis imperfecta: an introduction," *British Dental Journal*, vol. 212, no. 8, pp. 377–379, 2012.

[3] J. C. C. Hu, Y.-H. P. Chun, T. Al Hazzazzi, and J. P. Simmer, "Enamel formation and amelogenesis imperfecta," *Cells, Tissues, Organs*, vol. 186, no. 1, pp. 78–85, 2007.

[4] B. Backman and G. Holmgren, "Amelogenesis imperfecta: a genetic study," *Human Heredity*, vol. 38, no. 4, pp. 189–206, 1988.

[5] S. Sundell and G. Koch, "Hereditary amelogenesis imperfecta. I. Epidemiology and clinical classification in a Swedish child population," *Swedish Dental Journal*, vol. 9, no. 4, pp. 157–169, 1985.

[6] M. Nusier, O. Yassin, T. C. Hart, A. Samimi, and J. T. Wright, "Phenotypic diversity and revision of the nomenclature for autosomal recessive amelogenesis imperfecta," *Oral Surgery, Oral Medicine, Oral Pathology, Oral Radiology, and Endodontology*, vol. 97, no. 2, pp. 220–230, 2004.

[7] C. J. Witkop Jr., "Amelogenesis imperfecta, dentinogenesis imperfecta and dentin dysplasia revisited: problems in classification," *Journal of oral pathology*, vol. 17, pp. 547–553, 1989.

[8] M. J. Aldred, R. Savarirayan, and P. J. Crawford, "Amelogenesis imperfecta: a classification and catalogue for the 21st century," *Oral Diseases*, vol. 9, no. 1, pp. 19–23, 2003.

[9] M. Koruyucu, M. Bayram, E. B. Tuna, K. Gencay, and F. Seymen, "Clinical findings and long-term managements of patients with amelogenesis imperfecta," *European journal of dentistry*, vol. 8, no. 4, pp. 546–552, 2014.

[10] M. J. Aldred and P. J. Crawford, "Variable expression in Amelogenesis imperfecta with taurodontism," *Journal of Oral Pathology*, vol. 17, no. 7, pp. 327–333, 1988.

[11] A. Pavlic, T. Battelino, K. TrebusakPodkrajsek, and M. Ovsenik, "Craniofacial characteristics and genotypes of amelogenesis imperfecta patients," *European Journal of Orthodontics*, vol. 33, no. 3, pp. 325–331, 2011.

[12] K. M. Ayers, B. K. Drummond, W. J. Harding, S. G. Salis, and P. N. Liston, "Amelogenesis imperfecta - multidisciplinary management from eruption to adulthood. Review and case report," *The New Zealand Dental Journal*, vol. 100, no. 4, pp. 101–104, 2004.

[13] P. J. Crawford, M. Aldred, and A. Bloch-Zupan, "Amelogenesis imperfecta," *Orphanet Journal of Rare Diseases*, vol. 2, no. 1, p. 17, 2007.

[14] V. Gisler, N. Enkling, J. Zix, K. Kim, N. M. Kellerhoff, and R. Mericske-Stern, "A multidisciplinary approach to the functional and esthetic rehabilitation of amelogenesis imperfecta and open bite deformity: a case report," *Journal of Esthetic and Restorative Dentistry*, vol. 22, no. 5, pp. 282–293, 2010.

[15] B. C. Yaman, F. Ozer, C. S. Cabukusta, M. M. Eren, F. Koray, and M. B. Blatz, "Microtensile bond strength to enamel affected by hypoplastic amelogenesis imperfecta," *The Journal of Adhesive Dentistry*, vol. 16, no. 1, pp. 7–14, 2014.

[16] A. L. Faria-e-Silva, R. R. De Moraes, M. U. De Sousa Menezes, R. R. Capanema, A. S. De Moura, and H. E. Martelli-Júnior, "Hardness and microshear bond strength to enamel and dentin of permanent teeth with hypocalcified amelogenesis imperfecta," *International journal of paediatric dentistry*, vol. 21, no. 4, pp. 314–320, 2011.

[17] C. F. Chen, J. C. C. Hu, M. R. P. Estrella, M. C. Peters, and E. Bresciani, "Assessment of restorative treatment of patients with amelogenesis imperfecta," *Pediatric Dentistry*, vol. 35, no. 4, pp. 337–342, 2013.

[18] R. D. Venezie, G. Vadiakas, J. R. Christensen, and J. T. Wright, "Enamel pretreatment with sodium hypochlorite to enhance bonding in hypocalcified amelogenesis imperfecta: case report and SEM analysis," *Pediatric Dentistry*, vol. 16, no. 6, pp. 433–436, 1994.

[19] I. Şaroğlu, Ş. Aras, and D. Öztaş, "Effect of deproteinization on composite bond strength in hypocalcified amelogenesis imperfecta," *Oral Diseases*, vol. 12, no. 3, pp. 305–308, 2006.

[20] I. S. Sönmez, S. Aras, E. S. Tunç, and C. Küçükeşmen, "Clinical success of deproteinization in hypocalcified amelogenesis imperfecta," *Quintessence International*, vol. 40, no. 2, pp. 113–118, 2009.

[21] G. Pousette Lundgren and G. Dahllof, "Outcome of restorative treatment in young patients with amelogenesis imperfecta. A cross-sectional, retrospective study," *Journal of Dentistry*, vol. 42, no. 11, pp. 1382–1389, 2014.

[22] L. Ortiz, A. Pereira, and L. Jahangiri, "Management of amelogenesis imperfecta in adolescent patients: clinical report," *Journal of Prosthodontics*, vol. 28, no. 6, pp. 607–612, 2019.

[23] O. Krieger, G. Matuliene, J. Hüsler, G. E. Salvi, B. Pjetursson, and U. Brägger, "Failures and complications in patients with birth defects restored with fixed dental prostheses and single crowns on teeth and/or implants," *Clinical Oral Implants Research*, vol. 20, no. 8, pp. 809–816, 2009.

[24] G. Pousette Lundgren, G. I. MorlingVestlund, M. Trulsson, and G. Dahllof, "A randomized controlled trial of crown therapy in young individuals with amelogenesis imperfecta," *Journal of Dental Research*, vol. 94, no. 8, pp. 1041–1047, 2015.

[25] A. Lindunger and J. I. Smedberg, "A retrospective study of the prosthodontic management of patients with amelogenesis imperfecta," *The International Journal of Prosthodontics*, vol. 18, no. 3, pp. 189–194, 2005.

[26] G. S. P. Cheung, "A preliminary investigation into the longevity and causes of failure of single unit extracoronal restorations," *Journal of Dentistry*, vol. 19, no. 3, pp. 160–163, 1991.

[27] N. J. Walton, F. M. Gardner, and J. R. Agar, "A survey of crown and fixed partial denture failures: Length of service and reasons for replacement," *The Journal of prosthetic dentistry*, vol. 56, no. 4, pp. 416–421, 1986.

[28] C. Novelli and A. Scribante, "Minimally invasive diastema restoration with prefabricated sectional veneers," *Dentistry Journal*, vol. 8, no. 2, p. 60, 2020.

[29] E. M. Canger, P. Celenk, M. Yenisey, and S. Z. Odyakmaz, "Amelogenesis Imperfecta, hypoplastic type associated with some dental abnormalities: a case report," *Brazilian Dental Journal*, vol. 21, no. 2, pp. 170–174, 2010.

[30] M. Kida, T. Ariga, T. Shirakawa, H. Oquchi, and Y. Sakiyama, "Autosomal-dominant hypoplastic form of amelogenesis imperfecta caused by an enamel in gene mutation at the exon-intron boundary," *Journal of Dental Research*, vol. 81, no. 11, pp. 738–742, 2002.

[31] American Academy on Pediatric Dentistry Council on Clinical Affairs, "Guideline on oral heath care/dental management of heritable dental development anomalies," *Pediatric Dentistry*, vol. 30, pp. 196–201, 2009.

[32] W. K. Seow, "Clinical diagnosis and management strategies of amelogenesis imperfecta variants," *Pediatric dentistry*, vol. 15, no. 6, pp. 384–393, 1993.

[33] A. Hashem, A. Kelly, B. O'Connel, and B. O'Sullivan, "Impact of moderate and severe hypodontia and amelogenesis imperfecta on quality of life and self-esteem of adult patients," *Journal of dentistry*, vol. 41, no. 8, pp. 689–694, 2013.

[34] S. Poulsen, H. Gjørup, D. Haubek et al., "Amelogenesis imperfecta – a systematic literature review of associated dental and oro-facial abnormalities and their impact on patients," *Acta Odontologica Scandinavica*, vol. 66, no. 4, pp. 193–199, 2008.

[35] M. Patel, S. T. McDonnell, S. Iram, and M. F. W.-Y. Chan, "Amelogenesis imperfecta - lifelong management. Restorative management of the adult patient," *British Dental Journal*, vol. 215, no. 9, pp. 449–457, 2013.

[36] S. McDonald, N. Arkutu, K. Malik, K. Gadhia, and S. McKaig, "Managing the paediatric patient with amelogenesis imperfecta," *British Dental Journal*, vol. 212, no. 9, pp. 425–428, 2012.

[37] K. D. Coffield, C. Phillips, M. Brady, M. W. Roberts, R. P. Strauss, and J. T. Wright, "The psychosocial impact of developmental dental defects in people with hereditary amelogenesis imperfecta," *The Journal of the American Dental Association*, vol. 136, no. 5, pp. 620–630, 2005.

[38] A. Alqadi and A. O'Connell, "Parental perception of children affected by amelogenesis imperfecta (AI) and dentinogenesis imperfecta (DI): a qualitative study," *Dental Journal*, vol. 6, no. 4, p. 65, 2018.

[39] S. Parekh, M. Almehateb, and S. J. Cunningham, "How do children with amelogenesis imperfecta feel about their teeth?," *International Journal of Paediatric Dentistry*, vol. 24, no. 5, pp. 326–335, 2014.

[40] C. Novelli, "Restoration of gingival recession with periodontal preformed composite veneers," *Clinical Case Reports*, vol. 9, no. 3, pp. 1135–1145, 2021.

[41] H. Javidi, M. Tickle, and V. R. Aggarwal, "Repair _vs_ replacement of failed restorations in general dental practice: factors influencing treatment choices and outcomes," *British Dental Journal*, vol. 218, no. 1, pp. E2–E5, 2015.

[42] M. Ozcan, "The use of chairside silica coating for different dental applications: a clinical report," *The Journal of Prosthetic Dentistry*, vol. 87, no. 5, pp. 469–472, 2002.

[43] G. Moncada, E. Fernandez, J. Martin, C. Arancibia, I. A. Mjor, and V. V. Gordan, "Increasing the longevity of restorations by minimal intervention: a two-year clinical trial," *Operative Dentistry*, vol. 33, no. 3, pp. 258–264, 2008.

[44] F. H. van de Sande, R. R. Moraes, R. V. Elias et al., "Is composite repair suitable for anterior restorations? A long-term practice-based clinical study," *Clinical oral investigations*, vol. 23, no. 6, pp. 2795–2803, 2019.

[45] A. Postiglione, S. Pereira, L. C. Delgado, and B. C. Phillipini, "Color stability evaluation of aesthetic restorative materials," *Brazilian Oral Research*, vol. 22, pp. 3–9, 2008.

[46] J. L. Drummond, "Degradation, fatigue and failure of resin dental composite materials," *Journal of Dental Research*, vol. 87, no. 8, pp. 710–719, 2008.

[47] S. Tasin, G. Celik, A. Usmatullaev, and A. Usumez, "The effect of artificial accelerated aging on the color stability, microhardness, and surface roughness of differentdental laminate veneer materials," *Journal of Esthetic and Restorative Dentistry*, vol. 1, pp. 1–7, 2020.

[48] D. Dietschi and A. Devigus, "Prefabricated composite veneers: historical perspectives, indications and clinical application," *The European Journal of Esthetic Dentistry*, vol. 6, no. 1, pp. 2–11, 2011.

[49] K. Malik, K. Gadhia, N. Arkutu, S. McDonald, and F. Blair, "The interdisciplinary management of patients with amelogenesis imperfecta - restorative dentistry," *British Dental Journal*, vol. 212, no. 11, pp. 537–542, 2012.

[50] D. Markovic, B. Petrovic, and T. Peric, "clinical findings and oral rehabilitation of patients with amelogenesis imperfecta," *European Archives of Paediatric Dentistry*, vol. 11, no. 4, pp. 201–208, 2010.

[51] H. G. Ohrvik and C. Hjortsjö, "Retrospective study of patients with amelogenesis imperfecta treated with different bonded restoration techniques," *Clinical and experimental dental research*, vol. 1, pp. 1–8, 2019.

[52] S. Ardu, O. Duc, I. Krejci, and R. Perroud, "Amelogenesis imperfecta: a conservative and progressive adhesive treatment concept," *Operative Dentistry*, vol. 38, no. 3, pp. 235–241, 2013.

[53] S. Shibata, C. Taguchi, R. Gondo, and L. N. Baratieri, "Ceramic veneers and direct-composite cases of amelogenesis imperfecta rehabilitation," *Operative Dentistry*, vol. 41-3, pp. 233–242, 2016.

11

Macroabrasion and/or Partial Veneers: Techniques for the Removal of Localized White Spots

Ubiracy Gaião,[1] Ana Carolina Portes Pasmadjian,[2] Gabriela Resende Allig,[2] Liliana Vicente Melo de Lucas Rezende,[2] Vitória Beatriz Souza da Silva,[2] and Leonardo Fernandes da Cunha[2]

[1]Positivo University, Curitiba, Brazil
[2]Department of Dentistry, School of Health Sciences, University of Brasília, DF, Brazil

Correspondence should be addressed to Leonardo Fernandes da Cunha; cunha_leo@yahoo.com.br

Academic Editor: Andrea Scribante

Macroabrasion is a technique for the removal of localized white spots using a high-speed, intermittent high speed turbine finishing diamond tip. It is fast, safe, efficient, and an alternative to enamel microabrasion. However, when the stain is deeper, these localized intrinsic stains or defects can be treated with partial direct veneers. A conservative preparation should be done and that allows stratification of the resin to mask the hypoplasia and provide naturalness to the tooth. Thus, the objective of this work is to demonstrate, through a clinical case, macroabrasion and a partial veneer from the preparation, restoration, to the finishing and polishing to remove hypoplastic stains.

1. Introduction

According to Sturdevant [1], a technique for removing localized white spots, not subject to remineralizing therapy, is called macroabrasion. Macroabrasion simply uses a finishing diamond tip or multilaminated drill on a high turbine to remove the defect. Light and intermittent pressure should be used carefully when removing the dental structure to avoid the formation of a cavity unnecessarily [1].

During macroabrasion, irrigation is recommended to keep the tooth in a hydrated state to facilitate the assessment of stain and/or defect removal. This is because teeth that have white stain defects are particularly susceptible to dehydration, resulting in other apparent white stains that are not normally seen when the tooth is hydrated. Dehydration exaggerates the appearance of white spots and makes it difficult to assess the removal of defects [1].

Macroabrasion is considerably fast, safe, and efficient. It is an alternative to enamel microabrasion and can be associated with procedures such as whitening, closing of diastemas, and cosmetic remodeling [2, 3].

However, when the stain is deeper, a cavity can be generated in the buccal surface of the teeth. In such cases, small spots or localized intrinsic defects that are surrounded by healthy enamel can be ideally treated with partial direct veneers [1].

The professional should use a thick, elliptical, or spherical diamond tip with air-water cooling to prepare the tooth to an extent and depth sufficient to mask the defect or stain with the restorative material without generating overcontour and, normally, does not involve an area subgingival or incisal angle. In addition, finishing the cavo-superficial angle is recommended and essential to remove the outer layer of enamel that may be more resistant to acid etching, to create

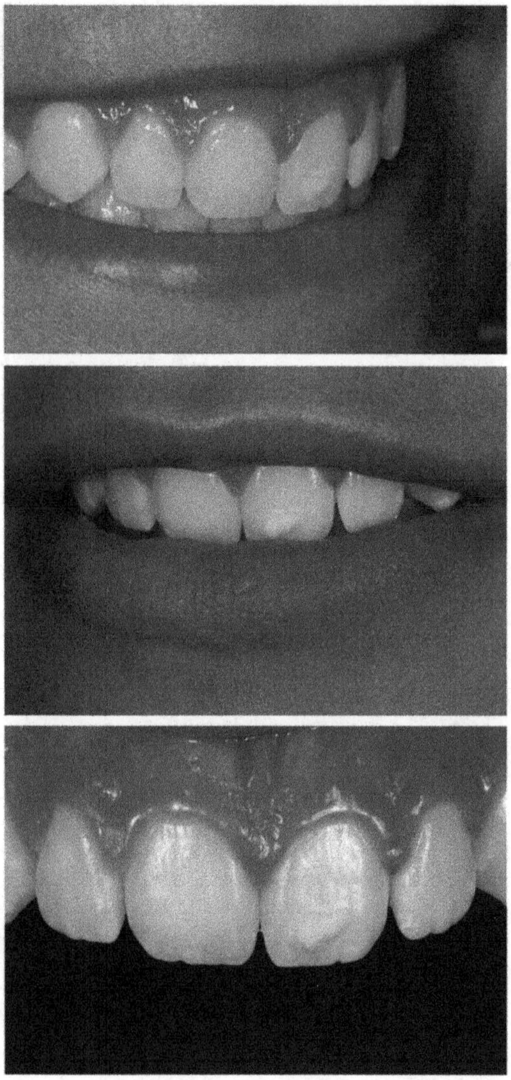

Figure 1: Initial smile and upper anterior teeth. Note the hypoplasia spots on the incisal third of the upper central incisors in the form of streaks and hypoplasia opaque white spot on the upper left central incisor.

a favorable surface for adhesion, and to establish a transition between the restoration/tooth.

Thus, the objective of this work is to demonstrate, through a clinical case, macroabrasion and a partial facet from preparation, restoration, to finishing and polishing to remove hypoplastic stains.

2. Case Report

A 16-year-old female patient sought dental care with small hypoplastic spots on the upper incisors in the form of stretch marks on the incisal third of the upper central incisors and a wider white spot on the upper left central incisor, which generated the patient's discontent in her smile (Figure 1). After anamnesis and clinical examination, the enamel macroabrasion and partial veneer technique with direct composite resin were proposed as a treatment.

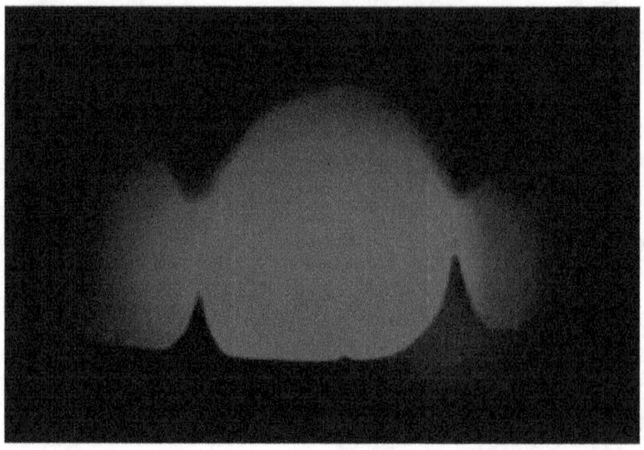

Figure 2: Transillumination to evaluate the spots. An LED unit positioned close to the palatal face of the tooth can help the clinician to examine the enamel stains.

An LED photopolymerization unit was placed on the palatal or lingual surface of the incisors to help examine the enamel stains (Figure 2) (Radii Xpert, SDI, Victoria, Australia), and the depth of the lesion can be estimated, since a darker color with more defined edges indicates a deeper stain.

Prophylaxis was performed, and then, macroabrasion was performed with a fine diamond tip (JOTA do Brasil, São Paulo, São Paulo, Brasil) in high rotation with refrigeration in the incisal third of the central incisors to decrease the small hypoplastic spots in the form of stretch marks. With the teeth still hydrated, the Essentia GC (GC Corporation, Tokyo, Japan) resin color was selected (Figure 3). The dentin colors LD (light dentin) and MD (medium dentin) were positioned to check the color, the LD being selected. Next, the enamel colors were positioned LE (light enamel) and DE (dark enamel), with LE being selected.

The absolute isolation of the operative field was performed using rubber and kept in position with dental floss. The white spot located dictates the shape of the contour by the extent of the defect and must include all discolored areas. High rotation with a spherical diamond tip (Figure 4) with air/water cooling was used to prepare the tooth to a depth that the stain could no longer be observed, being hydrated as can be seen in Figures 4(b) and 4(c). During preparation, high rotation irrigation is recommended to keep the tooth in a hydrated state to facilitate assessment of stain removal because teeth that have white stain defects are particularly susceptible to dehydration [1]. Dehydration exaggerates the appearance of white spots and makes it difficult to assess the removal of defects. When the stain is no longer seen, it means that the restorative material will be effective in masking the stain without having to prepare the tooth further.

After preparation, the cavo-superficial angle was finished with a coarse-grained sanding disc (OptiDisc, Kerr Corporation, Orange, California, USA) at low speed (Figure 5). The buccal surface of the incisor enamel was conditioned with 37% phosphoric acid to avoid the application of resin over an unconditioned area; then, the surface was dried, and the G-Premium Bond (GC) adhesive was applied. Polymerization was carried out according to the manufacturer's instructions (Radii Xpert, SDI, Victoria, Australia) (Figure 6).

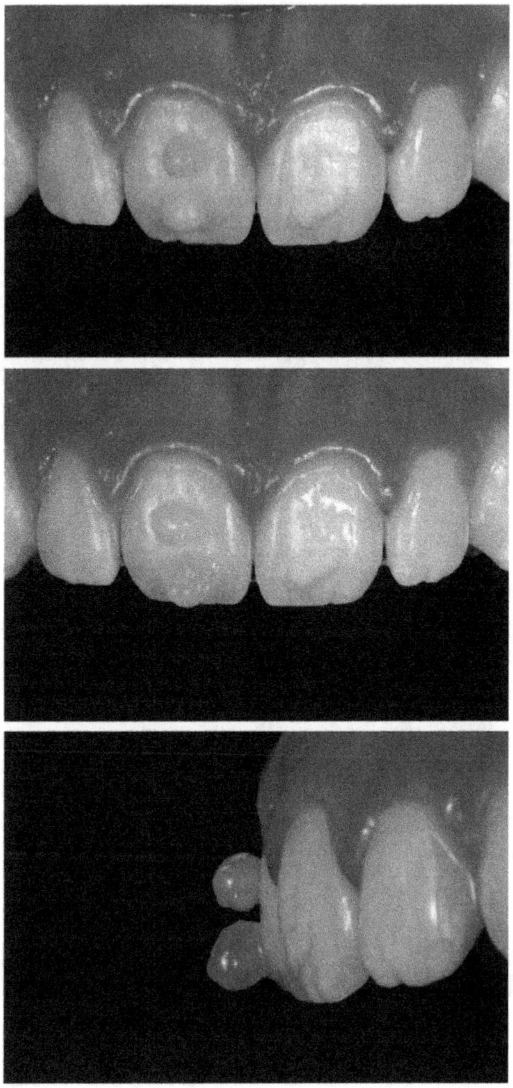

FIGURE 3: Macroabrasion was performed with high rotation and fine diamond tip for finishing to remove stains in the form of streaks, superficial enamel defects. Positioning of dentin (a) and enamel (b) resin increments on the tooth for color selection.

The stratification of the composite resin was initiated by the resin layer in the dentin LD color (Essentia, GC), and a single layer of LE resin (Essentia GC) was applied over the vestibular surface to provide a more harmonic contour (Figure 7). The increments were polymerized for the time recommended by the manufacturer with an LED-based device (Radii Xpert - SDI).

In the next clinical session, finishing and final polishing were performed (Figure 8). The contour of the restorations was delimited with abrasive discs with sequential granulometry (OptiDisc) and resin rubbers (JOTA do Brasil, São Paulo, São Paulo, Brasil).

The final aspect can be seen in Figure 9.

3. Discussion

Macroabrasion, as demonstrated in the case presented, is a technique for the removal of localized superficial white

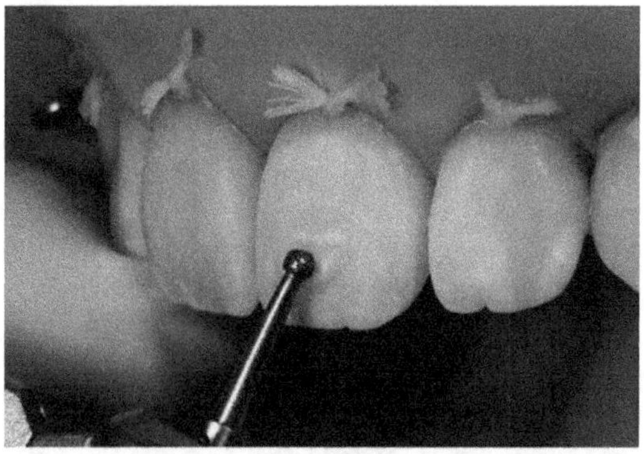

(a)

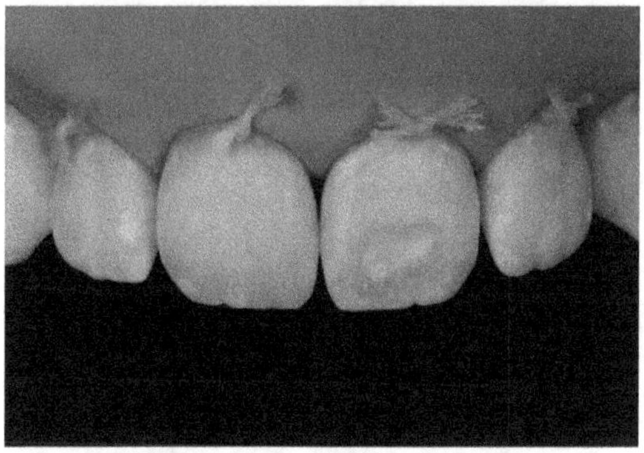

(b)

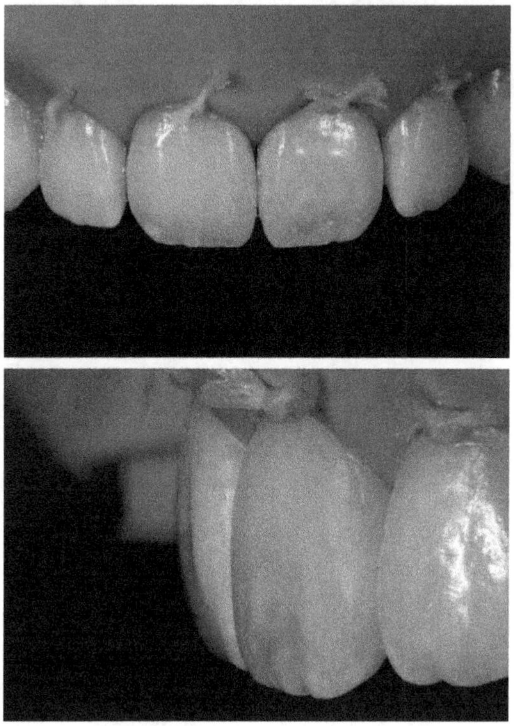

(c)

FIGURE 4: Absolute isolation was done with a rubber dam. The defect was removed with a spherical diamond tip. Lateral view of the central incisor after removal of the hypoplastic stain.

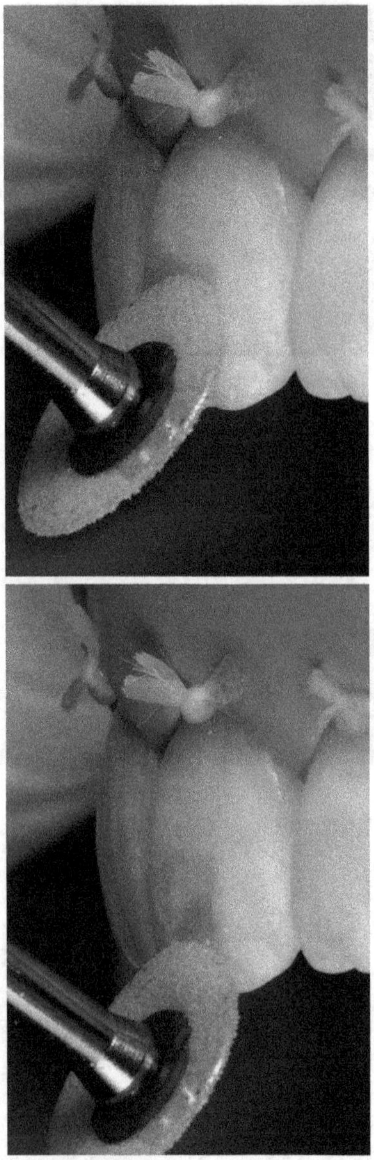

Figure 5: The finish of the bevel was made with coarse-grained sanding discs (OptiDisc, Kerr), thus eliminating fragile marginal prisms.

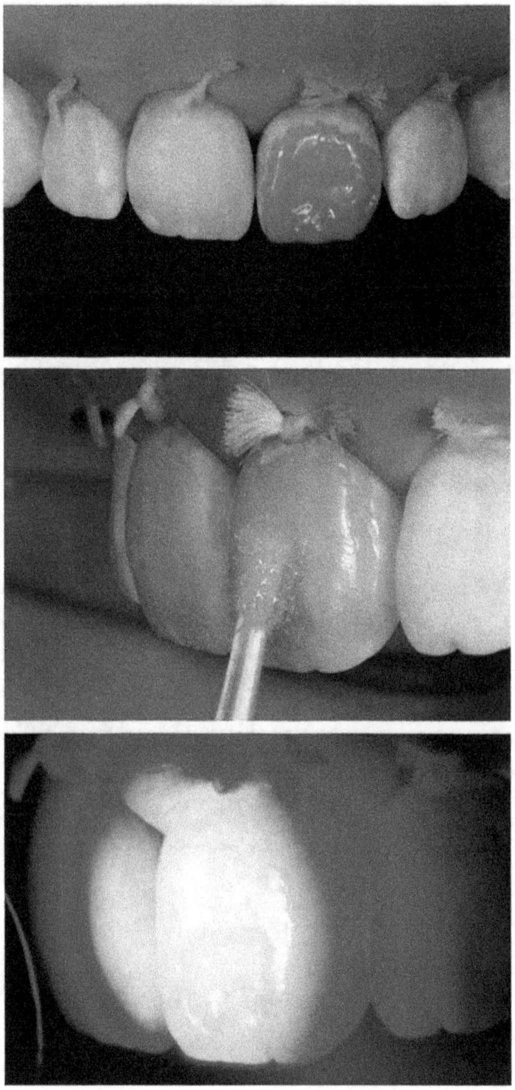

Figure 6: Application of the adhesive system.

stains, simply and quickly using simply a high-speed fine-grained diamond tip to remove the defect. Because it is high speed, care must be taken to use light and intermittent pressure to carefully monitor the removal of the tooth structure. It is an alternative to the enamel microabrasion technique that uses low speed, thus allowing greater control of the worn structure to avoid irreversible damage to the tooth [1, 3, 4, 5]. Another advantage is that it does not require absolute isolation to perform the procedure. Refrigeration during macroabrasion is essential, not only to avoid sensitivity due to heating but also to keep the tooth in a hydrated state to facilitate the assessment of defect removal. Teeth that have white stain defects are particularly susceptible to dehydration, resulting in other apparent white stains that are not normally seen when the tooth is hydrated [1]. To speed up the process, a combination of macroabrasion and microabrasion can also be considered. Most of the defect is removed with macroabrasion, followed by the final treatment with microabrasion. Additionally, biomimetic hydroxyapatite [6] and casein phosphopeptide-amorphous calcium phosphate have been recently introduced and showed promising remineralizing results, and further research is needed on the topic [7].

There are two types of aesthetic veneers: partial or total. Partial veneers are indicated for the restoration of localized defects, as in the case presented. Total veneers are indicated for the restoration of generalized defects or areas of intrinsic staining that involve most of the buccal surface of the tooth [3, 8, 9]. Therefore, important factors, including the patient's age, extent, and oral hygiene, must be evaluated before seeking facets as a treatment option. In the case presented, preparation was necessary to remove the altered structure that caused dissatisfaction for the patient. This is necessary to provide space for the opaque increment of dentin and then enamel, thus achieving aesthetics without excess material that

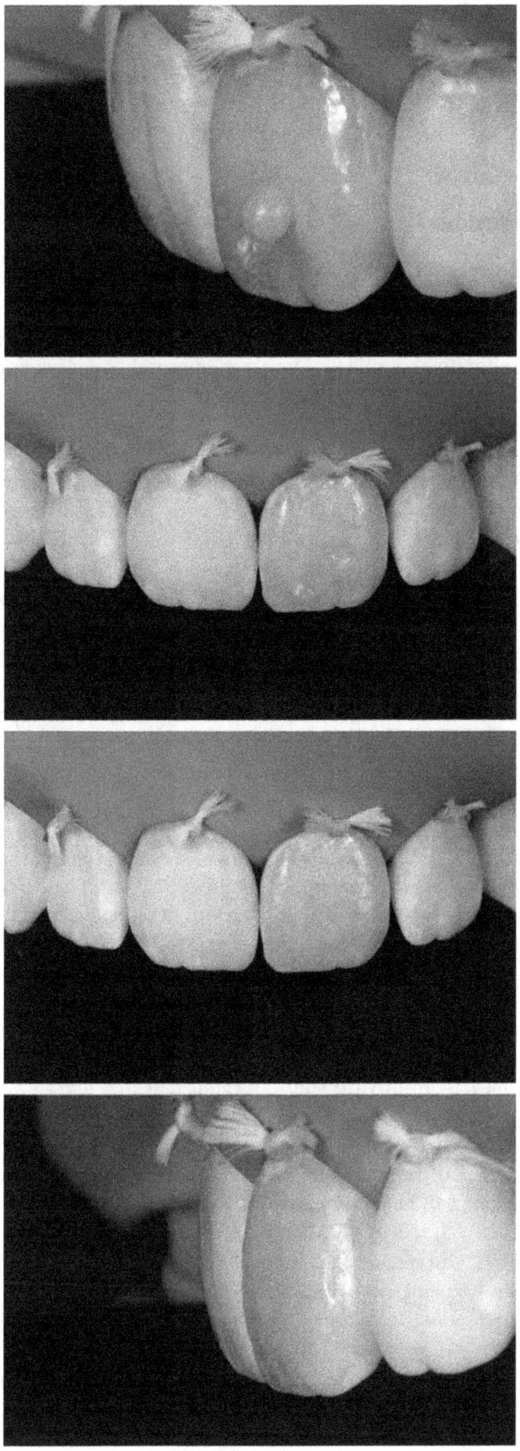

FIGURE 7: The first increment of the composite resin was applied in the color LD Essentia-GC. Then, the resin color LE Essentia-GC was applied, corresponding to the enamel region.

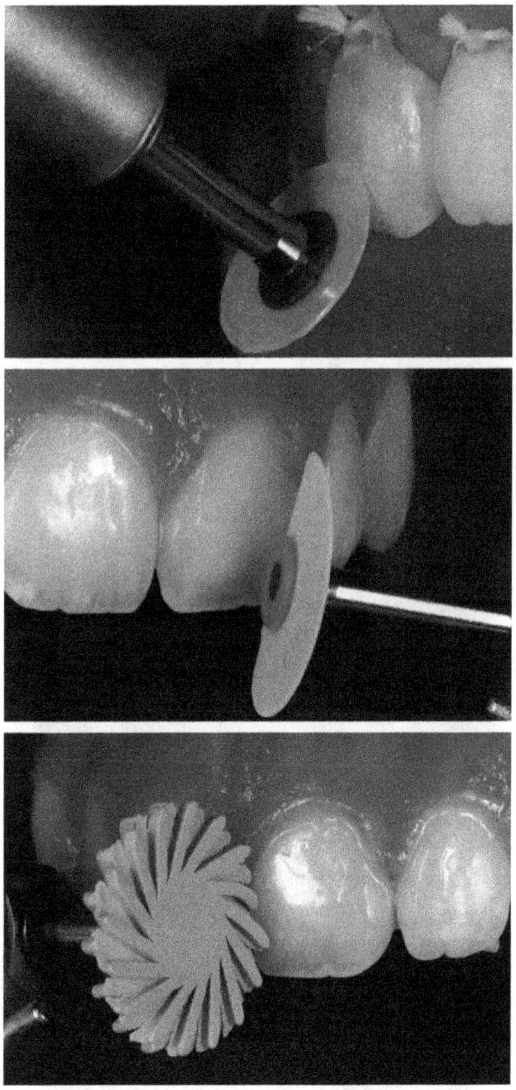

FIGURE 8: Resin finishing and polishing with discs (OptiDisc, Kerr) and resin rubbers (Jota do Brasil).

would generate overcontour. In the case presented, absolute isolation was carried out; however, the relative isolation would also allow for a restoration of excellence. It is not necessary to remove all the altered enamel in the pulp direction, because even with a small thickness, it is possible to mask the effect of this structure with composite resin. In peripheral areas, however, it is necessary to completely remove the altered structure so that a line between tooth/restoration does not remain [1]. Thus, in the case presented, part of the altered structure was not removed in the back wall but completely removed in the contour areas, as seen in Figure 4. The resin was placed in increments with a slight excess to allow freedom in the contour during finishing and polishing. The partial veneer is more conservative when compared to the total veneer; however, more professional skills are required so that the tooth/restoration transition line does not appear.

Finally, cavity preparation can be considered a limitation of the present report. However, it is a low cost and more predictable when compared with treatment such as infiltration using fluid resin or biomimetic hydroxyapatite [6, 7, 10, 11]. These two treatments can be considered recent and need more researches. Thus, as demonstrated here,

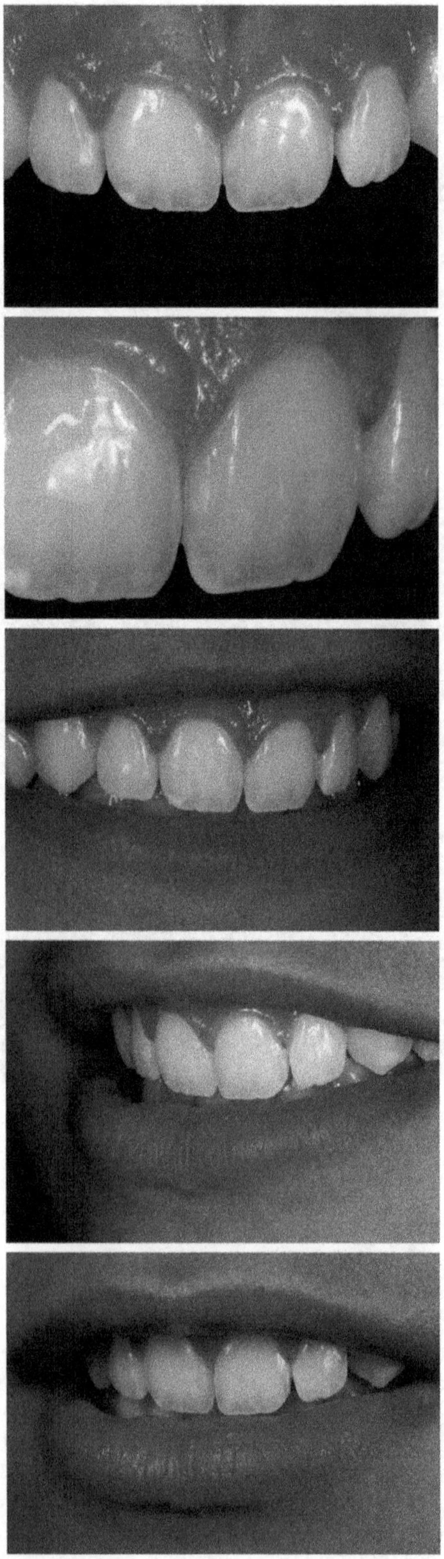

Figure 9: Final aspect of the upper anterior teeth. Note the color harmony provided by the association of enamel macroabrasion and partial veneer in composite resin.

direct composite resin restorations are well recognized because of their satisfactory esthetics and minimal wear of tooth structure [12].

4. Conclusion

The association of enamel macroabrasion and partial veneer in composite resin is conservative, fast, and aesthetic alternatives for removing localized hypoplasia stains.

References

[1] H. Heymann, E. Swift Jr., and A. Ritter, *Sturdevant's art and science of operative dentistry*, Mosby, 6th edition, 2012.

[2] L. Giannetti and R. Apponi, "Combined orthodontic and restorative minimally invasive approach to diastema and morphology management in the esthetic area. Clinical multidisciplinary case report with 3-year follow-up," *Case Reports in Dentistry*, vol. 2020, Article ID 3628467, 5 pages, 2020.

[3] G. Sammarco, "Combined minimally invasive treatment of white and brown fluorotic discolorations in a teenager: a case report," *The International Journal of Esthetic Dentistry*, vol. 14, no. 2, pp. 148–155, 2019.

[4] N. I. Pini, D. Sundfeld-Neto, F. H. Aguiar et al., "Enamel microabrasion: an overview of clinical and scientific considerations," *World Journal of Clinical Cases*, vol. 3, no. 1, pp. 34–41, 2015.

[5] C. C. Pavani, L. R. Vieira, T. C. Schott et al., "Case reports of enamel microabrasion associated with at-home dental bleaching after orthodontic bracket removal," *Operative Dentistry*, vol. 46, no. 3, pp. 237b–2245, 2021.

[6] A. Butera, M. Pascadopoli, S. Gallo et al., "SEM/EDS evaluation of the mineral deposition on a polymeric composite resin of a toothpaste containing biomimetic Zn-carbonate hydroxyapatite (microRepair®) in oral environment: a randomized clinical trial," *Polymers (Basel)*, vol. 13, no. 16, p. 2740, 2021.

[7] N. Khanduri, D. Kurup, and M. Mitra, "Quantitative evaluation of remineralizing potential of three agents on artificially demineralized human enamel using scanning electron microscopy imaging and energy-dispersive analytical X-ray element analysis: an in vitro study," *Dental Research Journal*, vol. 17, no. 5, pp. 366–372, 2020.

[8] M. M. M. Gresnigt, M. S. Cune, J. Schuitemaker et al., "Performance of ceramic laminate veneers with immediate dentine sealing: an 11 year prospective clinical trial," *Dental Materials*, vol. 35, no. 7, pp. 1042–1052, 2019.

[9] H. G. Ohrvik and C. Hjortsjö, "Retrospective study of patients with amelogenesis imperfecta treated with different bonded restoration techniques," *Clinical and Experimental Dental Research*, vol. 6, no. 1, pp. 16–23, 2020.

[10] A. Ndokaj, M. Jedlinski, D. Pasqualotto, C. Stamegna, M. Capocci, and F. Rinaldo, "Treatment of developmental defects of enamel," *La Clinica Terapeutica*, vol. 171, pp. 55-56, 2021.

[11] R. S. Rocha, M. Y. de Souza, L. C. F. Meirelles et al., "Effectiveness of home bleaching treatment after resin infiltrant application," *Oral Health & Preventive Dentistry*, vol. 18, pp. 549–554, 2020.

[12] B. Korkut and C. Turkmen, "Longevity of direct diastema closure and recontouring restorations with resin composites in maxillary anterior teeth: A4-yearclinical evaluation," *Journal of Esthetic and Restorative Dentistry*, vol. 33, no. 4, pp. 590–604, 2021.

12

The Replanting of a 1.1 from an Ectopic Position during the Course of Orthodontic Therapy: Follow-Up at 8 Years

Michele M. Figliuzzi,[1] Maria Altilia,[1] Simone Altilia,[1,2] Amerigo Giudice,[1] and Leonzio Fortunato[1]

[1]*School of Dentistry, Department of Periodontics and Oral Sciences, Magna Græcia University, Catanzaro, Italy*
[2]*Dentistry School, Tor Vergata University of Rome, Rome, Italy*

Correspondence should be addressed to Michele M. Figliuzzi; michelefigliuzzi@libero.it

Academic Editor: Maddalena Manfredi

The case that is reported here describes the replanting of a 1.1 from an ectopic position during orthodontic therapy. The 9-year-old patient suffered from class 2 type malocclusion with the upper maxilla contracted, right-left posterior cross-bite. The clinical case presented the following details: in the upper incisor group, the 1.1 was overlapping the 1.2 and was distalised and completely vestibularised, whilst in the place of the 1.1, a 1.1 supernumerary persisted in occlusion. Following several medical investigations, such as OPT and, most importantly, TC cone beam investigation, the dangerous position of the dental element became clear. This did not present vestibular cortical bone but only gingival mucosa. Following these investigations, the difficulty in bringing the dental element into its natural position through orthodontic treatment became obvious since the natural position was without sufficient bone support. From this, it became obvious that surgery and replanting of the 1.1 immediately after the extraction of the supernumerary 1.1 was the only choice available.

1. Introduction

Ectopia is a dental anomaly caused by an alteration of the eruption process in which the element erupts away from its normal seat, in a vestibular, lingual, or palatal position. Dental anomalies can be of genetic, congenital, or acquired origin. The etiopathogenesis can be found in an anomalous position of the dental germ, in the lack of space in the arch where it should lie, and in physiological limits of the deciduous teeth, a precocious loss of a deciduous tooth with subsequent loss of space for the permanent tooth or a basal-dental disharmony. An important aesthetic deficit occurs when ectopia occurs in the anterior section leading to the necessity of orthodontic treatment. Orthodontic dental movement occurs as a result of the remodelling of the bone alveolar and the modification of the periodontal ligaments. The limits of orthodontics are tied to the individual conditions which may modify the success of the treatment; one of these is found in the lack of an adequate connection between the dental element and the alveolar.

2. Replanting

The term replanting refers to the insertion of an extracted dental element into an alveolar with consequent temporary splinting. This procedure can be carried out following a trauma which causes the complete extraction of the element or as an intentional surgical operation. In the latter case, an atraumatic extraction is carried out on a dental element which is immediately repositioned in the previously prepared alveolar. In the year 1990, Andersson and Bodin have published a long-term clinical follow-up study [1]. Another study of hypodontia has been published by Symons et al. in 1993 in anomalies associated with hypodontia [2]. In the years 1994 and 1996, Pitt Ford et al. and Bakland and Andreasen identified other influential factors such as postsurgical complications,

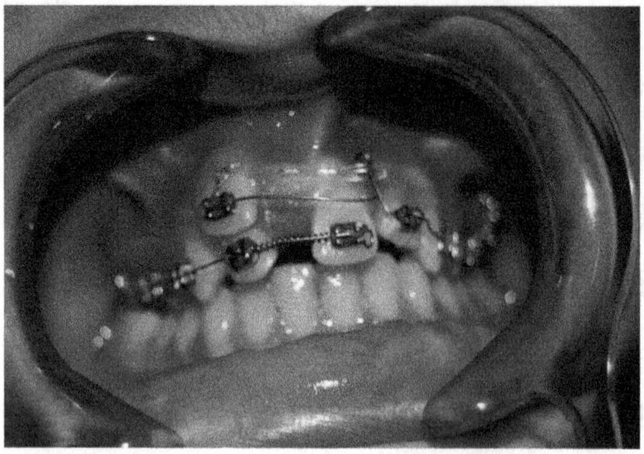

Figure 1: Ectopic permanent 1.1, distalised, vestibularised, and overlapping the 1.2.

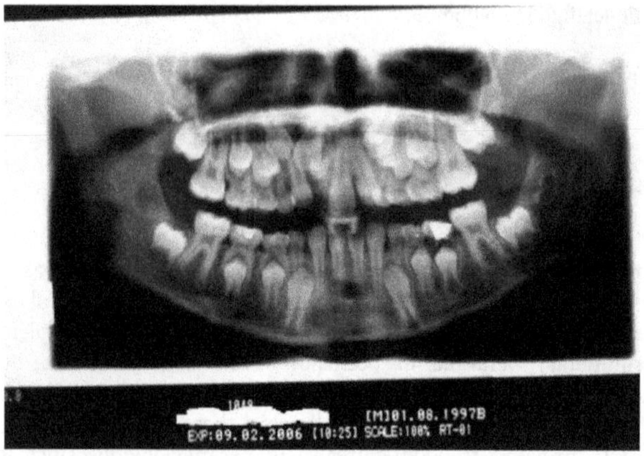

Figure 2: OPT shows the mixed dentition and the presence of the supernumerary 1.1.

endodontic healing, periodontal healing, and radicular reabsorption [3, 4].

Barrett and Kenny demonstrated the possibility of success in long-term natural tooth reimplant [5].

Andreasen et al. have published the study of the effect of treatment factors such as treatment delay, repositioning, splinting type, and period and antibiotics [6].

A minimally invasive surgery was proposed by Figliuzzi et al. for the management of impacted maxillary canines [7].

3. The Case

The 9-year-old male patient (M.G.) presented a class 2 type malocclusion with the upper maxilla contracted and posterior right-left cross-bite as well as an ectopia of the 1.1 that was distalised, vestibularised, and overlapping the 1.2 (Figure 1). The X-rays (Figure 2) showed an intraosseous inclusion of a supernumerary 1.1 in a mixed dentition situation. The presence of the 1.1 supernumerary in bone inclusion determined the ectopia of the permanent 1.1 tooth. Following clinical examination and X-rays, a TC cone beam was requested in order to study the topography of the ectopic element and its relationship with the surrounding structures. The results of the TC cone beam investigation showed the absence of the vestibular bone wall for the dental element (Figure 3) which turned out to be covered only by gingival mucosa. The lack of an adequate relationship between the alveolar and the dental element prevented successful orthodontic therapy; for this reason, the patient was referred for an intentional surgical replanting. The treatment was divided into three phases:

(1) *Initial Orthodontic Treatment.* The first phase of the treatment involved orthodontic therapy using a functional arch for 10 to 12 months, a rapid palatal expander, and fixed upper and lower braces (Figure 4).

(2) *Immediate Intentional Replanting.* After local infiltration with mepivacaina 1 : 100000 (Figure 5), a vestibular incision was made starting from the central incisor on the right side to the central incisor on the left. The incision, carried out using a Beaver 64, was intrasulcular type, partial depth without vertical release since this system guarantees a better closure of the flap at the end of the operation (Figure 6). After lifting the flap, the supernumerary 1.1 was extracted and the alveolar was suitably prepared to receive the permanent 1.1 (Figure 7). This phase was carried out using a surgical spoon in order to remove any residual bony fragments. At this point, the permanent 1.1 was extracted (Figure 8) and it was immediately replanted in the now empty alveolar which once held the supernumerary 1.1 (Figure 9). The replanted dental element was suitably splinted in order to keep it in place, and the flap was repositioned and sutured after the surgical site was accurately swabbed (Figure 10).

(3) *Final Orthodontic Treatment.* Having repositioned the ectopic element in the dental arch, the orthodontic therapy continued with the refining phases to close the case (Figure 11).

After approximately 1 year, the patient returned for a follow-up checkup and the replanted dental element (1.1) showed signs of necrosis. This was then treated endodontically and followed over a period of time. At the 6-year checkup, the patient was found to have excellent stability of the replanted dental element that had been subsequently treated endodontically (Figure 12).

4. Discussion

The biological mechanisms at the basis of intentional replanting are the preservation of the integrity of the periodontal ligament (the main factor in promoting clinical success), atraumatic extraction (fundamental for maintaining the vitality of the element), reduction of the extraoral stay time, and reduction of any osmotic shock of the ligament. Swabbing with water (rather than physiological solution) and lengthened time outside of the alveolar are associated

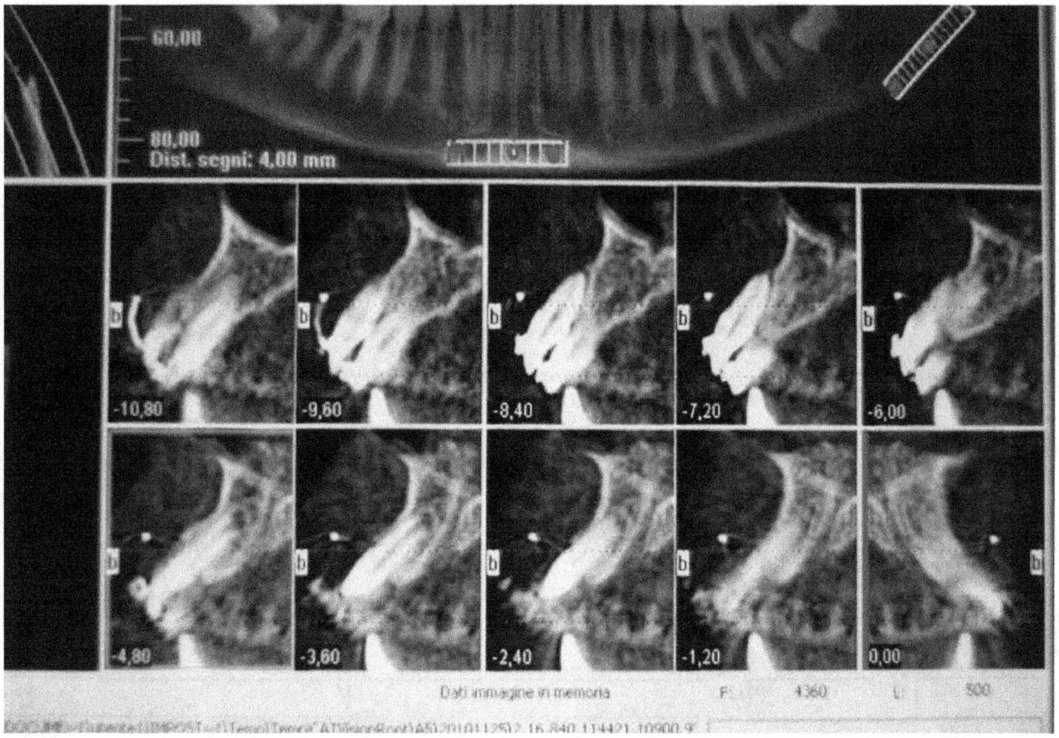

FIGURE 3: TC cone beam shows the lack of vestibular bone tissue around the permanent 1.1.

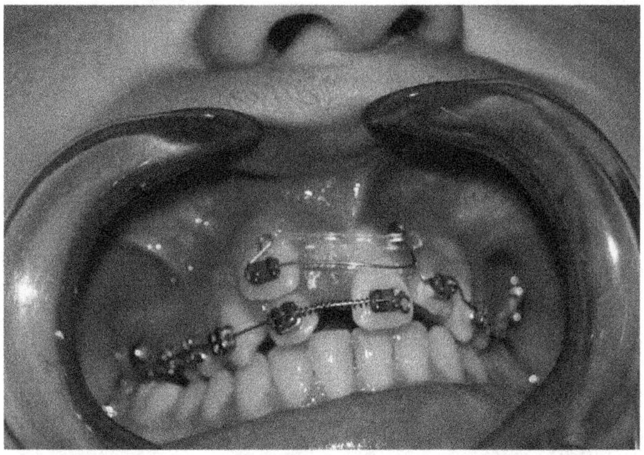

FIGURE 4: Initial orthodontic treatment.

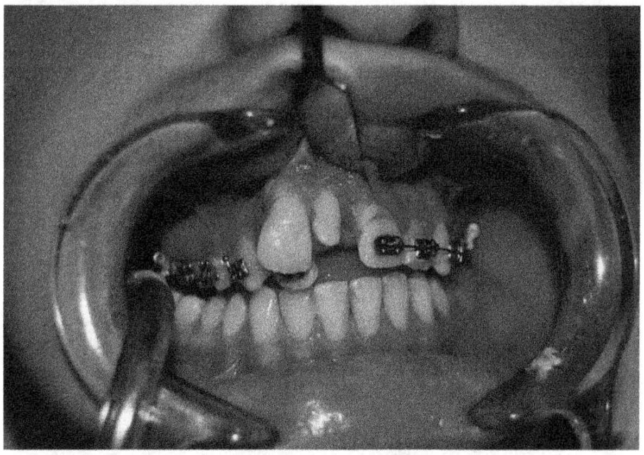

FIGURE 6: Envelope flap, intrasulcular partial depth from 1.1 to 2.1.

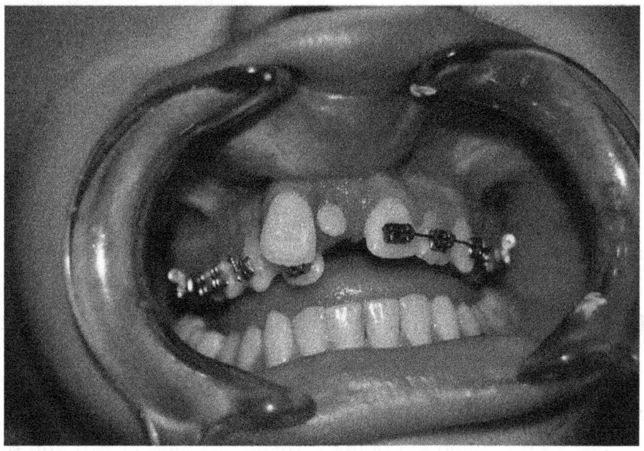

FIGURE 5: Local anaesthetic.

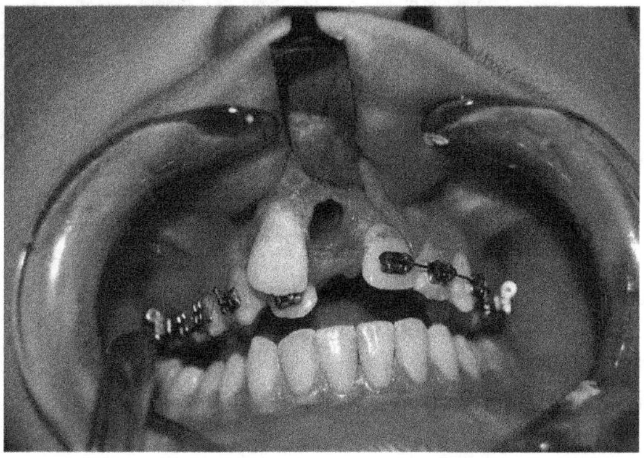

FIGURE 7: Extraction of the supernumerary 1.1 and preparation of the alveolar.

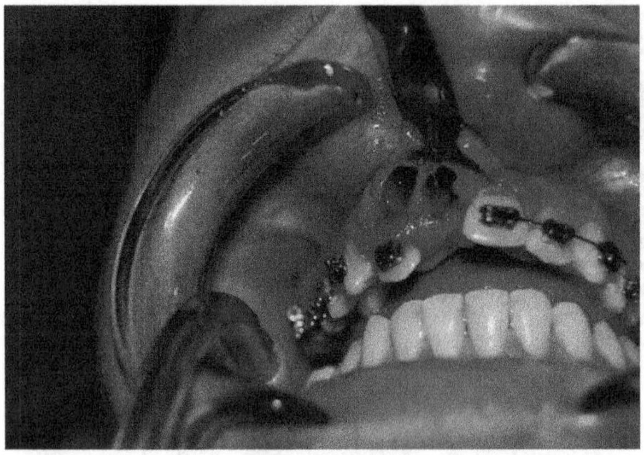

FIGURE 8: Extraction of the permanent 1.1.

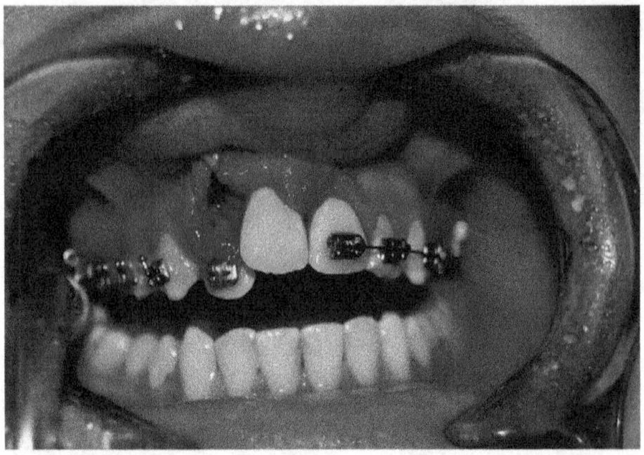

FIGURE 9: Replanting of the permanent 1.1 in the alveolar of the supernumerary 1.1.

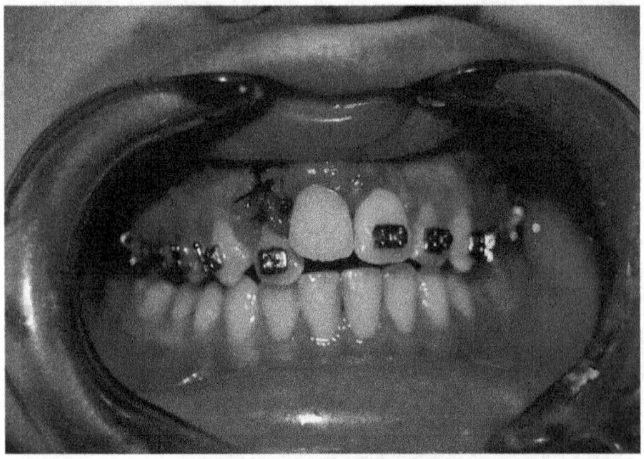

FIGURE 10: Sutured flap.

with a greater percentage of radicular reabsorption. Known side-effects of dental replanting are the presence of a complex radicular morphology, lesions to the furcation, periodontal lesions associated with class 3 dental mobility, and radicular caries. The advantages given by the success of replanting are aesthetic and functional recovery, reduced bone loss, absence of postoperative oedema, precise retrograde treatment, short timescale, and reduced risk of complications.

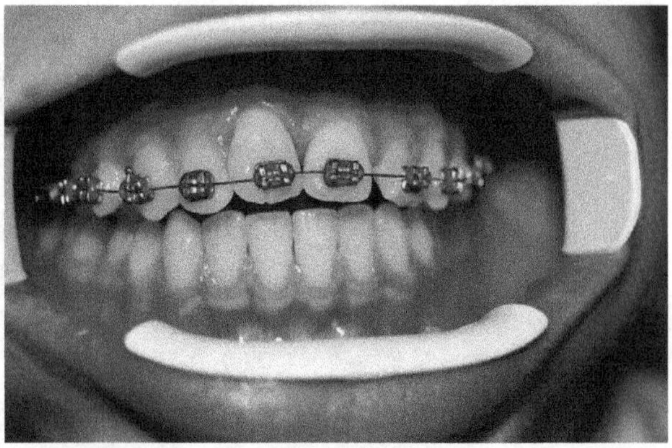

(a)

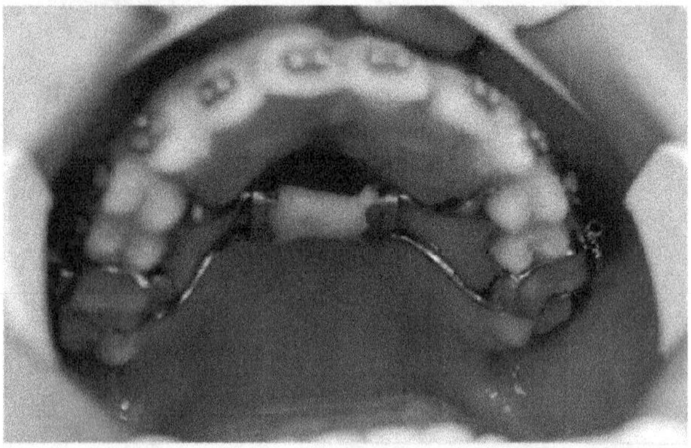

(b)

FIGURE 11: Final orthodontic treatment (a, b).

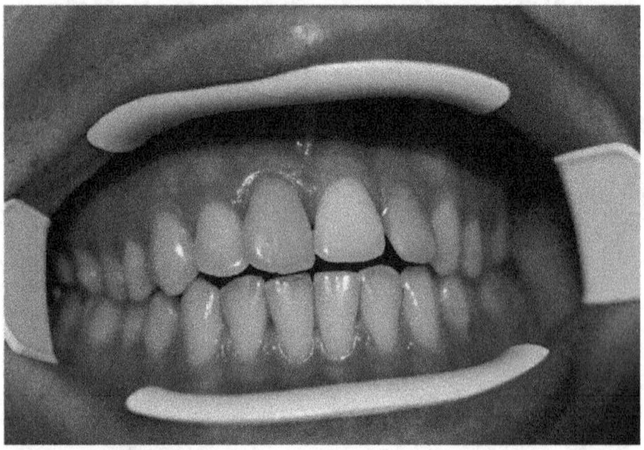

FIGURE 12: 6-year follow-up.

References

[1] L. Andersson and I. Bodin, "Avulsed human teeth replanted within 15 minutes - a long-term clinical follow-up study," *Endodontics & Dental Traumatology*, vol. 6, no. 1, pp. 37–42, 1990.

[2] A. L. Symons, F. Stritzel, and J. Stamation, "Anomalies associated with hypodontia of the permanent lateral incisor and second premolar," *The Journal of Clinical Pediatric Dentistry*, vol. 17, no. 2, pp. 109–111, 1993.

[3] T. R. Pitt Ford, J. O. Andreasen, S. O. Dorn, and S. P. Kariyawasam, "Effect of IRM root end fillings on healing after replantation," *Journal of Endodontia*, vol. 20, no. 8, pp. 381–385, 1994.

[4] L. K. Bakland and J. O. Andreasen, "Examination of the dentally traumatized patient," *Journal of the California Dental Association*, vol. 24, no. 2, pp. 35–37, 1996.

[5] E. J. Barrett and D. J. Kenny, "Survival of avulsed permanent maxillary incisors in children following delayed replantation," *Endodontics & Dental Traumatology*, vol. 13, no. 6, pp. 269–275, 1997.

[6] J. O. Andreasen, F. M. Andreasen, I. Mejaré, and M. Cvek, "Healing of 400 intra-alveolar root fractures. 2. Effect of treatment factors such as treatment delay, repositioning, splinting type and period and antibiotics," *Dental Traumatology*, vol. 20, no. 4, pp. 203–211, 2004.

[7] M. M. Figliuzzi, M. Altilia, L. Mannarino, A. Giudice, and L. Fortunato, "Minimally invasive surgical management of impacted maxillary canines," *Annali Italiani di Chirurgia*, vol. 89, pp. 443–447, 2018.

13

Challenges in the Dental Management of Rett Syndrome under General Anesthesia: A Rare Disease

Wisam Al-Hathlol,[1] Raed Bokhari,[1] Nada Alzahrani,[2] and Elaf Alkuwaiti[2]

[1]*Department of Pediatrics, National Guard Hospital, Dammam, Saudi Arabia*
[2]*College of Dentistry, Imam Abdulrahman Bin Faisal University, Dammam, Saudi Arabia*

Correspondence should be addressed to Wisam Al-Hathlol; wisam.hathlol@gmail.com

Academic Editor: Sreekanth Kumar Mallineni

Rett syndrome is a neurodevelopmental genetic X-linked disorder. It is predominantly found in females with a prevalence rate of 1 : 9000. Rett syndrome patients are usually healthy the first months of their lives. The syndrome goes into a deceleration phase where motor, behavioral, and cognitive skills are impaired. Regarding their oral health, bruxism is one of the common oral manifestations found among Rett syndrome patients. We present a case of an 8-year-old patient with Rett syndrome who presented to the dental clinic for oral rehabilitation. The patient was evaluated and treated under general anesthesia with multiple extractions, restorations, and crown installments. Oral rehabilitation of Rett syndrome is important for those patients, and proper evaluation and treatment are the most efficient when performed under general anesthesia.

1. Introduction

Rett syndrome (RS) is a rare neurological X-linked disorder caused by a dominant mutation in the MECP*2* gene, which exclusively affects females with a prevalence of 1 to 9000 (1, 2). Rett was the first to define the disease in 1966 (3), and Hagberg et al. provided comprehensive clinical characteristics of the syndrome in 1983 (4). In RS, patients are usually healthy for the first 6-18 months of life. Afterward, they begin to exhibit deceleration of head growth and muscular hypotonia which is followed by loss of motor coordination, acquired communication, and social skills (5). Furthermore, patients go through a period of stagnation between 2 and 10 years of age followed by a rapid regression in motor, behavioral, and cognitive skills. They are characterized by autistic-like behaviors such as mental retardation, hand tremors, and epileptic seizures. Other features including hyperventilation, apnea, kyphosis, development of osteoporosis, gastrointestinal problems, and weight loss can be found in RS (5–8). Moreover, around 50% of the affected patients may develop orthopedic deformities in late stages including scoliosis and/or multiple joint contractures as well as vascular and arterial malformations which can impede venous access (9).

RS patients can develop some oral manifestations including high arched palate, anterior open bite, bruxism, gingivitis, periodontitis, gingival hyperplasia, xerostomia, glossitis, erythema multiform, lingual paralysis, dental anomalies, and delayed eruption (10–14). Bruxism in RS is the most frequently observed oral habit, especially the diurnal bruxism that ranges from (53-95%) (15–17), followed by tongue thrusting (11), digits sucking (13), and oral breathing (11, 15). Many of the oral manifestations are linked with the anxiolytics and anticonvulsants therapies taken (10, 18).

RS diagnosis is mostly clinically based with no cure or specific treatment available to date (19, 20). Their management requires an interdisciplinary approach that covers pharmacological, symptomatic therapy, physiotherapy, social work, and speech therapy (21). Dental treatment and sedation used for such a complex syndrome differ. Some use nitrous oxide alone (22) or combined with sublingual midazolam (15), while some investigators prefer to use general anesthesia since the patients are considered at a high medical risk and are difficult to cooperate (10, 23). In this

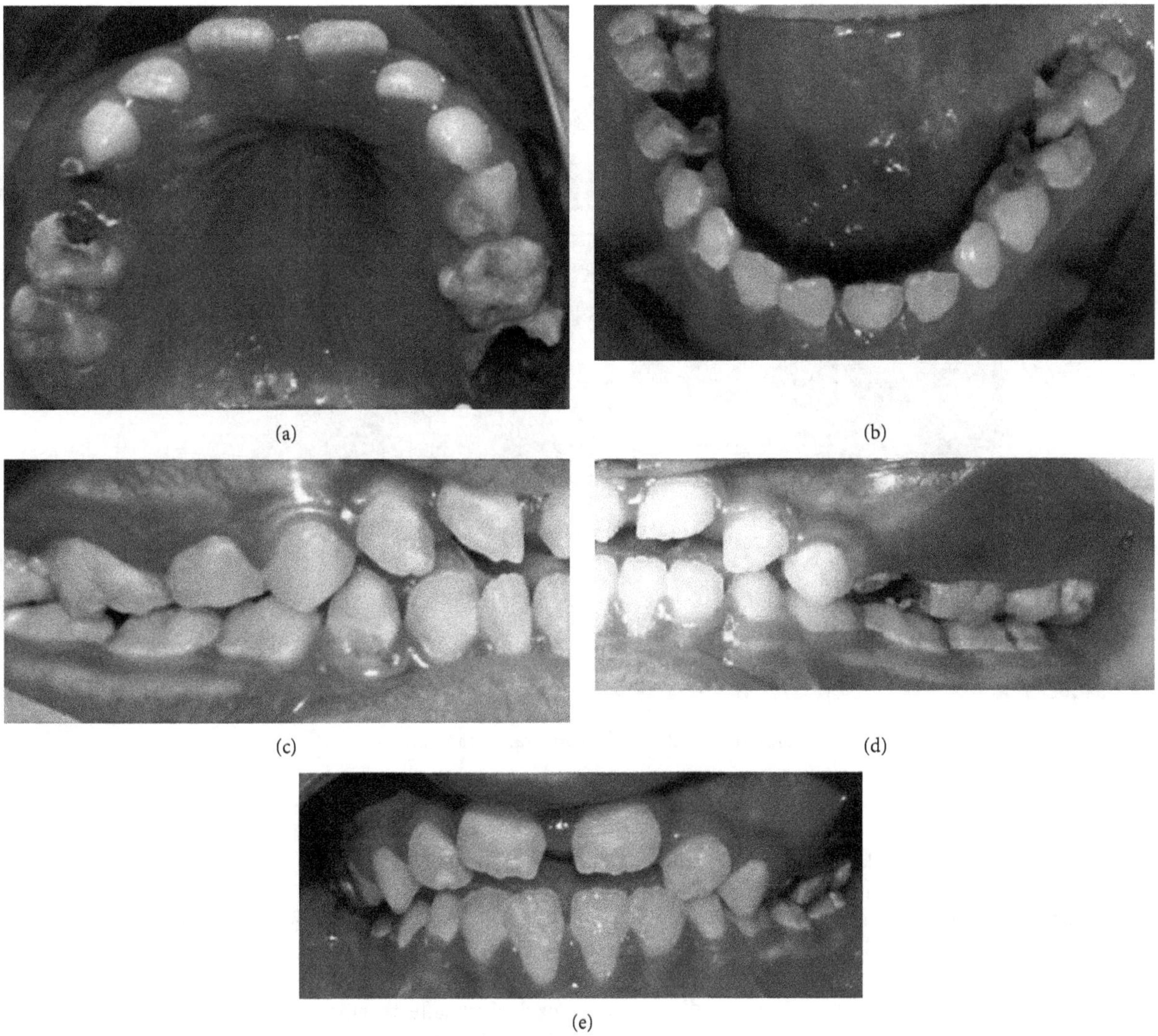

FIGURE 1: Intraoral preoperative photographs showing (a) maxillary occlusal view. (b) Mandibular occlusal view. (c) Right lateral view. (d) Left lateral view. (e) Frontal view.

case report, we aim to stress the challenges in the dental management of RS during general anesthesia.

2. Case Report

An eight-year-old female patient with Rett syndrome was scheduled to undergo oral rehabilitation under general anesthesia. She came to the dental clinic complaining of several cavities and discomfort in the posterior teeth. Preoperative examination showed mental retardation, normal consciousness, and lack of cooperation and orientation. Stiffness of the lower extremities, inability to stand, and the need for support to sit were noted. The patient was diagnosed with Rett syndrome after having multiple seizures and stereotypic hand movement at the age of two and a genetic blood test confirmed the presence of MECP2 mutation. Regarding her medication, the patient was not on any medication and was using herbal medication only. Meanwhile, her clinical examination including cardiac, respiratory, and gastrointestinal was normal. Her hemoglobin level was 138 gm/L, and serum electrolytes were within normal limits.

In regard to her dental examination, extraoral examination was insignificant. The patient had symmetrical face, and the lips were incompetent and dry. On the other hand, her intraoral examination was remarkable. Soft tissue examination showed normal alveolar mucosa, macroglossia, with generalized gingivitis with no abnormality in the floor of the mouth. The hard tissue examination showed mixed dentition stage matching chronological age, generalized enamel hypomineralization, multiple carious teeth, malocclusion, and anterior open bite (Figure 1).

Preoperatively, the patient received 1 mg of midazolam intravenously (IV). Regarding her vitals, her heart rate was 99/min, blood pressure was 112/64 mmHg, respiratory rate was 25/min, and peripheral oxygen saturation (SpO_2) was 99%. Before starting the operation, an administration of

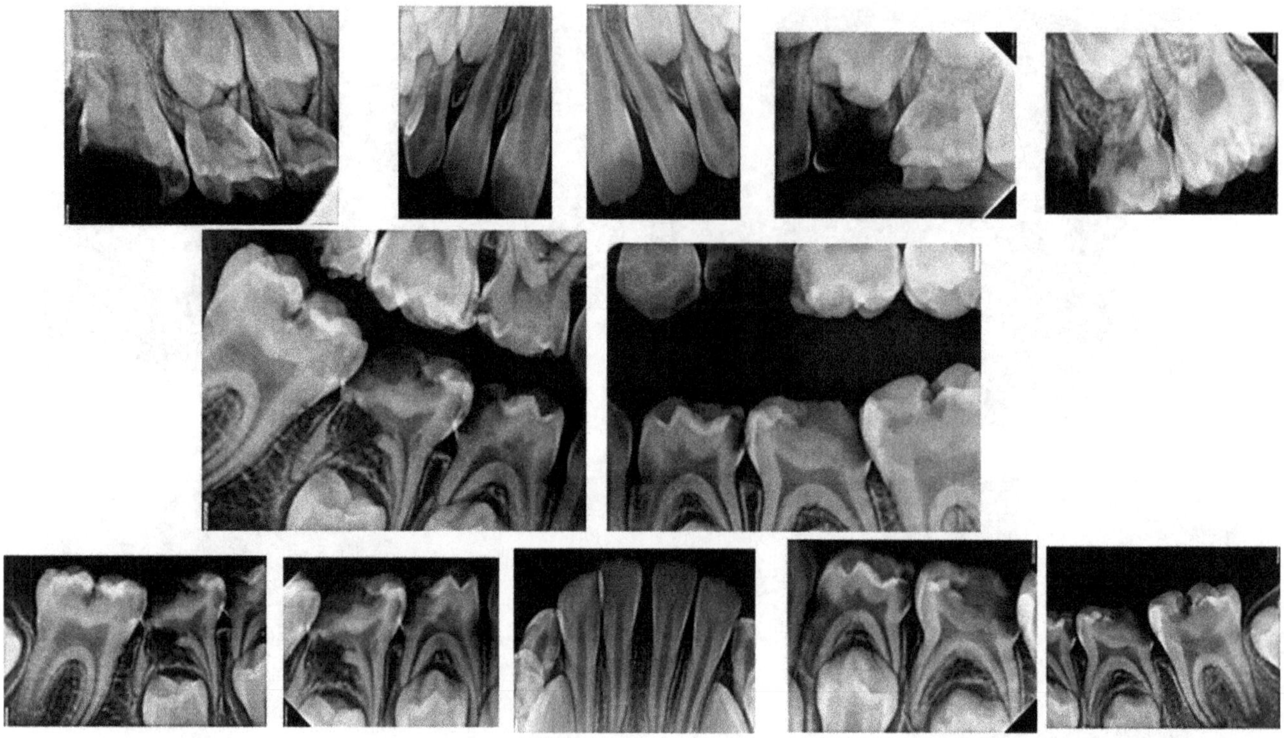

Figure 2: Full mouth preoperative radiographs.

20 mcg/kg of fentanyl, 40 mg/kg propofol, remifentanil 10 mcg/kg, and 2 mg/kg of dexamethasone was given IV. During the operation, administration of 10 mcg/kg of fentanyl, 80 mcg/kg remifentanil, and 12.5 mg/kg of diclofenac sodium was added. After initiating of general anesthesia through nasotracheal intubation, an intraoral radiographs and photographs showed multiple caries in the primary and permanent teeth with some pulpal involvement (Figure 2).

Therefore, the treatment plan was set to extract the decayed permanent teeth #16, #26, #36, and #46 as well as #64 and #85 primary teeth. A formacrsol pulpotomy was performed on teeth #65, #75, and #84 followed by Resin modified glass ionomer filling. Afterwards, the occlusal seal was achieved using stainless steel crowns. Stainless steel crowns were a superior treatment choice on teeth #55, #54, and #74 due to the patient's high risk for caries. A buccal composite restoration was done on tooth #83 along with prophylaxis and topical fluoride (Figures 3 and 4).

The operation took three hours and 24 minutes. The patient was taken to the recovery room afterwards and was monitored until she regained full motor function. She was discharged the next day and was given acetaminophen 24 mg/ml, elixir (LASA) of 160 mg oral QID every 6 hours PRN for mild pain for a total of five days, penicillin (250 mg/5 ml) suspension BID, and q12h for a duration of five days. Her discharge instructions were given to brush the teeth twice daily, reduce sugar intake, and undertake a healthy diet with regular follow-ups in the clinic.

3. Discussion

Rett was the first to define the disease in 1966 (3). RS is a rare developmental X-linked disorder caused by a dominant mutation in the MECP*2* gene (16). However, this syndrome exclusively affects females with a prevalence of 1 to 9000 (2). The Rett syndrome is categorized in detective phases into an initial phase of early normal development, followed by a regression phase, appearing as severe intellectual disability. Moreover, another study categorized RS into four conventional phases starting from a delayed developmental milestone to further regression with loss of acquired communication and signs of mental retardation. These were followed by neuromotor challenges such as walking, followed by a later phase of motor deterioration which is characterized by weight loss and skeletal deformities (24). In our case, inability of cooperation and orientation was noted along with stiffness of the lower extremities, inability to stand, and the need for support to sit that were noted. Other researchers reported the most common oral findings were bruxism, masseteric hypertrophy, anterior open bite mouth breathing, tongue thrusting, digital sucking, and high arch palate (25). In our case, there were no clinical signs of attrition or masseteric hypertrophy, but there was nonnutritive sucking habit.

In 2018, Lai et al. reviewed the Australian Rett Syndrome Database (ARSD) which was established in 1993. The registry includes all female RS patients born since 1976. They found that around two third of the population of RS attended the dental clinic with slightly higher proportion

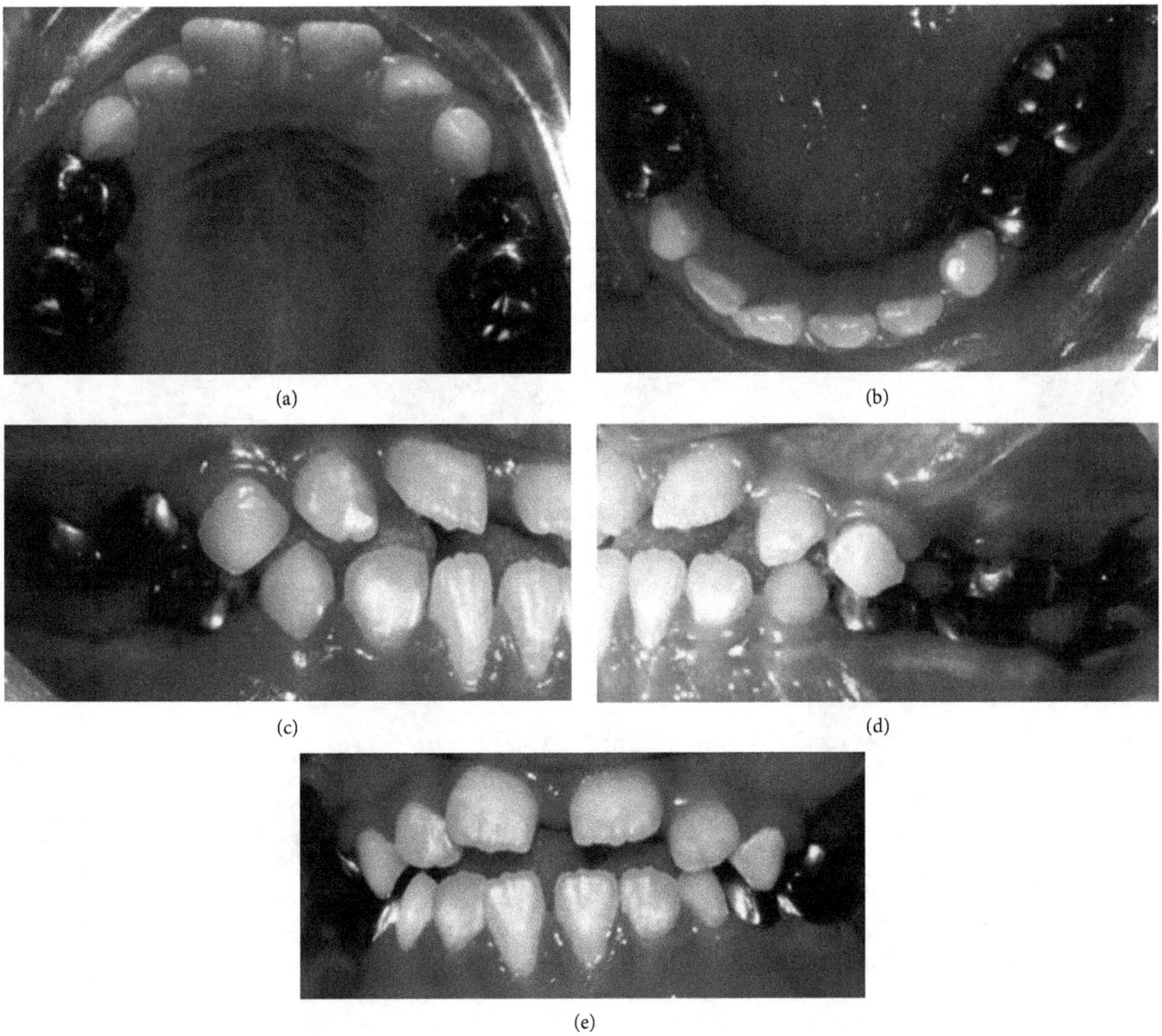

FIGURE 3: Intraoral postoperative photographs. (a) Maxillary occlusal view. (b) Mandibular occlusal view. (c) Right lateral view. (d) Left lateral view. (e) Frontal view.

with those having epileptic seizures. In addition, 75% of those with gastroesophageal reflux disease attended the dental clinic compared to 56% to those without the disease. Moreover, dental procedures that was done under general anesthesia were reported in 24 patients out of 77. It is worth mentioning that general anesthesia was performed on small procedures such as one tooth extraction. The authors also found that patient who underwent general anesthesia was reported higher in those living in inner regions compared to those living in major cities (26). This can be attributed to the epileptic, noncompliant nature of RS. In addition, proper evaluation would be performed more efficiently to diagnose any other dental disease. In our case, the patient underwent full investigatory panel under general anesthesia where multiple carries were discovered with pulp involvement.

According to Mahdi et al., the most common dental finding among RS patients is bruxism. Other findings include masseteric hypertrophy, anterior open bite, and nonphysiological tooth wear (16). This was also found in an older study by Magalhães et al. where they studied a total of 13 patients with RS and found that bruxism was the most common dental manifestation (27). However, our patient did not report bruxism or any masseteric hypertrophy. Meanwhile, Bianco and Rota stated that some extraoral manifestation may appear which are related to pharmacological therapy. These include xerostomia, glossitis, erythema multiforme, gingival hyperplasia, dysphagia, and lingual paralysis. In our patient, there were no oral manifestation present, however, she was not on any pharmaceutical therapy and was only treated by herbal medications.

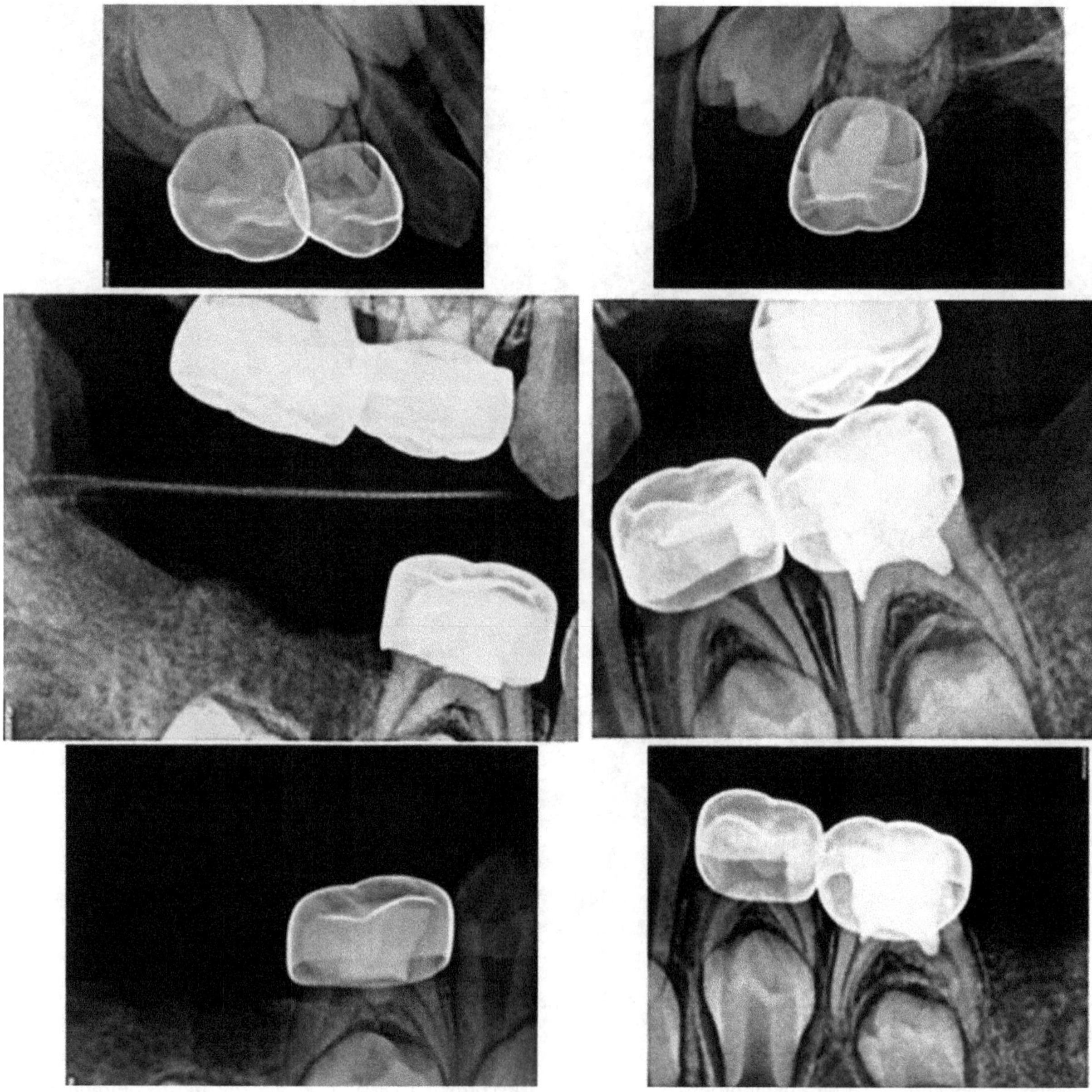

Figure 4: Postoperative radiographs.

4. Conclusion

Rett syndrome is a neurodevelopmental disorder which presents with a constellation of clinical findings. Based on the clinical representation, it is possible to diagnose a case of Rett syndrome. Early detection of the disease is important. A suitable multidisciplinary approach for management should be well established to improve the quality of life. Proper dental evaluation and management under general anesthesia are recommended due to the noncompliance nature of the patient.

Consent

An informed consent was obtained from the patient's guardians as well as the hospital to publish this work.

References

[1] R. E. Amir, I. B. Van den Veyver, M. Wan, C. Q. Tran, U. Francke, and H. Y. Zoghbi, "Rett syndrome is caused by mutations in X-linked _MECP2_ , encoding methyl- CpG-binding protein 2," *Nature Genetics*, vol. 23, no. 2, pp. 185–188, 1999.

[2] S. Fehr, A. Bebbington, N. Nassar et al., "Trends in the diagnosis of Rett syndrome in Australia," *Pediatric Research*, vol. 70, no. 3, pp. 313–319, 2011.

[3] A. Rett, "On a unusual brain atrophy syndrome in hyperammonemia in childhood," *Wiener Medizinische Wochenschrift (1946)*, vol. 116, no. 37, pp. 723-726, 1966.

[4] B. Hagberg, J. Aicardi, K. Dias, and O. Ramos, "A progressive syndrome of autism, dementia, ataxia, and loss of purposeful hand use in girls: Rett's syndrome: report of 35 cases," *Annals of Neurology*, vol. 14, no. 4, pp. 471–479, 1983.

[5] A. Janas and P. Osica, "Dental issues in Rett syndrome," *Developmental period medicine.*, vol. 19, no. 4, pp. 478–481, 2015.

[6] A. L. Jefferson, H. J. Woodhead, S. Fyfe et al., "Bone mineral content and density in Rett syndrome and their contributing factors," *Pediatric Research*, vol. 69, no. 4, pp. 293–298, 2011.

[7] K. J. Motil, E. Caeg, J. O. Barrish et al., "Gastrointestinal and nutritional problems occur frequently throughout life in girls and women with Rett syndrome," *Journal of Pediatric Gastroenterology and Nutrition*, vol. 55, no. 3, pp. 292–298, 2012.

[8] R. Cianfaglione, A. Clarke, M. Kerr, R. P. Hastings, C. Oliver, and D. Felce, "Ageing in Rett syndrome," *Journal of intellectual disability research: JIDR.*, vol. 60, no. 2, pp. 182–190, 2016.

[9] H. Zoghbi, "Genetic aspects of Rett syndrome," *Journal of Child Neurology*, vol. 3, 1_suppl, pp. S76–S78, 1988.

[10] A. H. Friedlander, J. A. Yagiela, V. I. Paterno, and M. E. Mahler, "The pathophysiology, medical management and dental implications of fragile X, Rett, and Prader-Willi syndromes," *Journal of the California Dental Association*, vol. 31, no. 9, pp. 693–702, 2003.

[11] L. Stojanović, "Etiological aspects of anterior open bite," *Medicinski Pregled*, vol. 60, no. 3-4, pp. 151–155, 2007.

[12] P. L. Anders and E. L. Davis, "Oral health of patients with intellectual disabilities: a systematic review," *Special care in dentistry: official publication of the American Association of Hospital Dentists, the Academy of Dentistry for the Handicapped, and the American Society for Geriatric Dentistry.*, vol. 30, no. 3, pp. 110–117, 2010.

[13] P. Carter, J. Downs, A. Bebbington et al., "Stereotypical hand movements in 144 subjects with Rett syndrome from the population-based Australian database," *Movement disorders: official journal of the Movement Disorder Society.*, vol. 25, no. 3, pp. 282–288, 2010.

[14] V. Massimo, H. Joseph, L. Guido et al., "ODONTOSTOMATOLOGIC anomalies associated with RETT syndrome in 216 patients," *International Journal of Clinical Dentistry*, vol. 5, no. 4, 2012.

[15] M.-C. Fuertes-González and F.-J. Silvestre, "Oral health in a group of patients with Rett syndrome in the regions of Valencia and Murcia (Spain): a case-control study," *Medicina Oral, Patología Oral y Cirugía Bucal*, vol. 19, no. 6, pp. e598–e604, 2014.

[16] S. S. Mahdi, H. A. Jafri, R. Allana, F. Amenta, M. Khawaja, and S. S. B. Qasim, "Oral manifestations of Rett syndrome-a systematic review," *International Journal of Environmental Research and Public Health*, vol. 18, no. 3, p. 1162, 2021.

[17] Y. Y. L. Lai, J. A. Downs, K. Wong, S. Zafar, L. J. Walsh, and H. M. Leonard, "Oral parafunction and bruxism in Rett syndrome and associated factors: an observational study," *Oral Diseases*, 2021.

[18] S. Chattopadhyay and R. Arora, "The ironies of human mind: a case of Rett syndrome," *Ethiopian Journal of Health Sciences*, vol. 24, no. 2, pp. 171–174, 2014.

[19] S. J. Moser, P. Weber, and J. Lütschg, "Rett syndrome: clinical and electrophysiologic aspects," *Pediatric Neurology*, vol. 36, no. 2, pp. 95–100, 2007.

[20] J. L. Neul, W. E. Kaufmann, D. G. Glaze et al., "Rett syndrome: revised diagnostic criteria and nomenclature," *Annals of Neurology*, vol. 68, no. 6, pp. 944-950, 2010.

[21] E. M. Lai and S. H. Wei, "A Chinese girl with Rett syndrome," *Hong Kong Dental Journal*, vol. 3, pp. 48–51, 2006.

[22] A. R. Alpoz, N. Ergul, and O. Oncag, "Bruxism in Rett syndrome: a case report," *The Journal of clinical pediatric dentistry.*, vol. 23, no. 2, pp. 161–163, 1999.

[23] M. A. Buccino and J. A. Weddell, "Rett syndrome–a rare and often misdiagnosed syndrome: case report," *Pediatric Dentistry*, vol. 11, no. 2, pp. 151–157, 1989.

[24] S. Cocca, M. Viviano, M. Loglisci et al., "Correlation between <i>dysphagia</i> and malocclusion in Rett syndrome: a preliminary study," *Sultan Qaboos University Medical Journal*, vol. 18, no. 4, pp. e489–e493, 2018.

[25] R. A. Ribeiro, A. Romano, E. Birman, and M. Mayer, "Oral manifestations in Rett syndrome: a study of 17 cases," *Pediatric Dentistry*, vol. 19, no. 5, pp. 349–352, 1997.

[26] Y. Y. L. Lai, K. Wong, N. M. King, J. Downs, and H. Leonard, "Oral health experiences of individuals with Rett syndrome: a retrospective study," *BMC Oral Health*, vol. 18, no. 1, p. 195, 2018.

[27] M. H. Magalhães, J. Y. Kawamura, and L. C. Araújo, "General and oral characteristics in Rett syndrome," *Special care in dentistry: official publication of the American Association of Hospital Dentists, the Academy of Dentistry for the Handicapped, and the American Society for Geriatric Dentistry*, vol. 22, no. 4, pp. 147–150, 2002.

14

Ameloblastic Carcinoma in a 2-Year-Old Child: A Case Report and Review of the Literature

Ngoc Bao Vu,[1,2] Ngoc Tuyen Le,[3] Risa Chaisuparat,[4] Pasutha Thunyakitpisal,[5] and Ngoc Minh Tran[6]

[1]*Dental Biomaterials Science Program, Graduate School, Chulalongkorn University, Bangkok 10330, Thailand*
[2]*Department of Maxillofacial and Plastic Surgery, Hanoi National Hospital of Odonto-Stomatology, Hanoi 100000, Vietnam*
[3]*Department of Maxillofacial Reconstructive Surgery, Hanoi National Hospital of Odonto-Stomatology, Hanoi 100000, Vietnam*
[4]*Department of Oral Pathology, Faculty of Dentistry, Chulalongkorn University, Bangkok 10330, Thailand*
[5]*Research Unit of Herbal Medicine, Biomaterial, And Material for Dental Treatment, Department of Anatomy, Faculty of Dentistry, Chulalongkorn University, Bangkok 10330, Thailand*
[6]*Department of Pathology, Hanoi Medical University, Hanoi 100000, Vietnam*

Correspondence should be addressed to Pasutha Thunyakitpisal; pthunyak@yahoo.com

Academic Editor: Anastasios Markopoulos

Ameloblastic carcinoma (AC) is a rare malignant odontogenic tumor in pediatric patients, only 22 cases have been reported in literature since 1932. We present an extremely rare case in which AC occurred in a 2-year-old girl, who had a tumor in the right mandible. Radiographic findings showed a multilocular, poorly defined, and mixed radiolucent-radiopaque lesion in the region of teeth #84 to #85, with bone and tooth root resorption. Computed tomography revealed buccal cortex destruction, tumor infiltration of soft tissue, and enlarged nodes. Incisional biopsy showed histomorphological features of AC. Immunohistochemical analysis exhibited a positive result for Cytokeratin (CK) 19 and overexpression of p53 and Ki67. The patient underwent right hemimandibulectomy and neck dissection. The final pathology was consistent with the initial diagnosis of AC. The patient did not exhibit signs of recurrence or metastasis within 2 years postoperatively. Given the rarity of this disease and the age of the patient, this report constitutes a valuable contribution to the current literature.

1. Introduction

Ameloblastic carcinoma, first described by Elzay in 1982, is a rare, malignant type of odontogenic tumor [1]. AC has features of both ameloblastoma and carcinoma, independent of the presence of metastasis; it should be distinguished from malignant (metastasizing) ameloblastoma (MA), which exhibits benign histological appearance of ameloblastoma in primary and metastatic lesions [2]. In 2005, the World Health Organization classification of odontogenic tumors included AC as a malignant tumor, in a manner similar to that for MA. However, in the most recent the World Health Organization classification (2017), MA was reclassified as a benign odontogenic tumor, whereas AC continues to be considered a rare and highly malignant odontogenic tumor [3–5].

AC involves the mandible more frequently than the maxilla. It most frequently affects adult men. However, a few pediatric cases have been reported, with a minimum age of 4 [6, 7]. In this report, we describe a 2-year-old girl who was diagnosed with right mandibular ameloblastic carcinoma.

2. Case Description

Written informed consent of the patient's mother was obtained prior to this paper's publication.

A 2-year-old girl presented with a painful mass in the right mandible, which had appeared 1 month prior. Her first examination was performed in a local hospital, and the initial diagnosis was gingivitis. Oral hygiene instruction and antibiotics were prescribed. One week later, the mass continued to increase in size and caused pain and fever; thus, the girl was admitted to the Department of Maxillofacial Surgery at Hanoi National Hospital of Odonto-Stomatology, Hanoi, Vietnam.

Clinical examination revealed a mass in the right body of the mandible that extended from the commissure of the lip to the angle of the mandible. It was approximately 1 × 1 cm in size and painful on palpation. No sign of lip paresthesia related to the mass was detected, and the overlying skin was normal in color and texture. The submandibular lymph nodes were palpable, tender but painless, and movable. Mouth opening was normal. Intraoral examination showed a swelling in the region of teeth #83 to #85, which obliterated the right buccal sulcus. Mobility and displacement of teeth #84 and #85 were detected. The lesion was soft in consistency and painful on intraoral palpation. The overlying mucosa exhibited overgrowth (covering the crown of #85), red color, and an ulcerated appearance.

2.1. Radiographic Findings. Orthopantomography showed a multilocular, mixed radiolucent, and radiopaque lesion with a poorly defined border affecting the region of teeth #84 and #85. The lamina dura, roots of #84 and #85, and furcation of #84 were resorbed (Figure 1). Axial and coronal computed tomography revealed a poorly defined lesion in the right body of the mandible. The tumor had destroyed the buccal cortex and infiltrated into the soft tissue; reactive lymph nodes may be observed. The lingual cortex was partially damaged (Figure 2). Computed tomography of the chest revealed no metastatic deposits.

2.2. Biopsy and Histological Findings. Incisional biopsy was performed at the intraoral vestibule, where the lesion had penetrated. Histologic examination revealed sheets and nests of odontogenic epithelium separated by fibrous tissue with inflammatory infiltration and stellate reticulum-like structure. The peripheral cells of the nests resembled preameloblasts with cuboid shape and nuclei polarization (Figure 3(a)). Dedifferentiated areas exhibited cytologic malignant cells with increased nucleocytoplasmic ratio and hyperchromatic nuclei; few mitotic figures were present (Figure 3(b)). Histomorphological analysis demonstrated an aggressive type of ameloblastoma, suggestive of AC.

Immunohistochemical stains were performed using CK19, Ki67, and p53. The ameloblastic epithelium showed a positive reactivity for CK19 (Figure 3(c)). High proliferation level of the neoplasm was confirmed by elevated expression of Ki67 and p53 (Figures 3(d) and 3(e)).

Based on these findings, the final diagnosis was ameloblastic carcinoma.

2.3. Surgery. The patient underwent right hemimandibulectomy, extending from the distal aspect of #71 to the angle of the right mandible, with safe osseous margins of 2 cm on each side of the tumor. The surrounding tissue was also excised. Complete supraomohyoid neck dissection was performed on the right side, combined with excision of the right submandibular gland. The patient recovered uneventfully, and the wound healed well after surgery. The histopathological examination of the resection specimens was performed, and the diagnosis of the primary tumor was consistent with the initial diagnosis of AC. The positive submandibular lymph nodes were identified, and the microscopic examination of the lymph nodes showed diffuse infiltration of neoplastic cells (Figure 4). The submandibular salivary gland was not involved (data not shown).

2.4. Follow-Up. The patient returned regularly for follow-up. Clinical and radiographic examination at 2 years postoperatively showed no sign of recurrence or metastasis (Figure 5).

3. Discussion

AC is considered a rare, malignant neoplasm of odontogenic origin. Patients of various ages can be affected, but the disease most commonly occurs during the fourth decade of life. Moreover, it appears more frequently in men than in women, and the mandible is affected more frequently than the maxilla [8].

AC shares some common clinical features with ameloblastoma, such as a mass in the jaw, resorption of bone, and mobility of teeth. However, its behavior is more aggressive, including rapid growth, pain, perforation of the cortical plate, soft tissue infiltration, and/or lower lip paresthesia [9]. Lymph node involvement has been reported as a dominant sign of metastasis [10]. The radiographic features of AC are comparable to those of ameloblastoma: unilocular or multilocular radiolucent lesions with lamina dura and tooth apex resorption. However, AC may exhibit focal radiopacities, dystrophic calcification, and a poorly defined lesion border [11].

Histologic features, such as cytologic atypia and increased mitotic figures, are important criteria for distinguishing AC from ameloblastoma [12]. When assessing carcinoma in the jaw, it is first necessary to exclude the metastasis or invasion of bone by neoplasm from adjacent tissue or the paranasal sinus, as well as metastasis in the jaw from visceral tumors [13]. The first consideration in differential diagnosis of AC is primary intraosseous carcinoma. In addition to epidemiologic and clinical differences, histological features of primary intraosseous carcinoma compared to AC include less differentiation and a lack of keratinization. Squamous cell carcinoma arising in the lining of an odontogenic cyst is another potential differential diagnosis, but its histological appearance more closely resembles that of oral squamous cell carcinoma [10].

Some immunohistochemical markers correlating with the diagnosis of AC have been identified. In our report, immunohistochemistry is employed for interpreting the tumor origin and biological behaviors. CK19 expression is detected in the epithelium of the dental germ, so it has been a good marker for odontogenic cysts and tumors, such as ameloblastoma. Ki67 is a nuclear protein which is presented in cellular proliferation. The immunoexpression of Ki67 has been considered as a prognostic tool to distinguish among benign and malignant tumor. p53, known as tumor suppressor gene, plays an important role in DNA repair and apoptosis initiation. The accumulation of p53 has been associated with increased cellular proliferation and malignant transformation. In Martínez et al.'s study comparing histological and immunohistochemical features of ameloblastoma and AC,

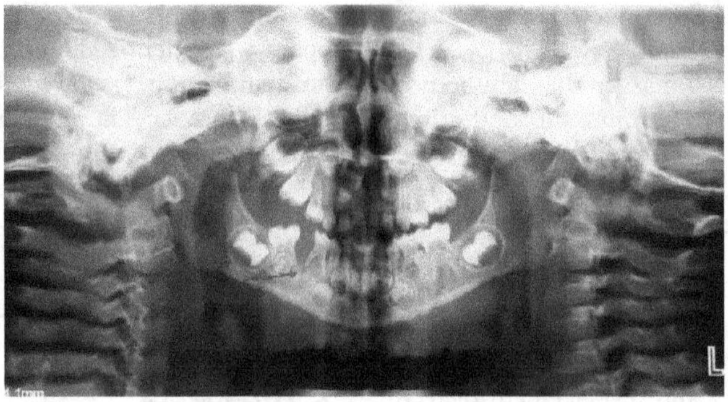

Figure 1: Orthopantomograph showing the presence of an ill-defined, mixed radiolucent-radiopaque lesion involving the #84 to #85 region. Bone and roots resorption can be observed (red arrow).

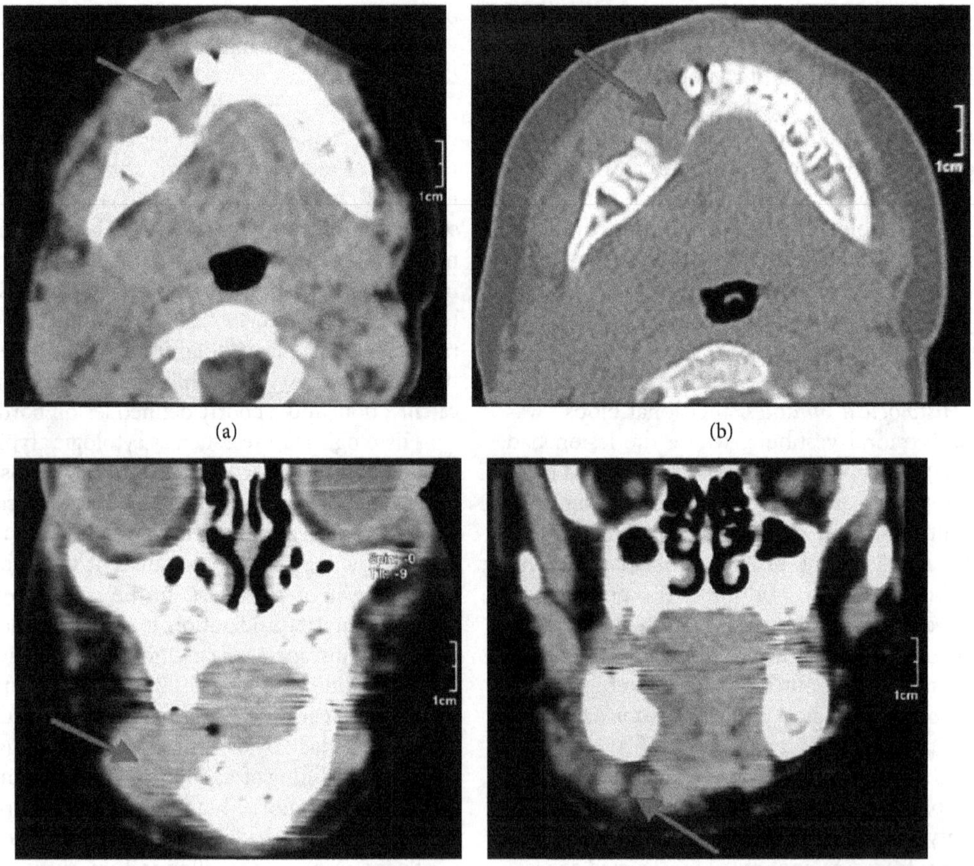

Figure 2: CT images showing a lesion with bony cortex perforation (red arrow, (a) and (b)) and soft tissue infiltration and lymph nodes involvement (red arrow, (c) and (d)).

they suggested that both Ki67 and p53 could be good markers of malignancy [14].

Little information regarding AC in pediatric patients is available. A review of the literature from 1932 to 2019 revealed 22 cases in pediatric patients, for whom age, sex, location, clinical signs, treatment, follow-up, recurrence, and metastasis status were collected [6]. However, a few details were unavailable (Table 1). Patient age ranged from 4 to 17 years, with a mean of 12.98 years; the male-to-female ratio was 3 : 1. In total, 64% of the patients had AC in the mandible. Swelling was the first symptom in 64% of the patients; other signs included pain, dysphonia, and trismus. Surgery was performed in 17 of 22 patients; three patients were treated with both surgery and radiotherapy because of the involvement of surgical margins. Chemotherapy alone was administered in one patient. Treatment details were not clear in 4 patients before 1979. The follow-up duration ranged from 0.5 to 24 years (mean of 6.4 years). In the review, we noted that recurrence occurred after an extended interval, from 1 to 16.3 years posttreatment, and was detected in 24% of the patients.

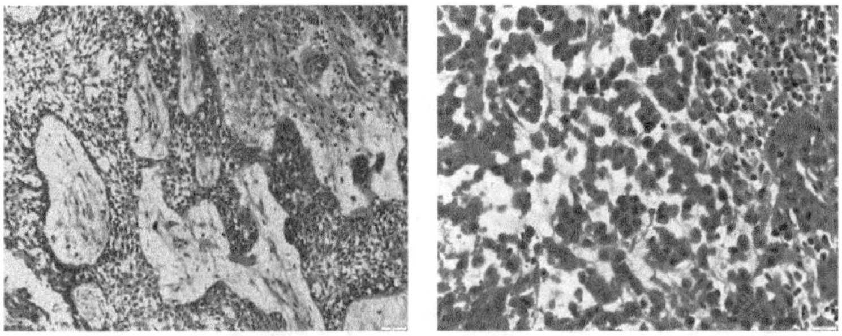

(a) (b)

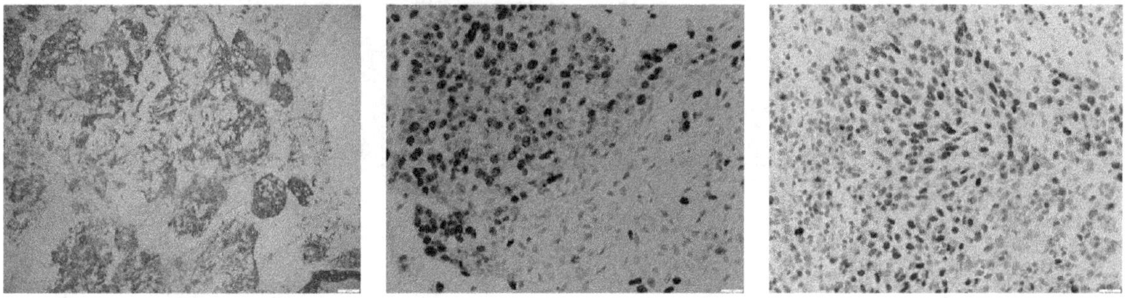

(c) (d) (e)

FIGURE 3: Photomicrographs showing sheets and nests of ameloblastic epithelium with inflammatory infiltration ((a) hematoxylin eosin); areas of tumor cells with hyperchromatism, nuclei pleomorphism, and some mitotic figures ((b) hematoxylin eosin); marked positive immunohistochemical expression of CK19 (c), Ki67 (d), and p53 (e).

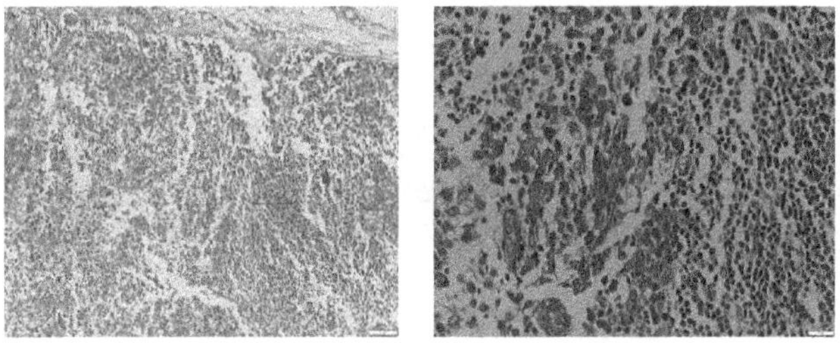

(a) (b)

FIGURE 4: Photomicrographs showing tumor infiltration in the submandibular lymph node: dedifferentiated area with infiltrated neoplastic cells ((a) hematoxylin eosin); higher power view of the infiltrated lymph node showing nuclear pleomorphism and hyperchromatism of the neoplastic cells ((b) hematoxylin eosin).

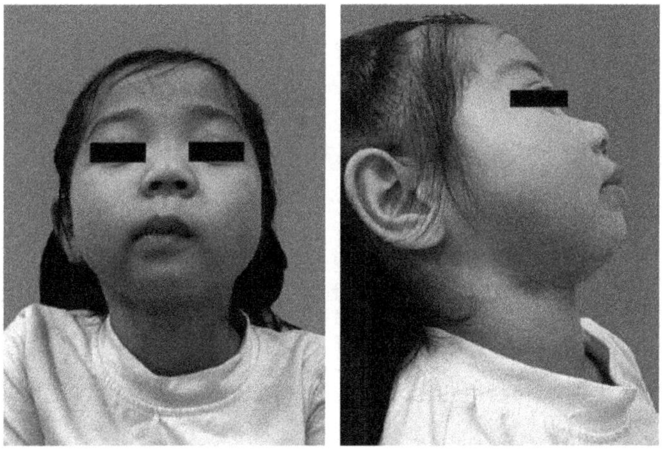

FIGURE 5: Photographs of the patient at 2-year postoperation.

Table 1: Published pediatric cases of AC (1932 to 2019).

Case	Authors	Age (y)	Gender	Site	Initial signs	Treatment	Follow-up (mo)	Metastasis/recurrence	Dead/alive
1	Spring (1932) [17]	5	Male	Mandible	Not mentioned	Not mentioned	168	Bone	Dead
2	Villa (1958) [18]	17	Male	Mandible	Swelling	Not mentioned	0		Alive
3	Herceg and Harding (1972) [19]	9	Male	Mandible	Not mentioned	Not mentioned	121	Lung+liver+lymph node	Dead
4	Höltje and Donath (1977) [7]	4	Male	Mandible	Not mentioned	Not mentioned	36		Dead
5	Krempien et al. (1979) [20]	5.5	Male	Maxilla	Swelling	Surgery	144	Lung	Alive
6	Nadimi et al. (1986) [21]	15	Female	Maxilla	Not mentioned	Surgery	0		Alive
7	Corio et al. (1987) [10]	15	Male	Maxilla	Swelling	Surgery	12		Alive
8	Corio et al. (1987) [10]	17	Male	Mandible	Pain, swelling, dysphonia	Surgery	12	Recurrence	Alive
9	Hall et al. (2007) [22]	15	Male	Maxilla	Swelling	Surgery	196	Recurrence	Alive
10	Hall et al. (2007) [22]	16	Male	Maxilla	Swelling	Surgery	288		Alive
11	Hall et al. (2007) [22]	7	Female	Maxilla	Swelling	Surgery	119	Recurrence	Alive
12	Hall et al. (2007) [22]	17	Female	Mandible	Swelling	Surgery	122	Recurrence	Dead
13	Yazici et al. (2008) [23]	10	Male	Maxilla	Swelling	Surgery+radiotherapy	6		Alive
14	Reid-Nicholson et al. (2009) [24]	15	Male	Mandible	Swelling	Surgery	Not mentioned	Lymph node	Not mentioned
15	Cherry et al. (2009) [25]	16	Male	Mandible	Swelling, pain	Surgery+radiotherapy	Not mentioned	Brain+lung	Alive
16	Ndukwe et al. (2010) [26]	16	Male	Mandible	Not mentioned	Surgery	Not mentioned		Not mentioned
17	Ndukwe et al. (2010) [26]	16	Female	Mandible	Not mentioned	Surgery	Not mentioned		Not mentioned
18	Devenney-Cakir et al. (2010) [27]	16	Male	Mandible	Swelling, trismus	Surgery+radiotherapy	48	Brain+lung	Alive
19	Horváth et al. (2012) [28]	8	Female	Mandible	Pain	Chemotherapy	8	Lung+bone	Dead
20	Yoshioka et al. (2013) [29]	17	Male	Mandible	Swelling	Surgery	39	Lung+recurrence	Dead
21	Sozzi et al. (2014) [6]	14	Male	Maxilla	Swelling	Surgery	24		Alive
22	Fahradyan et al. (2019) [30]	15	Male	Mandible	Swelling	Surgery	30		Alive

Metastasis was detected in eight patients (1 bone, 1 lymph node, 1 lung, and 5 patients with multiple metastases). Six of the 22 patients (27.3%) were reported to have died; four of these had metastasis.

The management of AC remains controversial, but surgical resection is always recommended. En bloc removal of the jaw with 2 cm of normal bone margin is indicated to assure a disease-free status. This approach results in a recurrence rate below 15% [15]. Cervical dissection should be considered when there is a sign of lymph node metastasis. Postoperative radiotherapy and chemotherapy may be useful; however, the outcomes of these therapies have not been well documented [16].

This report appears to describe the youngest patient with AC reported in the literature to date. The child had a rapidly growing and aggressive lesion, with bone destruction and suspected lymph node metastasis. The diagnosis was based on histopathologic and immunohistochemical features, including ameloblastic differentiation, nuclear pleomorphism, mitotic figures, and positive reactivities with specific immunomarkers. The treatments were segmental mandibulectomy (with safe bony margins of 2 cm) and neck dissection. No adjuvant therapy was applied. Regular check-ups were performed every 3 months, and the long-term prognosis for this patient is expected to be good.

4. Conclusion

To date, AC is still a rare, highly malignant odontogenic tumor, with a 5-year survival rate below 70%. Metastases to the lung, liver, lymph nodes, bone, and brain are the causes of death and may appear at 0.5 to 14 years postoperatively. Thus, radical treatment and meticulous long-term follow-up are essential, and sufficient time should be considered before reconstruction due to the potential for tumor recurrence.

References

[1] R. P. Elzay, "Primary intraosseous carcinoma of the jaws," *Oral Surgery, Oral Medicine, and Oral Pathology*, vol. 54, no. 3, pp. 299–303, 1982.

[2] P. J. Slootweg and H. Müller, "Malignant ameloblastoma or ameloblastic carcinoma," *Oral Surgery, Oral Medicine, and Oral Pathology*, vol. 57, no. 2, pp. 168–176, 1984.

[3] J. M. Wright and M. Soluk Tekkesin, "Odontogenic tumors: where are we in 2017?," *Journal of Istanbul University Faculty of Dentistry*, vol. 51, pp. 10–30, 2017.

[4] L. Barnes, J. W. Eveson, P. Reichart, and D. Sidransky, *World Health Organization Classification of Head and Neck Tumours*, WHO Classification of Tumours, 2005.

[5] W. H. Westra and J. S. Lewis, "Update from the 4th edition of the World Health Organization classification of head and neck tumours: oropharynx," *Head Neck Pathology*, vol. 11, no. 1, pp. 41–47, 2017.

[6] D. Sozzi, V. Morganti, G. M. Valente, F. Moltrasio, A. Bozzetti, and F. Angiero, "Ameloblastic carcinoma in a young patient," *Oral Surgery, Oral Medicine, Oral Pathology, and Oral Radiology*, vol. 117, no. 5, pp. e396–e402, 2014.

[7] W. J. Höltje and K. Donath, "Clinical aspects and histomorphology of malignant ameloblastoma," *Deutsche Zahnarztliche Zeitschrift*, vol. 32, no. 10, pp. 798–802, 1977.

[8] A. Benlyazid, M. Lacroix-Triki, R. Aziza, A. Gomez-Brouchet, M. Guichard, and J. Sarini, "Ameloblastic carcinoma of the maxilla: case report and review of the literature," *Oral Surgery, Oral Medicine, Oral Pathology, Oral Radiology and Endodontology*, vol. 104, no. 6, pp. e17–e24, 2007.

[9] R. Braimah, C. Uguru, and K. C. Ndukwe, "Ameloblastic carcinoma of the jaws: review of the literature," *Journal of Dental and Allied Science*, vol. 6, no. 2, pp. 70–73, 2017.

[10] R. L. Corio, L. I. Goldblatt, P. A. Edwards, and K. S. Hartman, "Ameloblastic carcinoma: a clinicopathologic study and assessment of eight cases," *Oral Surgery Oral Medicine Oral Pathology*, vol. 64, no. 5, pp. 570–576, 1987.

[11] S. L. Avon, J. McComb, and C. Clokie, "Ameloblastic carcinoma: case report and literature review," *Journal of the Canadian Dental Association*, vol. 69, no. 9, pp. 573–576, 2003.

[12] L. J. Slater, "Odontogenic malignancies," *Oral and Maxillofacial Surgery Clinics of North America*, vol. 16, no. 3, pp. 409–424, 2004.

[13] K. D. McClatchey, M. J. Sullivan, and D. R. Paugh, "Peripheral ameloblastic carcinoma: a case report of a rare neoplasm," *Journal of Otolaryngology*, vol. 18, no. 3, pp. 109–111, 1989.

[14] M. Martinez-Martinez, A. Mosqueda-Taylor, R. Carlos-Bregni et al., "Comparative histological and immunohistochemical study of ameloblastomas and ameloblastic carcinomas," *Medicina Oral, Patologia Oral y Cirugia Bucal*, vol. 22, no. 3, pp. 324–332, 2017.

[15] R. Datta, J. S. Winston, G. Diaz-Reyes et al., "Ameloblastic carcinoma: report of an aggressive case with multiple bony metastases," *American Journal of Otolaryngology*, vol. 24, no. 1, pp. 64–69, 2003.

[16] V. Maheshwari, M. Varshney, K. Alam et al., "Ameloblastic carcinoma: a rare entity," *BMJ Case Report*, vol. 2011, 2011.

[17] K. Spring, "Gibt es maligne adamantinome?," *Oesterreichische Zeitschrift für Stomatologie*, vol. 30, pp. 455–465, 1932.

[18] V. G. Villa, "A case of ameloblastoma evidently undergoing transformation to a new type of tumor," *Oral Surgery, Oral Medicine Oral Pathology*, vol. 11, no. 10, pp. 1148–1157, 1958.

[19] S. J. Herceg and R. L. Harding, "Malignant ameloblastoma with pulmonary metastases," *Plastic and Reconstructive Surgery*, vol. 49, no. 4, pp. 456–460, 1972.

[20] B. Krempien, W. E. Brandeis, and R. Singer, "Metastasierendes ameloblastom im kindesalter," *Virchows Archiv A Pathological Anatomy and Histology*, vol. 381, no. 2, pp. 211–222, 1979.

[21] H. Nadimi, P. D. Toto, E. Jaffe, and H. D. McReynolds, "Basement membrane defect in ameloblastic carcinoma: a case study," *Journal of Oral Medicine*, vol. 41, no. 2, pp. 79–81, 1986.

[22] J. M. Hall, D. R. Weathers, and K. K. Unni, "Ameloblastic carcinoma: an analysis of 14 cases," *Oral Surgery, Oral Medicine, Oral Pathology, Oral Radiology and Endodontics*, vol. 103, no. 6, pp. 799–807, 2007.

[23] N. Yazıcı, B. Karagöz, A. Varan et al., "Maxillary ameloblastic carcinoma in a child," *Pediatric Blood and Cancer*, vol. 50, no. 1, pp. 175-176, 2008.

[24] M. Reid-Nicholson, D. Teague, B. White, P. Ramalingam, and R. Abdelsayed, "Fine needle aspiration findings in malignant

ameloblastoma: a case report and differential diagnosis," *Diagnostic Cytopathology*, vol. 37, no. 8, pp. 586–591, 2009.

[25] B. Cherry, P. Mehra, V. Noonan, and D. Baur, "Radiolucent lesion of the posterior mandible," *Journal of Oral and Maxillofacial Surgery*, vol. 67, no. 4, pp. 862–866, 2009.

[26] K. C. Ndukwe, E. K. Adebiyi, V. I. Ugboko et al., "Ameloblastic carcinoma: a multicenter Nigerian study," *Journal of Oral and Maxillofacial Surgery*, vol. 68, no. 9, pp. 2111–2114, 2010.

[27] B. Devenney-Cakir, B. Dunfee, R. Subramaniam et al., "Ameloblastic carcinoma of the mandible with metastasis to the skull and lung: advanced imaging appearance including computed tomography, magnetic resonance imaging and positron emission tomography computed tomography," *Dentomaxillofacial Radiology*, vol. 39, no. 7, pp. 449–453, 2010.

[28] A. Horváth, E. Horváth, and S. Popşor, "Mandibular ameloblastic carcinoma in a young patient," *Romanian Journal of Morphology and Embryology*, vol. 53, no. 1, pp. 179–183, 2012.

[29] Y. Yoshioka, S. Toratani, I. Ogawa, and T. Okamoto, "Ameloblastic carcinoma, secondary type, of the mandible: a case report," *Journal of Oral and Maxillofacial Surgery*, vol. 71, no. 1, pp. 58–62, 2013.

[30] A. Fahradyan, L. Odono, J. A. Hammoudeh, and L. K. Howell, "Ameloblastic carcinoma in situ: review of literature and a case presentation in a pediatric patient," *The Cleft Palate-Craniofacial Journal*, vol. 56, no. 1, pp. 94–100, 2018.

15

Multidisciplinary Case Management in Mesiodens Impacted Cases with Calcifying Odontogenic Cyst

Tania Saskianti, Udijanto Tedjosaongko, Regina Ayu Pramudita, Nita Naomi, and Alit Rahma Restu

Department of Pediatric Dentistry, Faculty of Dentistry, Airlangga University, Surabaya 60132, Indonesia

Correspondence should be addressed to Tania Saskianti; tania-s@fkg.unair.ac.id

Academic Editor: Darko Macan

Calcifying odontogenic cyst (COC) is a cyst originating from odontogenic epithelium and has a characteristic ghost cell appearance. Clinically, COC is characterized by asymptomatic swelling, leading to lingual expansion, tooth migration, apical resorption, and perforation of cortical bone. COC is most often asymptomatic and is often only discovered during a routine radiological examination. This case report describes the clinical interventions to manage a patient with mesiodens impacted with COC. The procedure is aimed at evaluating the multidisciplinary management of COC at Universitas Airlangga Hospital, Surabaya. Multidisciplinary care has an important role in treating COC cases comprehensively.

1. Introduction

The calcifying odontogenic cyst is an uncommon benign cyst of odontogenic origin, characterized by an ameloblastoma-like epithelium with ghost cells that may calcify, first described by Gorlin et al. in 1962 [1].

Clinically, it is characterized by slowly growing asymptomatic swelling. It may have a central (intraosseous), or less frequently, a peripheral (extraosseous) localization. It may cause lingual expansion, displacement of teeth, root resorption, and perforation in the cortical bone [2].

On radiographs, COC appears as a well-limited unilocular radiolucent lesion of different sizes, shapes, and opacity levels. Impacted teeth may be associated. Root resorption, root divergence, or cortical blowing may be observed [3].

A definitive diagnosis of calcifying odontogenic cyst can be reliably made based on a histological examination. An abnormal form of keratinization in the form of the ghost cells is the most distinguishing feature of a COC. However, their presence does not confirm the diagnosis as other lesions show similar presentation. Hence, a diagnosis of COC should only be made for a lesion in which the formation of ghost cells takes place in a typical epithelial cyst lining, presenting a basal layer of cuboidal or short cylindrical cells and an overlying layer consisting of cells that bear resemblance to stellate reticulum-like cells [4].

The recommended treatment for COC consists of enucleation with curettage, which means enucleation followed by removal of a 1 to 2 mm layer of bone around the periphery of the cystic cavity with a sharp curette or a bone bur. This procedure is aimed at limiting the risk of recurrence. Decompression and marsupialization are conservative treatments used in large lesions with a high success rate [5].

In this case, the cyst has involved the apical part of the surrounding teeth, so multidisciplinary treatment is needed for comprehensive treatment to remove the cyst and preserve the tooth. The purpose of this report is to present an interesting and rare case of COC associated with impacted mesiodens and to highlight the importance of multidisciplinary management of COC.

2. Case Report

A 14-year-old boy came to the Pediatric Dental Clinic of Rumah Sakit Gigi dan Mulut Universitas Airlangga with a

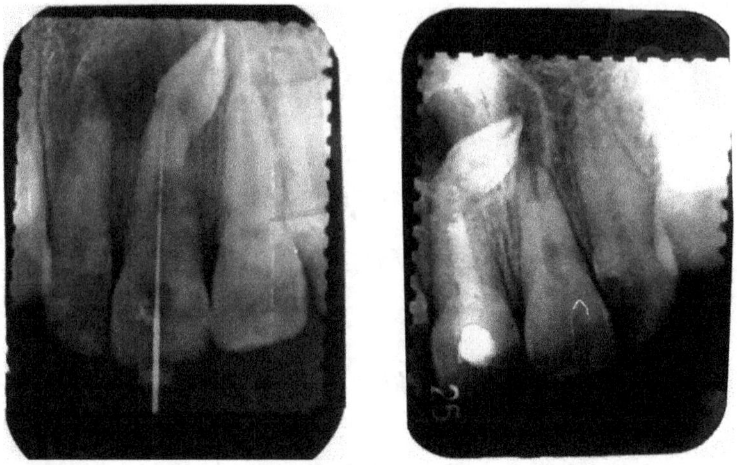

(a) (b)

Figure 1: Periapical radiograph: (a) #11 with open apex; (b) one year later found apexification material on root canal and closed apex. The impacted mesiodens shown surrounded with cyst between apical of #21 and #11.

history of fractured teeth due to an accident 5 years ago. The patient is currently on apexification treatment.

Periapical radiographic examination showed #11 with an open apex (Figure 1(a)), and the patient was scheduled for obturation. During treatment, the patient felt recurrent pain on #11. On clinical examination, #11 was found with an intact temporary restoration, negative percussion, and palpation test. Based on clinical examination, the provisional diagnosis is pulp necrosis with class III Ellis crown fracture classification (Figure 2). Radiograph examination revealed #11 with a closed apex and well-defined margin radiolucency area around mesiodens between apicals of #21 and #11 (Figure 1(b)).

Interpretation of CBCT radiographic examination showed inverted mesiodens impaction on the palate of #11 and #21; the lesion was demarcated, radiopaque, oval in shape, and causing a discontinuity in the base of the nasal cavity (Figure 3).

Based on periapical, panoramic, and CBCT, radiographs displayed unilocular, radiolucent, and well-delineated defect related to impacted mesiodens, suggesting a dentigerous cyst (Figure 4). The differential diagnoses are radicular cyst and nasopalatine duct cyst.

3. Case Management

Treatment was planned with a multidisciplinary approach with the oral and maxillofacial surgeon under general anesthesia for odontectomy of mesiodens impacted teeth and enucleation of the cyst, followed by apical resection of teeth involved teeth and closed with MTA plug.

Laboratory assessment and thorax radiographic examination were done before the procedure and found no negative symptoms. RT-PCR testing for SARS-CoV-2 detection from nasopharyngeal and oropharyngeal swabs to screen for both symptomatic and asymptomatic COVID-19 was done, and the result was negative. This test was mandatory for the preoperative procedure in the hospital. After confirming that the patient is completely anesthetized, an extraoral asepsis procedure was performed using 70% alcohol and 10% povidone-iodine intraorally. A vasoconstrictor consisting of 2 ampoules of pehacain diluted with 6 ml of saline, injected with a local infiltration technique using a 21 gauge syringe, was administered, and a full-thickness trapezium flap was elevated on a periapical area of #12, #11, #21, and #22 regions. A round carbide bur under constant irrigation for cooling was used to enlarge the bony defect to the buccal window to gain access to the periapical lesion and root end of the affected tooth (Figure 5(a)). Needle aspiration test showed mixed blood and cyst fluid; curettes were then used to remove the soft granulation tissue (Figure 5(b)), which further aided inadequate visualization of mesiodens to ensure complete extraction and no remaining dental follicle. Apex resection was initially planned for #11. However, the wall of the cyst was found extended to the adjacent teeth; hence, the apex resection was also performed on #21. The apical end of 2 mm was resected in faciolingual direction to the long axis of the tooth with a tapered fissured bur in a low-speed handpiece under constant irrigation (Figure 5(d)). The resected root surface was inspected, prepared, and then filled with mineral trioxide aggregate and glass ionomer cement on the periapical area (Figure 5(e)). Spongostan was then applied to the defect area, then sutured with silk Vicryl 4.0 (Figure 5(g)).

Surgical procedures also included germinectomy of 18, 28, 38, and 48 tooth buds.

Histopathological anatomy results obtained after cyst enucleation and mesiodens collection (Figure 6) confirmed the diagnosis in the form of COC.

The patient was recalled after one day to access the surgical site recovery and found no sign of pain, dizziness, nausea, and vomiting. On extraoral examination, there were no signs of edema, hyperemia, and tenderness. On intraoral examination, the postoperative wounds on #12, #11, #21, #22, #18, #28, #38, and #48 were well sewn and hyperaemic, and minimal debris was seen at the edges of the sutures (Figure 7).

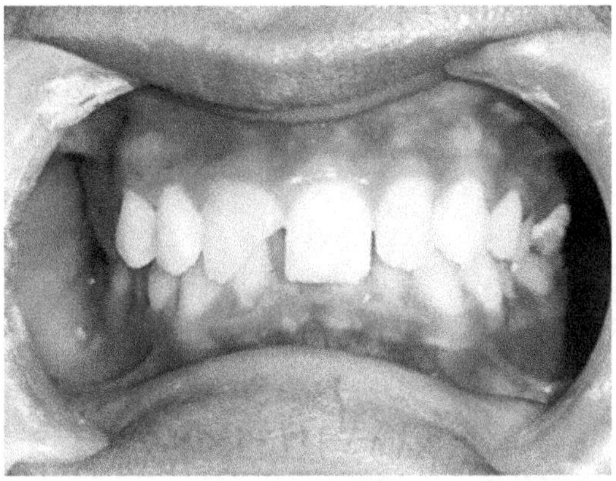

FIGURE 2: Clinical features. Intraoral photography highlighting #11 with class III Ellis crown fracture classification.

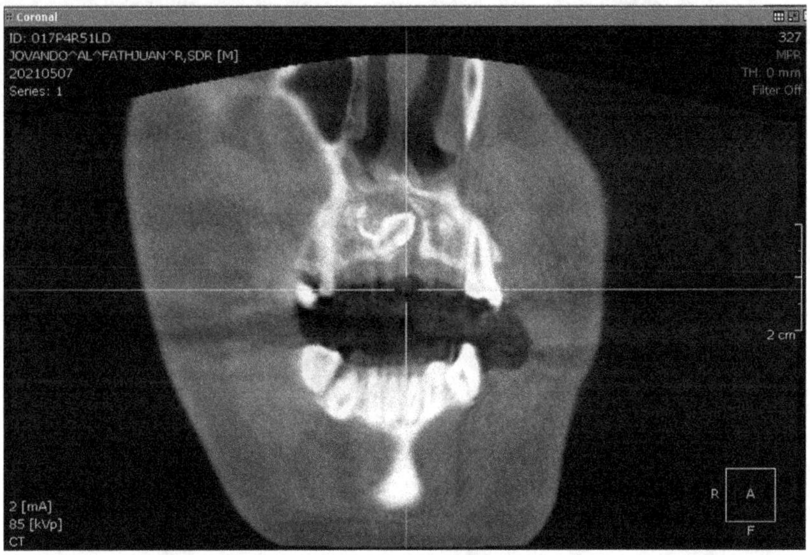

FIGURE 3: CBCT radiographic view. The mesiodens impacted tooth was seen between teeth 11 and 21 in an inverted position. Mesiodens tooth distance with the base of the nasal cavity: 3.93 mm. A mixed radiolucent-radiopaque image is seen around the crown of the mesiodens with a clear border with radiopaque edges and an oval shape. The lesion appears to cause a discontinuity of the palatal cortical bone, and the lesion is in contact with the floor of the nasal cavity.

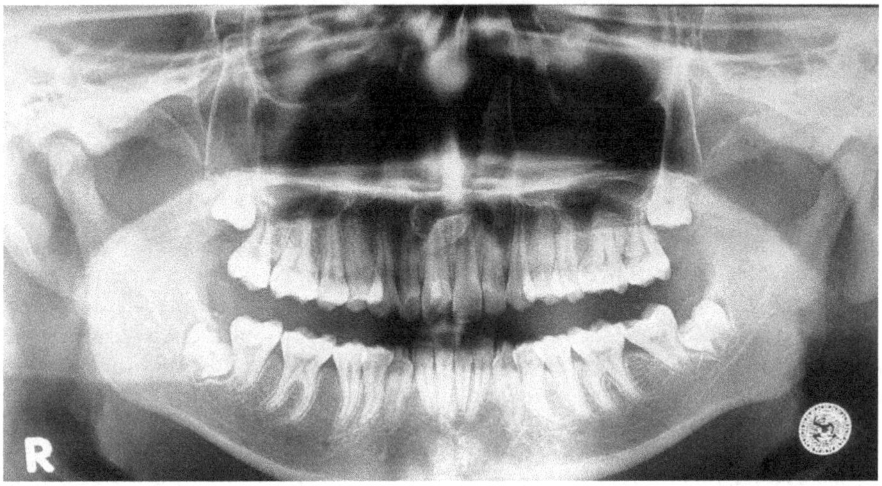

FIGURE 4: Panoramic radiographic view. Panoramic radiograph revealing a well-defined unilocular radiolucency around impacted mesiodens.

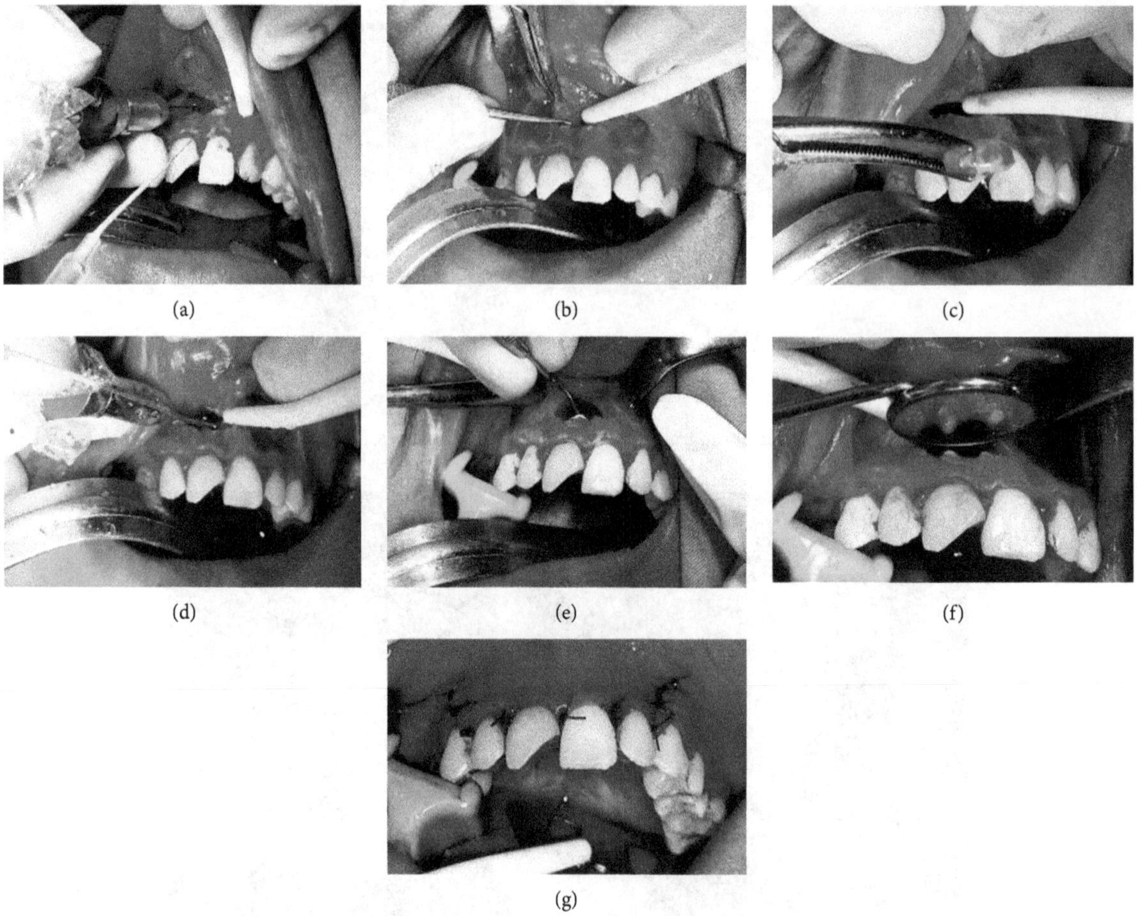

Figure 5: Surgical procedure: (a) buccal window; (b) curettes of granulation tissue; (c) extraction of mesiodens; (d) apex resection; (e) MTA and GIC application; (f) evaluation; (g) suturing.

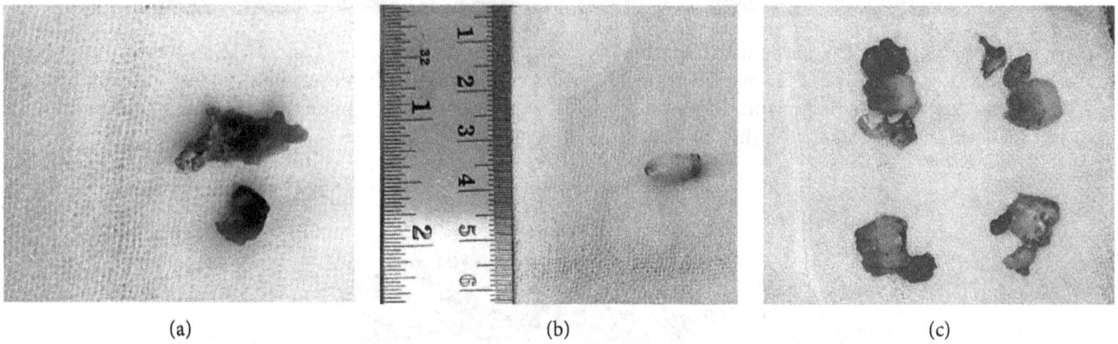

Figure 6: Specimen postoperative: (a) the cystic specimen after enucleation; (b) mesiodens; (c) tooth bud post germinectomy.

On palpation examination, the postoperative wound was palpated in the regions of #12, #11, #21, #22, #18, #28, #38, and #48, and there was minimal edema and tenderness at the edges of the sutures. On day 7 postoperative, the suture was removed. In #11, root canal access was completed without anesthesia and #21 with anesthesia. #11 and #21 were prepared up to sizes 40 and 50, respectively, 3 mm short of the apical foramen. In all teeth, the root canals were irrigated with 3 mL of 2.5% sodium hypochlorite (NaOCl), and distilled water at each change of file was used as an intracanal dressing. The quality of canal filling with the medication was confirmed radiographically. The teeth were temporarily restored with an intermediate restorative material.

After two times of sterilization, the intracanal dressing was removed, and the root canals of #11 and #21 were filled with gutta-percha and followed by composite resin restoration. Follow-up is scheduled at 3 months, 6 months, and 1 year to assess clinical and radiographic signs of healing.

The patient came after 3 and 6 months postoperative; there were no signs of swelling, redness, or tooth mobility of #11 and #21 and underwent an X-ray panoramic control which described a radiopaque area with several radiolucent

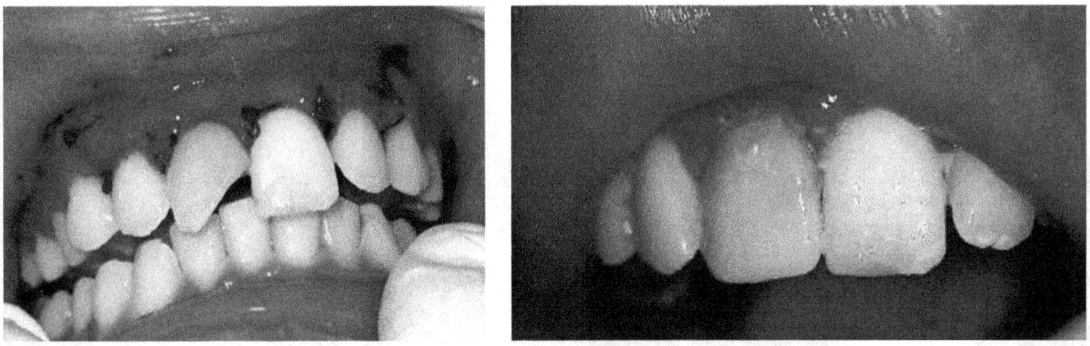

(a) (b)

Figure 7: Postoperative intraoral view: (a) one day postoperative; (b) composite restoration on #21 and #11.

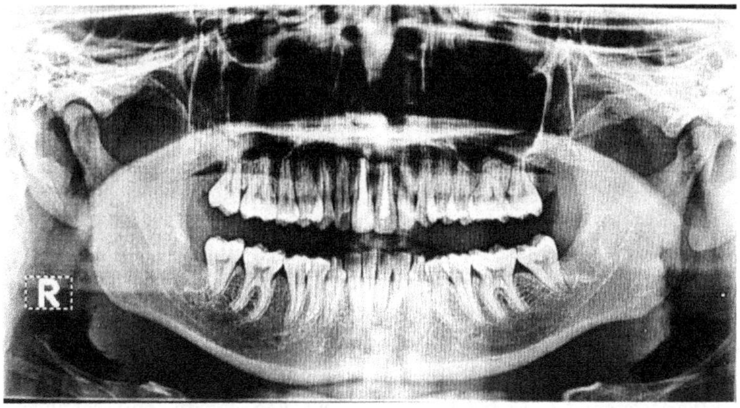

Figure 8: Radiographic examination 3 months postoperative.

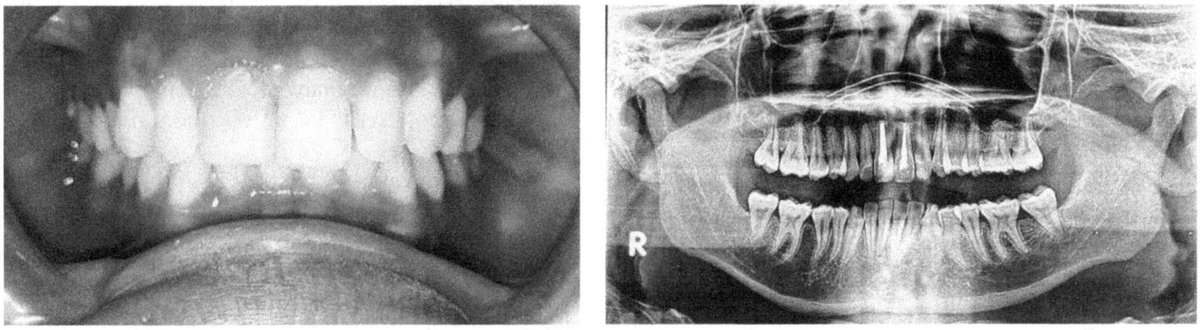

(a) (b)

Figure 9: 6 months postoperative recall: (a) intraoral view; (b) radiographic examination.

areas apical to #11; #12 with an impression of the bone ossification process showed a beginning bone regeneration. There are no signs of recurrence (Figures 8 and 9).

4. Discussion

The calcifying odontogenic cyst is an uncommon benign cyst of odontogenic origin [6]. Retrospective studies, case reports, or case series with a significant number of COC cases have been published [7–13].

The last 20 years from the following databases: PubMed, Medline Ovid, Web of Science, Scopus. The present systematic review revealed that COC patients' age ranged from two to 92 years, and the mean age at diagnosis was 30.7 (±21.0) years. Males made up 184 (51.8%) of the COC cases, while females made up 171 (48.2%) of the cases (male to female ratio: 1.0 : 1). Regarding anatomical location, a predilection for the maxilla (53.3%) was observed. The mandible was affected in 45.7% of cases, and information about the affected site was not available in only one case. COC was asymptomatic in 89.2% of patients. Symptom duration ranged from one to 180 months, with a mean of 18.1 (±29.8) months. Most cases exhibited a well-defined border (87.0%), with mixed (61.1%) and unilocular appearance

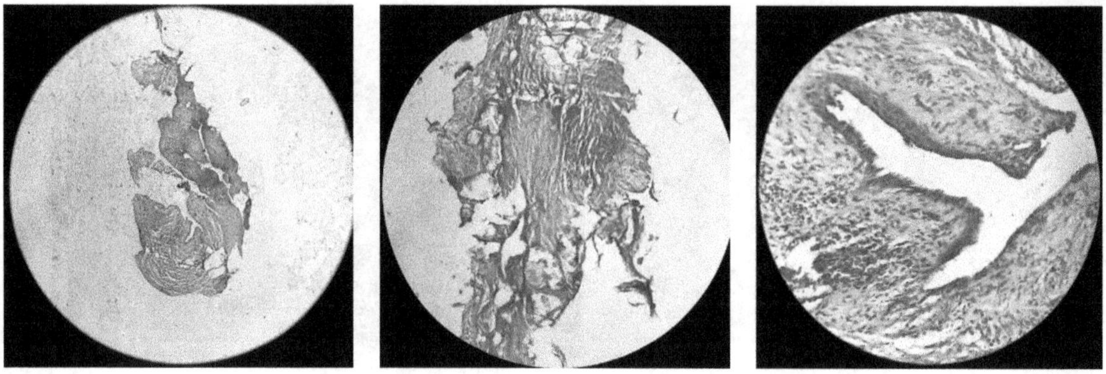

(a) (b) (c)

FIGURE 10: Histopathological examination: (a) showing cyst wall; (b) presence of ghost cells and calcification masses within the epithelium; (c) cuboidal and squamous epithelial cells.

(81.9%). The bone expansion was observed in 81.9% of cases. Lesion size ranged from 2.0 to 90.0 mm, with a mean of 29.5 (±20.8) mm. Regarding treatment, enucleation was the most common (69.9% of cases). In 194 cases (96.0%), no recurrence was reported. As regards the follow-up period, the mean duration of surveillance ranged from three to 264 months, with a mean of 42.2 (±43.6) months. Concerning treatment, enucleation was the modality of choice in most cases (85 cases, 77.1%) [14].

As regards treatment, conservative surgery was the main choice for COC. Herein, the two strategies most frequently reported for COC treatment were enucleation in 69.9% of cases and surgical removal or excisional biopsy in 18.5%. Furthermore, a two-stage approach was followed in 4.0% of cases. Uncommonly reported in COC therapy, this option is mainly chosen for other odontogenic cysts such as dentigerous or odontogenic keratocyst. Decompression or marsupialization is first performed to reduce intraluminal pressure and shrinkage of the cyst following a period of months. This allows bone growth and removal of the cyst in a second stage, with less risk of damage to important anatomical structures [15, 16].

The present review identified two COCs treated only by marsupialization. The recurrence rate after conservative COC management was low for both intraosseous and extraosseous lesions [14].

Considering the complexity of the case, we decided to manage the mesiodens impacted case with COC multidisciplinary [5]. Radiographically, COCs are well-circumscribed and present as a unilocular radiolucency with calcifications of varying density reported in one-third of cases [17].

In this case, radiographic examination revealed a solitary well-defined unilocular radiolucency around the impacted mesiodens. Based on the clinic-radiological findings, differential diagnosis of benign odontogenic lesions like a dentigerous cyst, radicular cyst, and nasopalatine duct cyst was considered. In the current case, with the presence of pericoronal radiolucency associated with unerupted mesiodens, the working diagnosis of the dentigerous cyst was made.

A definite diagnosis of calcifying odontogenic cyst can be reliably made based on a histological examination due to the lesion's lack of characteristic clinical and radiological features, as well as its variable biological behavior [19].

Histological features of the lesion show a fibrous capsule with a lining of odontogenic epithelium. The basal layer is made up of ameloblast-like columnar or cuboidal cells of 4–10 cell thickness. It is covered by loosely arranged epithelial cells bearing similarities to the stellate reticulum of the enamel organ. There are varying numbers of epithelial cells that are devoid of nuclei and eosinophilic and retain their basic cell outline (ghost cells). These ghost cells can calcify, and calcifications are constant but vary in number [6].

The results of the histopathological examination on this case show sections of cyst wall tissue lined with thin squamous cuboidal epithelium, consisting of round, mononucleated, and smooth chromatin cells. The stroma is a fibrous connective tissue with many foci of eosinophilic calcification resembling ghost cells. There were no signs of malignancy (Figure 10).

The patient came with a history of trauma and swelling. Traumatic dental injuries to the teeth and the maxillofacial structures are a common occurrence, with the majority affecting the dentoalveolar structures. The most common types of traumatic dental injuries are crown fractures in the permanent dentition. An accurate diagnosis is essential to facilitate prompt management, which is widely regarded to have a major influence on the prognosis of the outcome.

Radiographic examination is essential for the diagnosis of traumatic dental injuries. In addition to a thorough clinical examination, intraoral radiographs such as periapical radiographs and upper standard occlusal radiographs are routinely prescribed to identify the location and nature of traumatic dental injuries. The diagnostic radiographs also form part of the baseline records to allow objective assessment at the follow-up appointment [20].

The clinical parameters observed were the presence of symptoms in the traumatized tooth, coronary discoloration, degree of tooth mobility, and the health of surrounding soft tissues, through visual examination and palpation. The radiographic parameters were the presence or absence of periapical lesion, pulp canal obliteration, and pathological

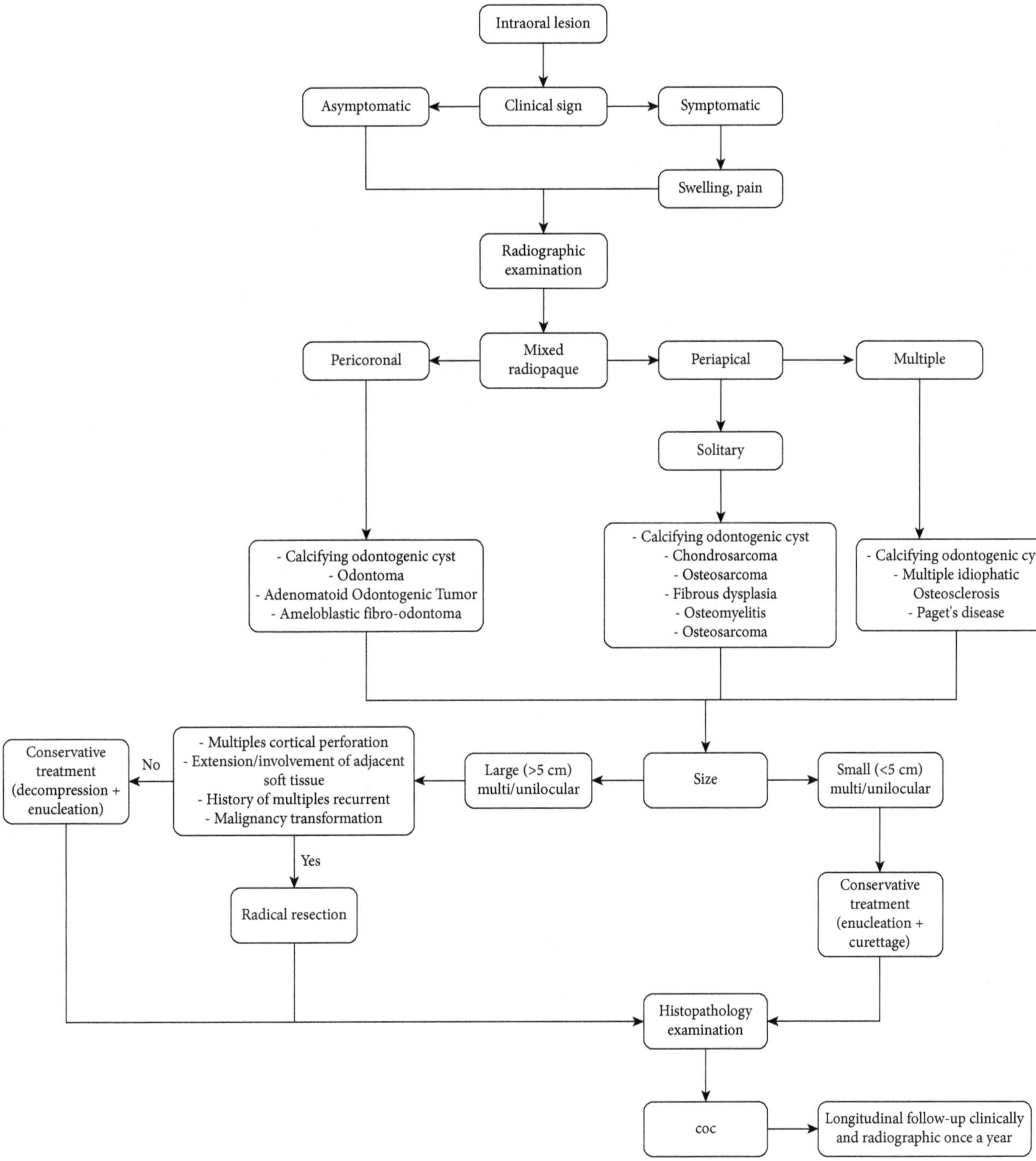

Figure 11: Algorithm to diagnose and manage cystic lesions [18].

root resorption, which was differentiated from physiological resorption by clinical history, patient age, and morphological characteristics of resorption. With both clinical and radiographic parameters, an analysis of both was performed to establish the condition of vitality or pulp necrosis [21].

Moreover, it has also been suggested that trauma diagnostics during childhood is more difficult than in grown-up persons. These authors reported that the sutures of the skull are wider and that more adipose tissue covers the bones, which will complicate the diagnostics accuracy. Fortunately, intraoral radiographs give a very low radiation dose if the correct technique and good X-ray equipment are used making it ethically indicated to prescribe intraoral radiographs for adults and children whenever the clinical examination indicates that a more severe dental injury might exist [22].

Recently, a new tomographic imaging method has started to be used, cone-beam CT (CBCT). CBCT has high diagnostic accuracy in cases of traumatic dental and maxillofacial injuries. But intraoral radiographs are a good start and are accurate enough if we only suspect dental injuries or minimally displaced bone fractures according to other researchers. In general, in dental trauma, CBCT should only be prescribed in selected cases, where conventional radiographs provide inadequate information for treatment planning [22].

In this case, after the periapical radiographic examination revealed mesiodens impaction on the apical of the maxillary anterior teeth, we referred the patient for a CBCT radiographic examination to help determine the diagnosis and location of the impacted tooth and appropriate treatment plan.

According to the periapical radiography, apical #11 was exposed with an open apical; then, apexification was performed by the pediatric dentist. Apexification is a method of treatment for immature permanent teeth in which root growth and development ceased due to pulp necrosis. Its purpose is to induce root-end closure with no canal wall thickening or continuous root lengthening. It can be achieved in two ways: (1) as a long-term procedure using calcium hydroxide dressing to allow the formation of a biologic hard tissue barrier or (2) as a short-term (more recent) procedure, creating an artificial apical plug of MTA or other bioceramic material [23].

The mechanism of action of calcium hydroxide in the induction of an apical barrier is still controversial, although it is formed by cells originating from the adjacent connective tissue. The calcified barrier, even when appearing radiographically and clinically complete, is histologically porous and may be composed of cementum, dentin, bone, or osteodentin. This procedure requires multiple visits and could take a year or more to achieve a complete apical barrier that would allow root canal filling using gutta-percha (GP) and sealer [24].

Cyst size is an important factor when formulating a treatment plan. The cystic lesions having a size < 5 cm can be managed with simple enucleation/curettage and submitted for pathologic examination (excisional biopsy) while preserving the strategic tooth or teeth involved. In the few cases that had clinical or radiographic evidence of multilocular lesions, extensive lesions with involvement of adjacent soft tissues or a history of multiple recurrent lesions should be considered to have aggressive behavior, and radical resection could be the first choice of treatment option depending on the surgeon's training, available resources, and the patient's preferences. Otherwise, conservative treatment methods such as decompression with a second surgical procedure (enucleation) and another aggressive approach than bone resection can be chosen, and the failures of this treatment must indicate the radical resection method as well as for extensive lesions without aggressive behaviors. Longitudinal follow-up should be considered [18, 25] (Figure 11).

The recommended treatment for COC, in general, is total excision in one step. Enucleation associated with curettage is the usual therapy when referring to the cystic variant. Hence, after removing the lesion, a layer of 1 to 2 mm of bone must be removed at the periphery of the cystic cavity [26].

The patient underwent cyst enucleation, mesiodens impacted tooth odontectomy, periapical exploration of #11 and #12, followed by apical resection of the teeth. Apical #11 and #21 were closed with MTA and GIC and planned orthograde root canal filling for tooth 11 and pulpectomy for #21 after surgery.

In this case, MTA was chosen because preclinical studies clearly showed that MTA has a high sealing capability, good material stability, and excellent biocompatibility. Multiple experimental studies in animals highlighted the mild tissue reactions observed adjacent to this material. Furthermore, histological analysis of the periapical regions demonstrated a frequent deposition of new cementum not only onto the resection plane (cut dentinal surface) but also directly onto MTA. For these reasons, MTA is considered a bioactive material.

In addition, germinectomy for tooth buds #18, #28, #38, and #48 was also performed under general anesthesia. General anesthesia was chosen because based on the CBCT interpretation, the lesion was in contact with the floor of the nasal cavity, and the patient also required the extraction of the four wisdom teeth.

Obturation of #11 was performed one week after surgery and was followed by root canal treatment on #21. In the three- and six-month follow-ups, there were no complaints subjectively. Objectively, there were no signs of swelling, redness, or tooth mobility in #11 and #21. Panoramic and periapical X-rays showed the hermetic filling of #11 and #21, radiopaque area with several radiolucent areas apical to #11, and #12 with an impression of the bone ossification process. There are no signs of recurrence.

The patient was scheduled for periodic follow-up appointments once a year to see if there are any complaints and if signs of healing have formed.

This study is expected to provide insight into how to determine the diagnosis of a lesion through clinical approaches and radiographic and pathological examinations, especially when the lesion involves surrounding structures such as adjacent tooth roots. Cross-sectoral collaboration is needed to be able to handle complex cases to achieve complete care for the patient.

5. Conclusion

Our case represents the classical features of the calcifying odontogenic cyst. The comprehensive and multidisciplinary approach is the best way to manage complex cases of mesiodens impaction with COC to relieve symptoms and assure total healing. A proper diagnostic setup is the starting point to develop an efficient treatment plan.

References

[1] A. Vatsyayan, A. K. Adhyapok, S. C. Debnath, and K. Malik, "Calcifying odontogenic cyst: case report and review of literature," *International Journal Dental Medical Research*, vol. 1, no. 4, pp. 69–75, 2014.

[2] T. Uzun and E. Çinpolat, "Calcifying odontogenic cyst associated with the impacted third molar: a case report," *The Pan African Medical Journal*, vol. 33, p. 151, 2019.

[3] A. K. Nagarajappa, A. Dhimole, S. Asrani, A. Agarwal, and A. Kakkad, "Calcifying cystic odontogenic tumor: a diagnostic challenge," *Journal of Advances in Medicine and Medical Research*, vol. 21, no. 3, pp. 1–5, 2017.

[4] R. Rojo, J. C. Prados-Frutos, I. Gutierrez Lázaro, and J. A. Herguedas Alonso, "Calcifying odontogenic cysts," *Journal of Stomatology, Oral and Maxillofacial Surgery*, vol. 118, no. 2, pp. 122–124, 2017.

[5] M. C. Samir, G. Lamiae, and C. Bassima, "Calcifying odontogenic cyst of anterior maxillary: Case report and review," *International Journal of Surgery Case Reports*, vol. 85, p. 106267, 2021.

[6] J. A. Arruda, L. V. Silva, L. Silva et al., "Calcifying odontogenic cyst: a 26-year retrospective clinicopathological analysis and immunohistochemical study," *Journal of Clinical and Experimental Dentistry*, vol. 10, no. 6, pp. e542–e547, 2018.

[7] C. Ledesma-Montes, R. J. Gorlin, M. Shear et al., "International collaborative study on ghost cell odontogenic tumours: calcifying cystic odontogenic tumour, dentinogenic ghost cell tumour and ghost cell odontogenic carcinoma," *Journal of Oral Pathology & Medicine*, vol. 37, no. 5, pp. 302–308, 2008.

[8] S. K. Lee and Y. S. Kim, "Current concepts and occurrence of epithelial odontogenic tumors: II. Calcifying epithelial odontogenic tumor versus ghost cell odontogenic tumors derived from calcifying odontogenic cyst," *Korean Journal of Pathology*, vol. 48, no. 3, pp. 175–187, 2014.

[9] T. J. Li and S. F. Yu, "Clinicopathologic spectrum of the so-called calcifying odontogenic cysts: a study of 21 intraosseous cases with reconsideration of the terminology and classification," *The American Journal of Surgical Pathology*, vol. 27, no. 3, pp. 372–384, 2003.

[10] B. R. Chrcanovic and R. S. Gomez, "Peripheral calcifying cystic odontogenic tumour and peripheral dentinogenic ghost cell tumour: an updated systematic review of 117 cases reported in the literature," *Acta Odontologica Scandinavica*, vol. 74, no. 8, pp. 591–597, 2016.

[11] G. Del Corso, M. L. Tardio, D. B. Gissi, C. Marchetti, L. Montebugnoli, and A. Tarsitano, "Ki-67 and p53 expression in ghost cell odontogenic carcinoma: a case report and literature review," *Oral and Maxillofacial Surgery*, vol. 19, no. 1, pp. 85–89, 2015.

[12] S. Irani and F. Foroughi, "Histologic variants of calcifying odontogenic cyst: a study of 52 cases," *The Journal of Contemporary Dental Practice*, vol. 18, no. 8, pp. 688–694, 2017.

[13] E. R. Fregnani, F. R. Pires, R. D. Quezada, I. Shih, P. A. Vargas, and O. P. de Almeida, "Calcifying odontogenic cyst: clinicopathological features and immunohistochemical profile of 10 cases," *Journal of Oral Pathology & Medicine*, vol. 32, no. 3, pp. 163–170, 2003.

[14] J. de Arruda, J. Monteiro, L. G. Abreu et al., "Calcifying odontogenic cyst, dentinogenic ghost cell tumor, and ghost cell odontogenic carcinoma: a systematic review," *Journal of Oral Pathology & Medicine*, vol. 47, no. 8, pp. 721–730, 2018.

[15] M. A. Pogrel, "Treatment of keratocysts: the case for decompression and marsupialization," *Journal of Oral and Maxillofacial Surgery*, vol. 63, no. 11, pp. 1667–1673, 2005.

[16] H. A. Emam, J. Smith, A. Briody, and C. A. Jatana, "Tube decompression for staged treatment of a calcifying odontogenic cyst–a case report," *Journal of Oral and Maxillofacial Surgery*, vol. 75, no. 9, pp. 1915-1920, 2017.

[17] S. Gamoh, H. Akiyama, C. Furukawa et al., "Calcifying cystic odontogenic tumor accompanied by a dentigerous cyst: a case report," *Oncology Letters*, vol. 14, no. 5, pp. 5785–5790, 2017.

[18] B. F. Nyimi, Z. Yifang, and B. Liu, "The changing landscape in treatment of cystic lesions of the jaws," *Journal of International Society of Preventive & Community Dentistry*, vol. 9, no. 4, pp. 328–337, 2019.

[19] E. Deliverska, "Calcifying odontogenic cyst – a case report and literature review," *Practice*, vol. 3, no. 2, pp. 422–431, 2016.

[20] S. Patel, T. Puri, F. Mannocci, and A. Navai, "Diagnosis and management of traumatic dental injuries using intraoral radiography and cone-beam computed tomography: an in vivo investigation," *Journal of Endodontics*, vol. 47, no. 6, pp. 914–923, 2021.

[21] D. M. C. Pugliesi, L. D. C. Araujo, V. E. S. Junior, and R. F. Cunha, "Clinical and radiographic analysis of traumatized primary teeth and permanent successors: longitudinal study," *Journal of the Indian Society of Pedodontics and Preventive Dentistry*, vol. 38, no. 3, pp. 232–237, 2020.

[22] L. Kullman and M. Al Sane, "Guidelines for dental radiography immediately after a dento-alveolar trauma, a systematic literature review," *Dental Traumatology*, vol. 28, no. 3, pp. 193–199, 2012.

[23] T. von Arx, "Mineral trioxide aggregate (MTA) meine erfolgsgeschichte in der apikalen chirurgie mineral trioxide aggregate (MTA) a success story in apical surgery," *Swiss Dental Journal*, vol. 126, no. 6, pp. 573–595, 2016.

[24] B. A. Fuks and E. Nuni, *Pulp Therapy for the Young Permanent Dentition*, Springer, Switzerland, 2016.

[25] B. E. Krishnamurthy, S. M. Panneerselvam, V. V. Kumar, and A. Rai, *Oral and Maxillofacial Surgery for the Clinician*, Springer, Singapore, 2021.

[26] N. B. de Siqueira, J. R. T. Costa Filho, J. V. S. Rodrigues, E. Hochuli-Vieira, R. Okamoto, and B. C. do Egito Vasconcelos, "Unusual treatment for calcifying odontogenic cyst using decompression tube to prevent pathological fracture," *Research, Society and Development*, vol. 10, no. 1, p. e40410111819, 2021.

16

Papillon-Lefèvre Syndrome: Diagnosis, Dental Management and a Case Report

Jean-Claude Abou Chedid,[1] Michel Salameh,[1] Abbass El-Outa,[2] and Ziad E. F. Noujeim[3]

[1]Department of Pediatric Dentistry, Faculty of Dental Medicine, Saint-Joseph University, Beirut, Lebanon
[2]Private Practice of Oral Medicine and Restorative Dentistry, Beirut, Lebanon
[3]Department of Oral Medicine and Maxillofacial Radiology and Imaging, Faculty of Dental Medicine, Lebanese University, Beirut, Lebanon

Correspondence should be addressed to Ziad E. F. Noujeim; ziadnari@hotmail.com

Academic Editor: Sukumaran Anil

Aim. This paper revisits Papillon-Lefèvre syndrome (PLS), addresses its diagnostic update and dental management, and reports a case of a 5-year-old Lebanese patient with consanguineously married parents. *Background.* PLS, also known as "keratoris palmoplantaris with periodontopathia" and "hyperkeratosis palmoplantaris with periodontosis," is an extremely rare autosomal-recessive trait that combines a diffuse palmoplantar hyperkeratosis and a severe generalized, progressive prepubertal form of a precocious form of juvenile, aggressive periodontitis. *Case Description.* We are reporting a 5-year-old boy that sustained a spontaneous loss of all his primary teeth. At consultation, he was under treatment for hyperkeratosis of his palms and soles. Detailed family history of the child revealed that the patient's parents, grandparents, and relatives were consanguineously married and two of his cousins displayed similar clinical signs (palmoplantar hyperkeratosis and premature loss of deciduous and most of the permanent teeth). *Conclusion.* PLS is an extremely rare disorder that usually becomes apparent from approximately 1-5 years of age. Genetic counseling should always be suggested to parents of affected children, informing them of chances of their offspring having the inherited disease.

1. Introduction

Papillon-Lefèvre syndrome (PLS) is a very rare genodermatosis of autosomal-recessive inheritance. It is an ectodermal dysplasia, and a type IV palmoplantar keratosis [1]. It was named, in 1924, by French physicians M.M. Papillon and Paul Lefèvre [1] and is characterized by a hyperkeratosis of soles of feet and palms of the hands (palmar-plantar) and extensive, severe, aggressive, and prepubertal periodontitis, leading to premature loss in both deciduous and permanent dentitions.

PLS prevalence is estimated between 1/250,000 and 1/1,000,000 in the general population [2, 3].

PLS disorder can be hereditary, acquired, or associated with other syndromes, but in most described cases, PLS is genetic, resulting from mutations on both alleles of the cathepsin C gene (CTSC) on chromosome 11q14.2. Most PLS patients are homozygous for CTSC mutations [4–7].

2. Case Report

A 5-year-old boy presented to the Department of Pediatric Dentistry of the Faculty of Dental Medicine at Saint-Joseph University of Beirut, Lebanon, with a chief complaint of loosening of all primary teeth, followed by their spontaneous loss. The patient's medical history showed that he was undergoing a dermatological treatment for the "hyperkeratosis of his palms and soles"; the treating dermatologist referred the patient to the dentist after having suspected PLS. A detailed family history revealed that the patient's

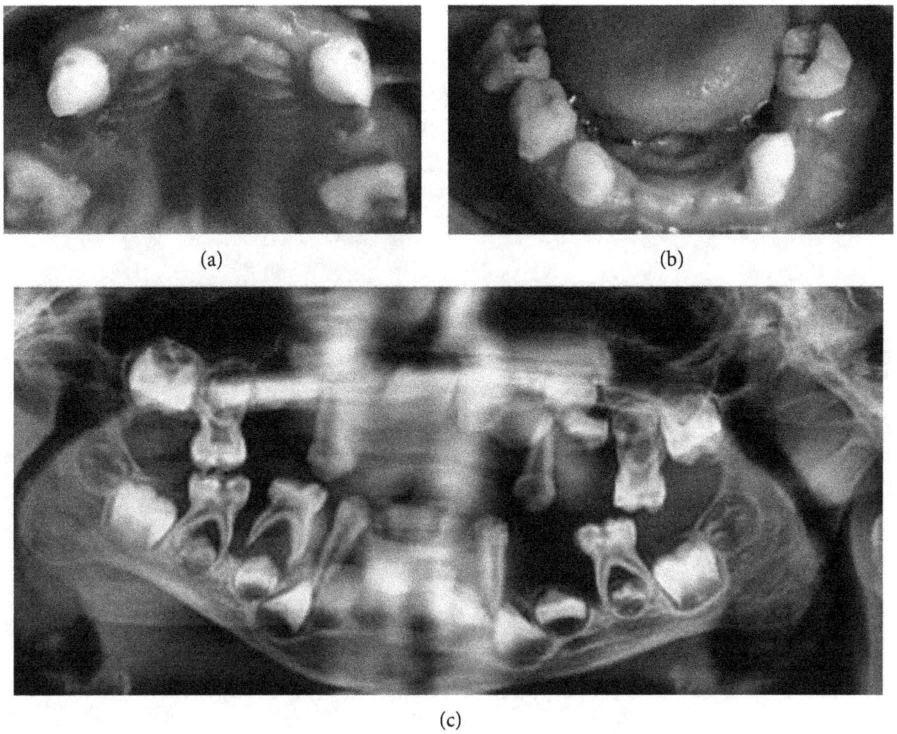

FIGURE 1: (a and b) Intraoral maxillary and mandibular aspects before multiple dental extractions. (c) Panoramic radiograph before extractions.

parents, grandparents, and relatives were consanguineously married and two of his cousins exhibited similar clinical signs (palmoplantar hyperkeratosis and premature loss of deciduous and permanent teeth).

Intraoral examination revealed that many primary teeth (teeth 54, 52, 51, 61, 62, 64, 74, 72, 71, 81, and 82) were missing while remaining teeth (teeth 85, 84, 83, 73, 75, 65, 63, 53, and 55) exhibited plaque accumulation, multiple caries, and generalized grade III mobility with the formation of periodontal pockets (Figure 1); gingival tissues surrounding these teeth were inflamed, edematous, and tender to palpation, while those of edentulous regions appeared normal and nontender to palpation. Dental and periodontal abscesses were noticed on teeth 85 and 75. Panoramic radiograph displayed several floating teeth with generalized horizontal and vertical bone loss (Figure 1).

Extraoral examination of the patient revealed hyperkeratosis on the dorsum surface of his hands (Figure 2) and feet (Figure 3).

Routine hematological examination (CBC and blood chemistry profile) and liver function tests were normal. In addition, a genetic test was performed at the Saint Joseph University Faculty of Medicine/Laboratory of Molecular Biology, Beirut; PCRs (polymerase chain reaction) followed by fluorescent Sanger sequencing of exons 3 to 7 of *CTSC* gene, for the affected child, revealed no mutation. However, PCR amplification of exons 1 and 2 did not result in any product, suggesting that affected child harbored a homozygous deletion of the $5'$UTR region and exons 1 and 2.

Level of patient's cooperation was assessed during the first clinical examination, and it was decided to implement the treatment under general anesthesia, at hospital. A written informed consent form was signed by the child's parents after having discussed with them all the steps of the treatment planning, from extraction of all remaining teeth to the fabrication of an immediate removable complete denture (RCD). The importance of oral hygiene was emphasized, and enforcement of oral hygiene habits was advocated.

At hospital, the first dose of amoxicillin (50 mg/kg) and clavulanic acid was administered through IV route before beginning the surgery and it was continued for the following postoperative seven days. In order to maintain a stable occlusion, two impressions of maxilla and mandible were taken with the remaining teeth in place using an addition silicon material. All remaining teeth were extracted, and all extraction sockets were irrigated with a 0.12% chlorhexidine digluconate solution. No sutures were needed, and impressions were directly transferred to the dental laboratory in order to be casted.

Two weeks after extractions, maxillary and mandibular RCDs were fabricated (Figure 4(a)) and inserted in the mouth (Figure 4(b)). No pressure spots were noticed, and occlusion showed no interferences. Patient and parents were taught the proper oral hygiene measures for RCDs; they were also informed of the need for regular dental visits (one week after the insertion and every three months afterwards) in order to reexamine the appliances and, when necessary, replace or reline them according to arch growth and eruption of the permanent teeth. Eight-month follow-up revealed the erupting mandibular central incisors (Figure 5).

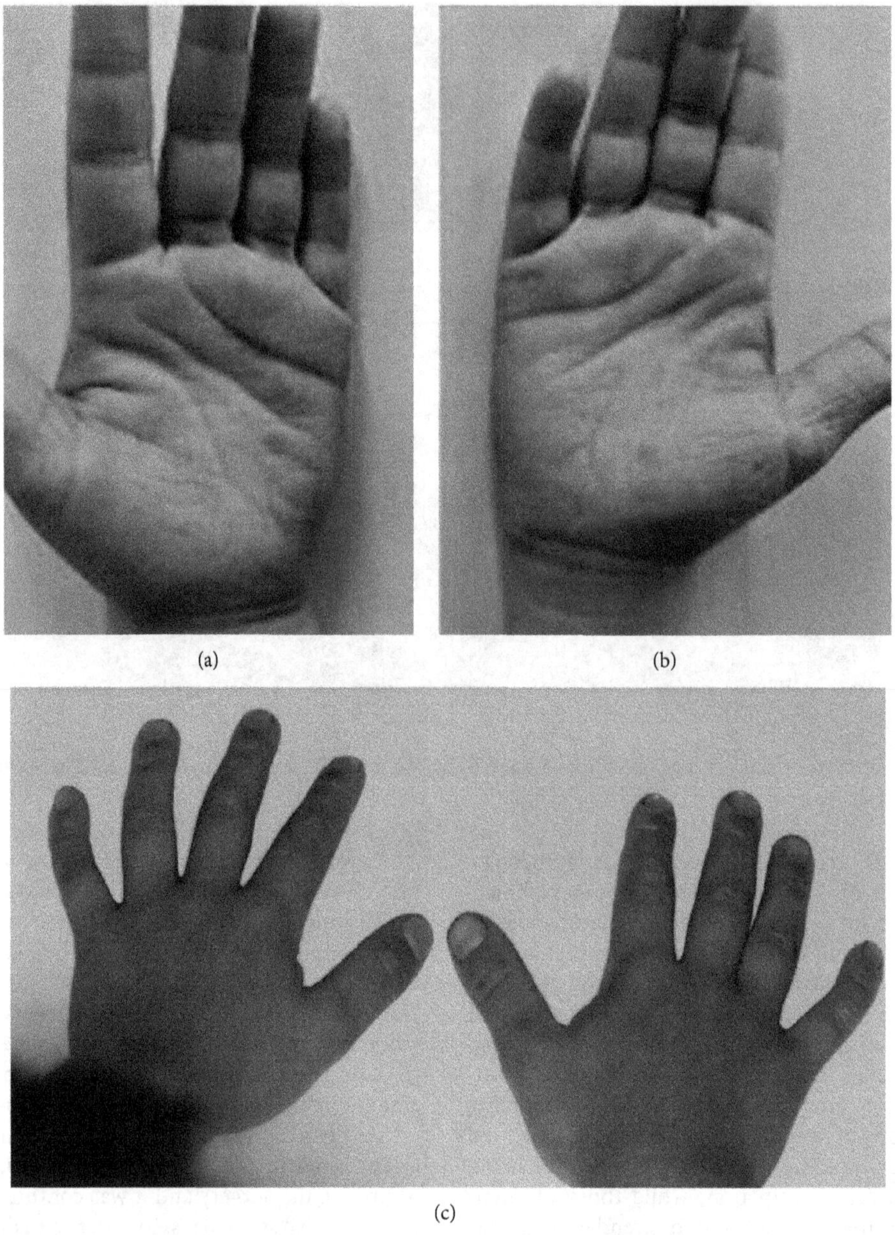

(a) (b) (c)

FIGURE 2: Hyperkeratosis on hand palms (a and b) and dorsal surfaces (c).

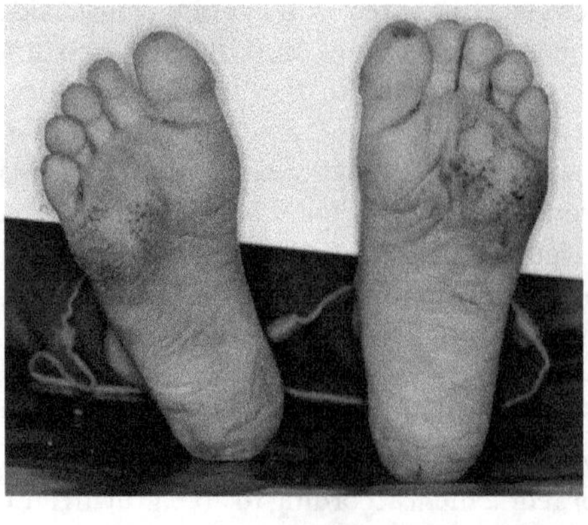

FIGURE 3: Hyperkeratosis of soles of feet (scaly and rough soles).

3. Discussion

3.1. Consanguinity in PLS. Consanguineous marriage [8] is matrimony between persons who are closely related. It is defined as a union between two individuals who are related as second cousins or closer, with an inbreeding coefficient (F) equal or higher than 0.0156; F representing a measure of the proportion of loci at which the offspring of a consanguineous union is expected to inherit identical gene copies from the father and mother. This includes unions termed first cousins and second cousins. In some Arab communities where unions occur between double first cousins, the highest inbreeding coefficients are reached, and in some regions of South India where uncle-niece marriages occur, F reaches 0.125 [8].

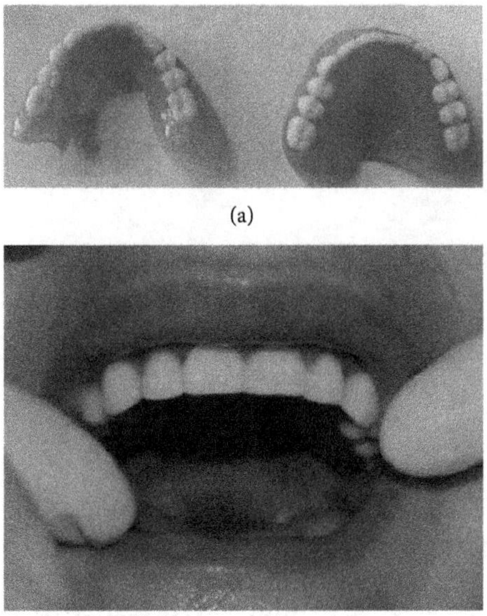

(a)

(b)

FIGURE 4: (a) Maxillary and mandibular removable complete dentures. (b) Insertion of maxillary denture in the mouth.

Increased genetic risks to the offspring represent the main negative impact of consanguineous marriages. Indeed, consanguineous unions may lead to an increased expression of autosomal-recessive disorders, and the closer the biological relationship between parents, the greater is the probability that their offspring will inherit similar copies of one or more detrimental recessive genes [9]. Consanguinity does not increase the risk for autosomal-dominant diseases when only one of the parents is affected nor for X-linked recessive conditions if neither parent is affected [8].

Premarital screening and preconception counseling programs are important in raising public's awareness of possible genetic diseases and their prevention by knowing more on consanguinity as a risk factor for the expression of recessive disorders. In Shiraz, Southern Iran, among 2,686 couples presenting for genetic counseling during a period of 4 years, 85% had consanguineous relationships and 74% were first cousins [10].

In preconception counseling for consanguinity, it is important to make the difference between families with no known genetic disorder and those with a known inherited or genetic one. Taking a detailed family history and constructing a four-generation pedigree (offspring, siblings, parents, aunts, uncles, grandparents, nieces, nephews, and first cousins) are obligatory [9]. Collection of information is implemented by addressing very specific questions that could lead to the detection of a genetic or hereditary disorder in the extended family; these questions should include any relevant information about any of the following pathologies in blood relatives:

(1) Congenital anomalies or birth defects

(2) Learning disability or mental retardation (or disability)

(3) Inherited blood disorder

(4) Undiagnosed severe condition or anomaly

(5) Early vision and/or hearing impairment

(6) Failure to thrive or developmental delay

(7) Epilepsy

(8) Unexplained infant (or neonatal) death in the offspring

Consanguinity is a deeply rooted social trend among one-fifth of the world population mostly residing in the Middle East, North Africa, and West Asia, as well among some emigrants from these regions now residing in Europe, North America, and Australia. In these highly consanguineous populations and communities, premarital counseling on consanguinity is almost absent. Around one billion of the current global population live in regions and communities with an obvious preference for consanguineous (blood relatives) marriages. In such communities and regions, though cousin marriages are customary, there are inconsistencies among healthcare providers in counseling for consanguinity possible consequences and sequelea [9].

When PLS is genetic, it is transmitted as an autosomal-recessive trait, and 20-40% of patients are children of consanguineously married parents [11].

In their original paper, back in 1924, Papillon and Lefèvre reported [1] the case of two siblings who were the products of a first-cousin mating, and the condition described in their paper featured two hallmarks which were a premature loss of deciduous and permanent dentitions and diffuse transgradient palmoplantar keratosis. Consanguinity is now recognized as a risk factor [12] for PLS, and many articles reported PLS cases in the same family [13–15]. Considering that consanguineous marriage is customary in Lebanese society, potential parents are to be warned that this leads to an increased birth prevalence of infant with severe recessive disorders; consequently, this kind of marriage should be discouraged, and genetic counseling should be advocated. Families at increased risk should be identified, and carrier testing should be implemented when feasible [16].

3.2. Clinical Manifestations. PLS becomes clinically apparent from the ages of 1 to 5; dry scaly patches of palms and soles (palmar-plantar hyperkeratosis) and severe, aggressive, and early-onset periodontitis are its main clinical features, but additional symptoms may be associated to it, such as pyogenic skin infections, nail dystrophies, and hyperhidrosis. Patches of the skin usually develop around the age of 1 to 5; they are mostly confined to the undersides of feet and hands, but they may appear on elbows and knees. In rare cases, upper portions of hands and feet, eyelids, and other parts of the body may be affected as well. Affected skin is often thick and red, but texture and color may vary; skin lesions may worsen during cold weather, and walking is often uncomfortable and painful.

Patients affected with PLS may also exhibit generalized hyperhidrosis (excessive perspiration), leading to unpleasant,

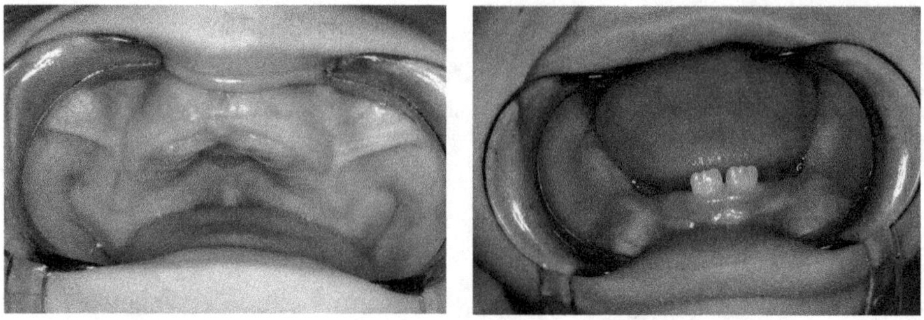

(a) (b)

FIGURE 5: The erupting mandibular central incisors.

malodorous odors. Most patients with PLS have hypotrichosis (sparse hair on the scalp and body), dirty colored skin, and very fragile nails that easily break off, but some of them may release excessive amounts of keratine in hair follicles, causing rough papules on the skin.

Only some individuals affected by PLS may experience other kinds of infections such as furunculosis, respiratory tract infections, and hidradenitis suppurativa (painful and swollen lesions in the breast, groin, and armpit).

3.3. Craniofacial, Oral, Dental, and Periodontal Aspects. Dental and periodontal manifestations [3] of PSL become apparent by the age of 2-3 years; they start with severe gingivitis and rapid periodontal destruction, followed by premature exfoliation of all deciduous teeth by the age of 4 to 5. The same sequence of events recurs as the permanent dentition erupts, leading to its early shedding, and without treatment, most of the permanent teeth may fall by the same mechanism by the age of 16 years. Consequences of this premature tooth loss will affect the patient's daily functions, such as mastication and speech.

Gingival and periodontal tissues are involved (gingivitis, gingival ulcers, periodontal pockets, and severe, aggressive periodontitis) in PLS. Aggregatibacter actinomycetemcomitans plays an important role in the progression of periodontal infections and inflammations. Treponema denticola, Porphyromonas gingivalis, and Fusobacterium nucleatum are also suggested as causative agents [17].

At eruption of deciduous teeth, gums appear red, inflamed, and sometimes bleedy and enlarged. In some cases, all oral mucosae may appear erythematous (stomatitis), with possible perioral lymphadenopathies. Halitosis may also develop in some individuals. Apart from that, discrepancies in the arch length and psychological problems may follow [18].

In rare people affected with PLS, dry scaly patches of the skin (hyperkeratosis) may appear on lips, cheeks, and eyelids, and in some rare adult patients, cysts may develop on eyelids and calcium may accumulate in the skull, causing intracranial calcifications [19, 20].

3.4. Differential Diagnosis. To distinguish between PLS and palmoplantar hyperkeratosis syndromes, occurrence of severe, aggressive, and early-onset destructive periodontitis has to be taken into consideration [21].

Many disorders share similar clinical and genetic features with PLS [22]:

(1) The association with severe, aggressive, and early-onset periodontitis is unique to PLS and Haim-Munk syndrome (HMS). HMS (known also as "palmoplantar keratoderma with periodontitis and arachnodactyly and acroosteolysis" or "Cochin Jewish disorder") is a skin condition caused by a cathepsin C gene mutation; it is an extremely rare disorder of keratinization of recessive inheritance that manifests with scaly, red, and thickened patches of the skin of soles of the feet and palms of the hands (palmoplantar hyperkeratosis), pes planus (flat foot), arachnodactyly (a peculiar deformity of terminal phalanges of hands and feet), acroosteolysis, atrophic changes of nails (onychogryphosis), a radiographic deformity of fingers, recurrent abscess formations, and a severe early-onset periodontitis. PLS cases were reported worldwide while HMS ones were only described among descendants of a religious isolate originally from Cochin, India. Consanguinity is a major feature of both conditions.

(2) Palmoplantar ectodermal dysplasia (PPED) is a skin condition that includes 8 types: PPED type 1 or pachyonychia congenita which is autosomal dominant, PPED type 2, PPED type 3 or acrokeratoelastoidosis, PPED type 4 which resembles the PLS, PPED type 5 or oculocutaneous tyrosinemia type II or Richner-Hanhart syndrome which is autosomal recessive, PPED type 6 or Olmsted syndrome, PPED type 7, and PPED type 8 or Meleda disease or "mal de Meleda" or "acral keratoderma" which is autosomal recessive.

(3) von Feer's disease (acrodynia, pink disease, mercurialism, erythredema, and Swift-Feer disease) affects children which is characterized by dusky pink discoloration in hands and feet, loss of teeth, hair, and nails, red lips, cheeks, and nose, transient rashes, hypotonia, photophobia, kidney dysfunction, peripheral neuropathy (paresthesia, itching, burning sensation, and pain), and neuropsychiatric symptoms (insomnia, emotional lability, and memory impairment). Mercury intoxication/poisoning is incriminated as a causative factor of this disease.

Other pathologies and syndromes sharing clinical features with PLS [22] include palmoplantar hyperkeratosis (Unna-Thost syndrome), palmoplantar hyperkeratosis-punctate, Vohwinkel's syndrome, Vörner's localized epidermolytic palmoplantar keratoderma, Howel-Evans syndrome, Gamborg-Nielsen syndrome, and Greither's transgrediens and progrediens palmoplantar keratoderma.

Some PLS patients were reported to have palmoplantar keratosis and periodontal destruction in their permanent dentition, with no periodontal destruction observed in their deciduous one [21, 23, 24].

A cohort study including 47 patients [25] supported the concept that the two major components of PLS (periodontal destruction and palmoplantar keratosis) appeared to be unrelated to each other; in this study, skin and oral changes developed early in life, with no exception. Dermatological involvement showed no correlation with age, while periodontal infection was significantly worse in young age with primary teeth. Finally, a strong correlation was found between feet and hand condition, although the scores for the feet were significantly higher, and no significant correlation could be demonstrated between the severity of skin affections and the level of periodontal destruction [25].

4. Conclusion

PLS periodontosis ultimately leads to premature loss of deciduous and permanent dentitions at a very young age. This devastating periodontitis is attributed to a point mutation of the cathepsin C gene. Prognosis of dentition in these patients is poor, and most of them ultimately become edentulous, except for third molars, and end up with a small maxilla and mandible. In almost half of the patients, PLS displays an enhanced susceptibility to systemic and cutaneous infections, such as skin abscesses, furunculosis, hidradenitis suppurativa, and respiratory tract infections. Patients may also sustain nail dystrophies, follicular hyperkeratosis, dural calcifications, and malodorous hyperhidrosis; on very rare occasions, PLS may be associated with squamous cell carcinoma and malignant melanoma.

Conventional treatment of PLS is mainly based on the use of oral retinoids which often attenuate signs of palmoplantar keratoderma and, somehow, slow the resorption of the alveolar bone on the remaining teeth. Etretinate, a synthetic retinoid, lately showed very promising results in the medical treatment of PLS. Antibiotics are also prescribed in treating recurrent infections.

A very good oral hygiene with concomitant use of chlorhexidine mouth rinses should also be recommended to patients in order to slow the aggressive progression of periodontitis. Finally, deciduous and remaining teeth are often extracted and replaced, either by conventional removable dentures or dental osseointegratable implants.

Successful periodontal management of PLS patients is the key to improve the prognosis of the dentition, preventing or delaying primary and permanent tooth loss. It is mandatory that all dental professionals be familiar and aware of this disease as well as the importance of its early diagnosis and management.

References

[1] M. M. Papillon and P. Lefèvre, "Deux cas de kératodermie palmaire et plantaire symétrique familiale (maladie de Meleda) chez le frère et la sœur. Coexistence dans les deux cas d'altérations dentaires graves," *Bulletin de la Société Française de Dermatologie et de Vénéréologie*, vol. 31, pp. 82–87, 1924.

[2] B. Dalgic, A. Bukulmez, and S. Sari, "Eponym: Papillon-Lefèvre syndrome," *European Journal of Pediatrics*, vol. 170, no. 6, pp. 689–691, 2011.

[3] P. J. Dhanrajani, "Papillon-Lefèvre syndrome: clinical presentation and a brief review," *Oral Surgery, Oral Medicine, Oral Pathology, Oral Radiology, and Endodontology*, vol. 108, no. 1, pp. e1–e7, 2009.

[4] T. C. Hart, P. S. Hart, D. W. Bowden et al., "Mutations of the cathepsin C gene are responsible for Papillon-Lefèvre syndrome," *Journal of Medical Genetics*, vol. 36, no. 12, pp. 881–887, 1999.

[5] A. Wani, N. Devkar, M. Patole, and Y. Shouche, "Description of Two New Cathepsin C Gene Mutations in Patients With Papillon-Lefèvre Syndrome," *Journal of Periodontology*, vol. 77, no. 2, pp. 233–237, 2006.

[6] N. A. Cagli, S. S. Hakki, R. Dursun et al., "Clinical, genetic, and biochemical findings in two siblings with Papillon-Lefèvre syndrome," *Journal of Periodontology*, vol. 76, no. 12, pp. 2322–2329, 2005.

[7] T. C. Hart, P. S. Hart, M. D. Michalec et al., "Haim-Munk syndrome and Papillon-Lefèvre syndrome are allelic mutations in cathepsin C.," *Journal of medical genetics*, vol. 37, no. 2, pp. 88–94, 2000.

[8] H. Hamamy, "Consanguineous marriages. Preconception consultation in primary health care settings," *Journal of Community Genetics*, vol. 3, no. 3, pp. 185–192, 2012.

[9] R. L. Bennett, A. G. Motulsky, A. Bittles et al., "Genetic counseling and screening of consanguineous couples and their offspring: recommendations of the national society of genetic counselors," *Journal of Genetic Counseling*, vol. 11, no. 2, pp. 97–119, 2002.

[10] M. Fathzadeh, M. A. Babaie Bigi, M. Bazrgar, M. Yavarian, H. R. Tabatabaee, and S. M. Akrami, "Genetic counseling in Southern Iran: consanguinity and reason for referral," *Journal of Genetic Counseling*, vol. 17, no. 5, pp. 472–479, 2008.

[11] F. Acun Kaya, Z. Seyfioglu Polat, E. Akuzum Baran, and G. G. Tekin, "Papillon-Lefèvre syndrome. 3 years follow up: a case report," *International Dental and Medical Disorders*, vol. 1, no. 1, pp. 24–28, 2008.

[12] A. F. Shah, P. Tangade, and S. Agarwal, "Papillon–Lefevre syndrome: Reporting consanguinity as a risk factor," *The Saudi Dental Journal*, vol. 26, no. 3, pp. 126–131, 2014.

[13] S. S. Pareek and A. K. Al-Aska, "Papillon-Lefevre syndrome. A report of six cases in one family," *International Journal of Dermatology*, vol. 25, no. 10, pp. 638–641, 1986.

[14] A. K. Valeshabad, A. Mazidi, R. K. Valeshabad et al., "Papillon-Lefèvre Syndrome: A Series of Six Cases in the Same Family," *ISRN Dermatology*, vol. 2012, Article ID 139104, 4 pages, 2012.

[15] Z. M. AlBarrak, A. S. Alqarni, E. P. Chalisserry, and S. Anil, "Papillon–Lefèvre syndrome: a series of five cases among siblings," *Journal of Medical Case Reports*, vol. 10, no. 1, pp. 260–265, 2016.

[16] B. Modell and A. Darr, "Genetic counselling and customary consanguineous marriage," *Nature Reviews Genetics*, vol. 3, no. 3, pp. 225–229, 2002.

[17] A. Stabholz, N. S. Taichman, and W. A. Soskolne, "Occurrence of Actinobacillus actinomycetemcomitans and anti-leukotoxin antibodies in some members of an extended family affected by Papillon-Lefèvre syndrome," *Journal of Periodontology*, vol. 66, no. 7, pp. 653–657, 1995.

[18] B. Sreeramulu, N. D. V. N. Shyam, P. Ajay, and P. Suman, "Papillon–Lefèvre syndrome: clinical presentation and management options," *Clinical, Cosmetic and Investigational Dentistry*, vol. 7, pp. 75–81, 2015.

[19] M. M. Brownstein and P. Skolnik, "Papillon-Lefèvre Syndrome," *Archives of Dermatology*, vol. 106, no. 4, pp. 533-534, 1972.

[20] E. F. Corson, "Keratosis palmaris et plantaris with dental alternation," *Archives of Dermatology and Syphilology*, vol. 40, p. 639, 1939.

[21] E. Haneke, "The Papillon-Lefèvre syndrome: keratosis palmoplantaris with periodontopathy: report of a case and review of the cases in the literature," *Human Genetics*, vol. 51, no. 1, pp. 1–35, 1979.

[22] T. C. Hart and L. Shapira, "Papillon-Lefèvre syndrome," *Periodontology 2000*, vol. 6, no. 1, pp. 88–100, 1994.

[23] T. Q. Nguyen, K. E. Greer, G. B. Fisher Jr, and P. H. Cooper, "Papillon-Lefèvre syndrome: report of two patients treated successfully with isotretinoin," *Journal of the American Academy of Dermatology*, vol. 15, no. 1, pp. 46–49, 1986.

[24] E. M. Rateitschak-Pluss and H. E. Schroeder, "History of periodontitis in a child with Papillon-Lefèvre syndrome. A case report," *Journal of Periodontology*, vol. 55, no. 1, pp. 35–46, 1984.

[25] C. Ullbro, C. G. Crossner, T. Nederfors, A. Alfadley, and K. Thestrup-Pedersen, "Dermatologic and oral findings in a cohort of 47 patients with Papillon-Lefèvre syndrome," *Journal of the American Academy of Dermatology*, vol. 48, no. 3, pp. 345–351, 2003.

17

TAD's for the Derotation of 90° Rotated Maxillary Bicuspids

Hasan Sabah Hasan[1] **Ayshan Kolemen**[2] **Mohamed Elkolaly**[3] **Anand Marya**[4] **Shreyas Gujjar**[5] **and Adith Venugopal**[4,6]

[1]*Orthodontic Department, Khanzad Teaching Center, General Directorate of Hawler-Ministry of Health, Erbil, Iraq*
[2]*Orthodontic Department, Al-Mustaqbal University College, Babel, Iraq*
[3]*Orthodontic Department, Royal Dental Center, Alexandria, Egypt*
[4]*Section of Orthodontics, University of Puthisastra, Phnom Penh, Cambodia*
[5]*Sri Balaji Dental College, Moinabad, Telangana, India*
[6]*Department of Orthodontics, Saveetha Dental College, Saveetha Institute of Medical and Technical Sciences, Saveetha University, Chennai, India*

Correspondence should be addressed to Adith Venugopal; avenugopal@puthisastra.edu.kh

Academic Editor: Andrea Scribante

It is undeniable that the advent of extra-alveolar mini-implants for anchorage purposes has revolutionized the field of Orthodontics. This case report sheds light on an innovative anchorage plan using TADs, to carry out treatment for a 15-year-old female patient. The patient reported to the clinic with a chief complaint of rotated second premolars, crowding, and a deep bite. On examination, it was seen that the patient had a Class I skeletal pattern, Class II subdivision molar relationship, 90-degree maxillary second premolar rotations, crowding in both the arches, and a deep bite. In this case, the clinicians decided to use TADs for premolar derotation as it not only provides a pure rotational couple without any deleterious effects on the adjacent teeth but also helps shorten the overall treatment time. The total treatment time for this case was 10 months.

1. Introduction

Any tooth rotation is considered a malocclusion that requires management by an orthodontist. A rotated premolar leads to not only occlusal problems but also esthetic concerns [1, 2]. Derotation of premolars must be carried out during the initial phase of fixed orthodontic mechanotherapy [3]. Derotation of posterior teeth provides for space that can be utilized to relieve crowding in the anterior region. Derotation of the teeth, if carried out with a continuous wire, can lead to unwanted iatrogenic effects on the anchor teeth. Therefore, such rotated teeth need to be derotated using couple mechanics that involve the use of equal and opposite forces that bring about pure rotational movement [3, 4].

Patients undergoing fixed orthodontic therapy desire timely completion of their treatment which is why it is essential for an orthodontist to correct the malocclusion without any associated iatrogenic problems. This is where the use of temporary anchorage devices (TADs) has revolutionized fixed orthodontic therapy. The judicious use of TADs for treating orthodontic patients allows an orthodontist to plan for a broader range of movements [5, 6]. This case report highlights the use of TADs to treat a 15-year-old patient that reported to the clinic with a Class I skeletal pattern, a Class II subdivision molar relationship, 90-degree maxillary second premolar rotations, crowding in the maxillary and mandibular arches, and an anterior deep bite.

2. Case Presentation

A 15-year-old patient reported to the clinic with a chief complaint of malaligned teeth and desired orthodontic treatment. Her previous dental history was unremarkable. On extraoral examination, she had a good facial form and proportion with a straight profile and a minimal display of buccal corridors on smiling. Intraoral examination showed mild crowding in

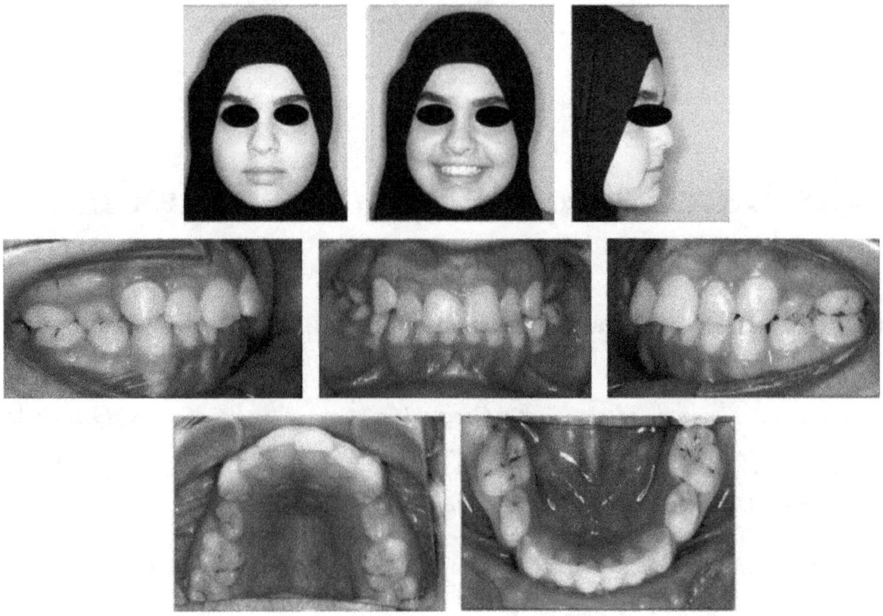

Figure 1: Pretreatment extra-oral and intra-oral pictures.

both the maxillary and the mandibular arches, a Class I molar relation on the right side, and a half-unit Class II relation on the left side. In addition, the canine relationships were half-unit Class II on both sides, the overjet was normal, there was a 4 mm anterior deep bite, there were missing upper and lower right/left first premolars due to previous extractions, and both the maxillary second premolars were present with 90-degree rotations (Figure 1).

The panoramic radiograph showed no abnormality except for missing upper and lower, right/left first premolars. Cephalometric analysis was carried out using WebCeph software (AssembleCircle Corp., Republic of Korea) and revealed a skeletal Class I relationship, a hypodivergent facial pattern, and proclined upper incisors (Figure 2).

3. Treatment Objectives

(1) Develop a unique anchorage design using TADs for derotation of the maxillary second premolars without compromising the anchorage units

(2) Apply a pure rotational couple force without effect on the adjacent teeth

(3) Reduce the overall treatment time

(4) Alleviate crowding in both the maxilla and the mandible

(5) Correct the anterior deep bite

(6) Correct the molar and canine relationships

4. Treatment Planning

The patient showed a Class I skeletal base, CI II subdivision molar relationship, mild crowding, deep bite, hypodivergent facial pattern, procline upper incisors, and missing upper and lower right/left first premolars and both upper second premolars with 90-degree rotation.

The treatment plan was proposed as follows:

(1) Leveling and alignment of the maxillary and mandibular arches using fixed orthodontic therapy

(2) Placement of two mini-implants, one in the buccal aspect and the other in the hard palate for derotation of rotated premolars simultaneously while leveling and aligning the arch in order to save time

(3) Closure of residual spaces

(4) After treatment completion, retention with the upper and lowered fixed bonded lingual retainers

5. Treatment Alternatives

Three alternatives were proposed to achieve treatment goals:

(1) The first option was to use a stiff.019 x.025″ SS base arch wire after leveling and alignment in the maxillary arch. Reinforcing the anterior anchorage from the canine to canine (joining the segment using tight ligature ties) as well as a posterior anchorage (by joining first and second molars together using a ligated wire). These anchorage units would be used to derotate the premolars using power chains from the buccal surface of the second premolars to the hook of the molar tube and from the lingual surface of the second premolars to the lingual surface of the upper canines (using lingual buttons). Bite turbos would be placed to disocclude the premolars during the alignment phase

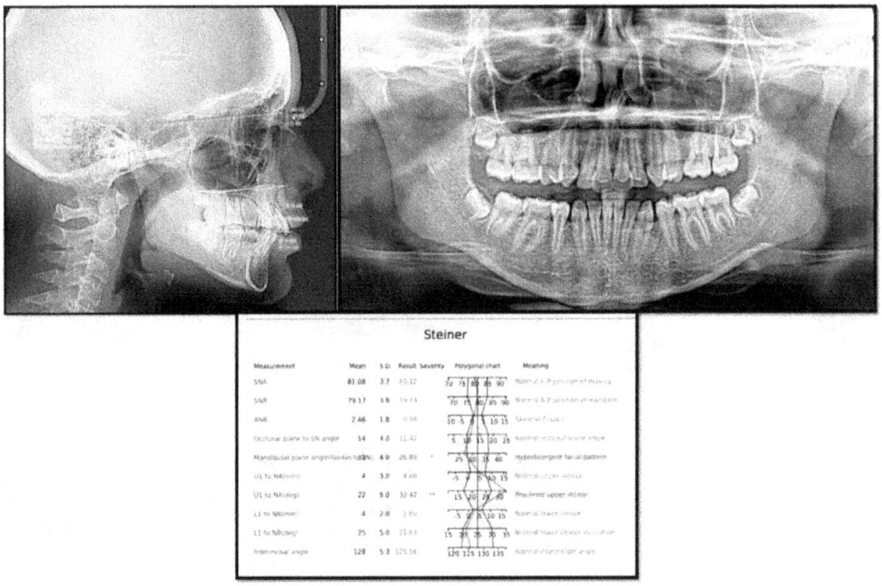

FIGURE 2: Pretreatment cephalogram and panoramic radiograph with analysis of the lateral cephalogram using the Steiner analysis.

(2) The second option was to again use a stiff.019 x.025″ SS wire as the base arch wire. The anterior anchorage would be the same as the first option, but in this case, the posterior anchorage would be reinforced using a Transpalatal arch bonded to the first maxillary molars. The derotation would be carried out using similar biomechanics to the first option

(3) The third option was to use TADs as maximum anchorage so that derotation of the premolars could be carried out at the same time as the leveling and alignment of the other teeth. Four TADs would be placed between the upper first molars and second premolars buccally, and two would be placed between the upper canine and second premolars on the palatal aspect in the hard palate without using bite turbos. The TADs would be utilized to derotate using couple mechanics and maintain an intrusive effect on the premolars

After careful consideration of all the three treatment options, the third option was chosen as it shortened the treatment time and helped achieve the derotation of the premolars without any adverse effects on the adjacent teeth.

6. Treatment Progress

Prior to bracket placement, impressions were taken for fabrication of study models, followed by oral prophylaxis. Fixed orthodontic appliance was bonded (slot 0.022-inch, Roth prescription, Discovery, Dentaurum, Germany) with four lingual buttons (Dentaurum, Germany) on the buccal and lingual aspects of second premolars. At the same time, four TADs (used as anchorage for derotation of the first premolars; 1.6 × 8 mm) (Gssem, Korea) were inserted: the first two were inserted in the left/right buccal aspects between the upper second premolars and first molars, and the other two were inserted in the hard palate between the canines and second premolars. Both TADs were positioned close to the occlusal surface to reduce the intrusion effect on premolars.

Leveling and alignment was started on a 0.014″ NiTi archwire and followed by a sequence of 0.016″, 0.018″, and 0.016 × 22″NiTi along with active power chains (clear continuous; Vimel, Koreas, changed every two weeks) from the TADs to the attached buttons on the second premolars. The elastic chains were placed to derotate the premolars using pure couple forces [7] (Figures 3(a), 3(b), 4(a), and 4(b)).

After completion of the derotation, the buttons were removed and brackets were bonded on the second premolars. A.016 x.022″ NiTi wire was placed in the bracket slots of the derotated premolars to align them. Once we were able to engage a.019 x.025″ SS wire in the slot, the palatal TADs were removed and the buccal screws were used as anchorage. Closure of remaining spaces was done with hooks placed between the canines and the lateral incisors and placement of 6 mm closed coil springs from the buccal TAD to the hook. The residual space left after premolar alignment was eventually closed and was helpful in the correction of the anterior deep bite. Additionally, inter-arch elastics were placed between the maxillary and mandibular premolars and first molars (1/4-inch, medium, Dentaurum, Germany) to settle the occlusion. (Figures 3(c), 3(d), 4(c), and 4(d)) Once the occlusion was well settled, the fixed appliance was debonded using a Carbide bur (TDF-6R, Brassler, USA) and retention was provided. Circumferential supracrestal fiberotomy (CSF) was performed on the second premolars to avoid any further chances of relapse (Figure 4(e)).

7. Results

The orthodontic treatment was completed in ten months. Class I molar and canine relationships were obtained on both

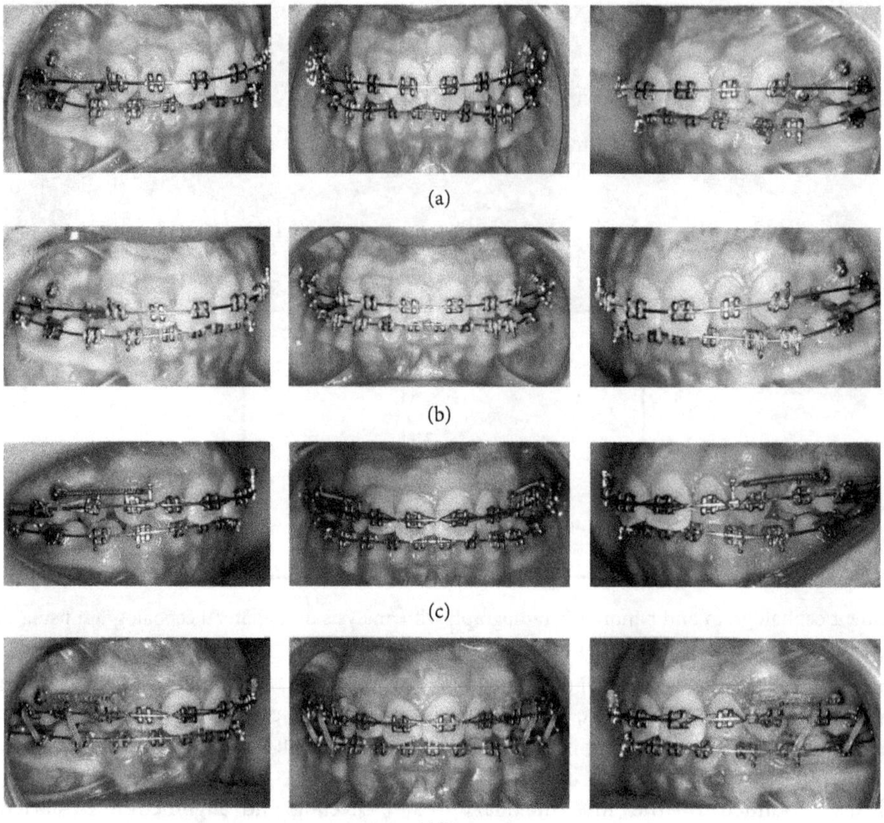

FIGURE 3: Showing treatment progress; (a, b) simultaneous leveling and alignment stage with derotation of the upper second premolars, (c) en masse retraction, (d) usage of elastic rings for maximum intercuspation.

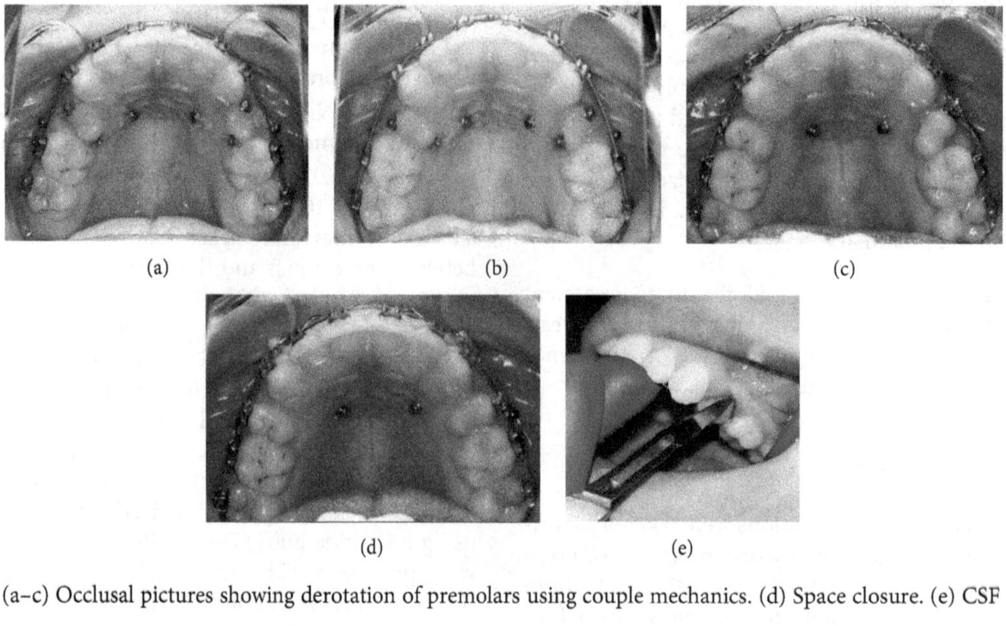

FIGURE 4: (a–c) Occlusal pictures showing derotation of premolars using couple mechanics. (d) Space closure. (e) CSF technique.

sides with ideal overbite, overjet, correct incisor inclinations, and well-aligned teeth (Figures 5 and 6). The upper and lower midlines were minimally off at the end of treatment (Figure 5). Upper right and left second premolar rotations were corrected by a customized TAD based approach. Circumferential supracrestal fiberotomy (CSF) was performed on the derotated premolars to reduce the chances of relapse. The result was retained using a fixed lingual bonded retainer using a braided stainless steel wire on the upper and lower arches (Figure 5). Additionally, clear Essex retainers were

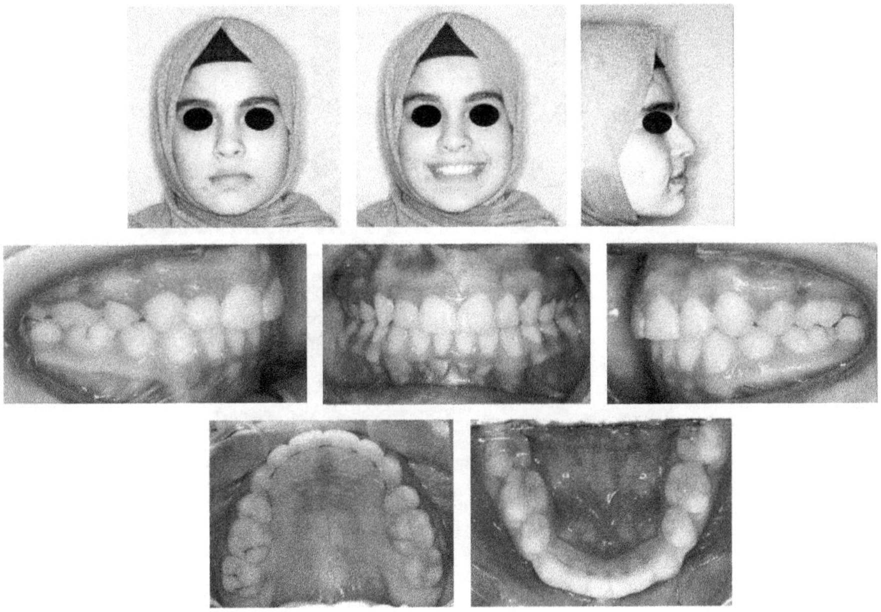

FIGURE 5: Posttreatment extra and intraoral images.

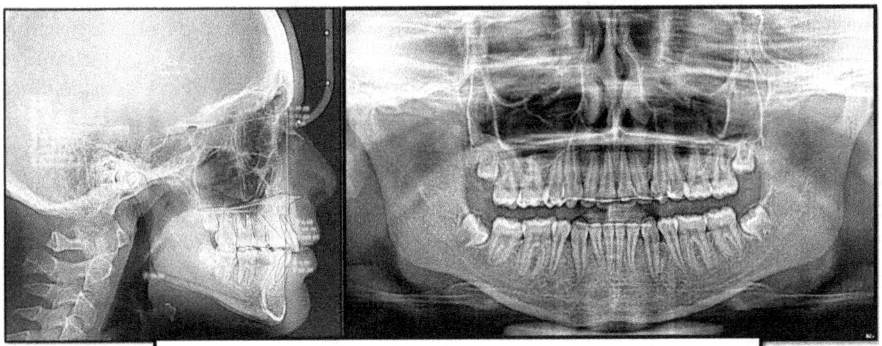

Steiner

Measurement	Mean	S.D.	Result	Severity	Polygonal chart	Meaning
SNA	81.08	3.7	79.38			Normal A-P position of maxilla
SNB	79.17	3.8	77.47			Normal A-P position of mandible
ANB	2.46	1.8	1.91			Skeletal Class I
Occlusal plane to SN angle	14	4.0	15.85			Normal occlusal plane angle
Mandibular plane angle(Go-Gn to SN)	33	4.0	28.82			Normodivergent facial pattern
U1 to NA(mm)	4	3.0	2.63			Normal upper incisor
U1 to NA(deg)	22	5.0	24.75			Normal upper incisor inclination
L1 to NB(mm)	4	2.0	3.26			Normal lower incisor
L1 to NB(deg)	25	5.0	23.80			Normal lower incisor inclination
Interincisal angle	128	5.3	129.53			Normal interincisor angle

FIGURE 6: Posttreatment cephalogram and panoramic radiograph with analysis of the lateral cephalogram using the Steiner analysis.

provided to the patient for full time wear. The posttreatment records demonstrate the completed case findings and follow-up after 5 years of treatment (Figure 7).

8. Discussion

Amongst the various treatment alternatives that have been suggested in this case report, the use of couple mechanics on adjacent teeth is most commonly preferred method. Unfortunately, due to poor control on the adjacent teeth, such mechanics lead to iatrogenic effects causing further delay in treatment.

Since TADs are being used as anchorage in clinical orthodontic treatment widely, there has been a change in treatment approach over the last few years [8–14]. Controlling anchorage in certain cases that demand strict anchorage requirements helps to avoid undesirable tooth movements. However, even a small reactive force can cause undesirable

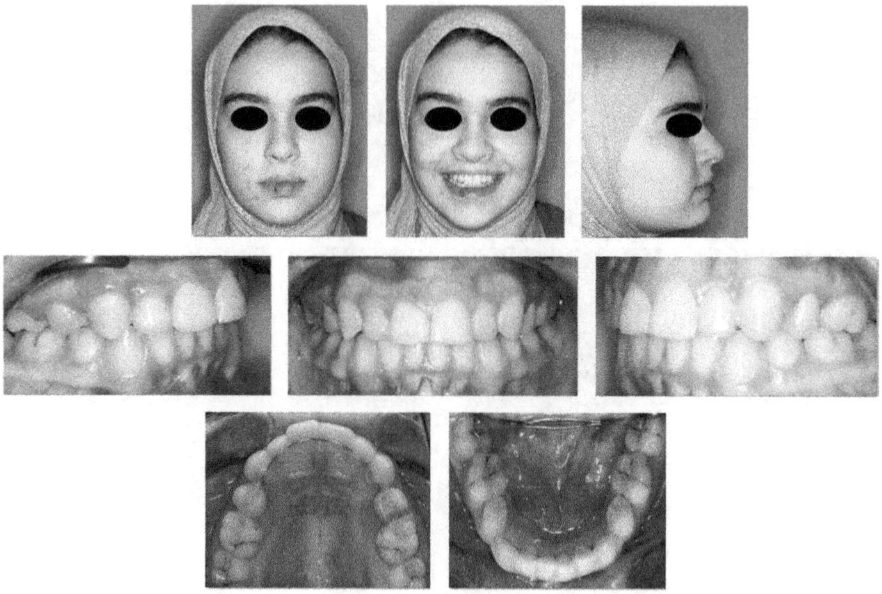

FIGURE 7: Posttreatment extra- and intraoral images 5 years posttreatment.

movements and so; it is important to have absolute anchorage to avoid them [15, 16]. Absolute or infinite anchorage is defined as zero anchorage loss due to the forces applied to move teeth [17]. It can only be obtained by using dental implants as anchors, relying on bone to inhibit movement. Anchorage provided by devices, such as implants or TADs fixed to bone, may be obtained by enhancing the reactive unit's support (indirect anchorage) or by fixing the anchor units (direct anchorage), thus facilitating skeletal anchorage. Orthodontic anchorage is an important factor in obtaining good treatment results. Stable anchorage is a prerequisite for orthodontic treatment with fixed appliances and especially for derotation of rotated posterior teeth [18].

A *couple* is a form of moment. It is created by a pair of forces with equal magnitudes but in opposite directions with a noncoincidental line of action. Because the forces have the same magnitude but are oppositely directed, this special force system's net potential to translate the body on which it acts is nil and there is only pure rotation. The magnitude of the couple's moment (MC) depends on both force magnitude and distance between the two forces. The moment created by a couple is the sum of the moments created by each of the two forces. If there are two forces of a couple system acting on opposite sides of the Cres, their effect to create a moment is additive. If they are on the same side of the Cres, they are subtractive [19]. Both TADs were placed in proximity to the occlusal surface reducing the intrusion on second premolars during derotation, which also allowed for disocclusion in the premolar region. The forces originating from bracket-wire interactions are transmitted to tooth structures causing displacement (unwanted tipping movement), in this case the TADs. The TADs not only provide anchorage but also help bring about pure rotational movement and minimizing the overall treatment time.

Successful orthodontic treatment depends a lot on the various strategies that are employed to prevent relapse of orthodontically treated teeth. There are many factors that may contribute to relapse of a successfully treated malocclusion. Growth in an unfavorable manner or tissue rebound may be some of the factors responsible [20]. Rotated teeth are known to relapse more commonly, and the role of the periodontium has been extensively studied in this regard [20, 21]. Reorientation and lack of reorganization of the supracrestal fibers are considered the main culprit for such relapse [22]. A surgical technique to sever these periodontal fibers was reported by Edwards [23] and was termed circumferential supracrestal fiberotomy (CSF). The theory behind this was that such a surgery would relieve the tension on the supra-alveolar fibers after derotating a tooth, reducing the chances of relapse [21]. Even with long-term retention using fixed retainers, these sets of fibers have poor reorientation or reorganizational capacity [24–26]. Many further studies have validated the efficacy of CSF as a standard to retain derotations in conjunction to other retentive measures [26–28].

Some degree of relapse appeared on upper right central incisor after five years. However, this corresponded with what Al-Jasser et al. [29]; Naraghi et al. [30] found, as they mentioned, that minor relapse in short-term follow-up (1 year) was noted in the maxillary anterior teeth after correction of irregularities compared to a 2 to 4-year period of bonded retention. This result could be attributed to failures that may occur during the retention period without any follow-up checkup of the patient. Other contributing factors to relapse are unfavorable skeletal growth as well as contact point discrepancy relative to the dental arch during the retention period. Changes in the arch form, which frequently occur during both the treatment and posttreatment periods, have also shown to influence retention [20].

Clear aligners (CAT) could also have been explored as one of the options for treating this case. However, several studies have demonstrated that auxiliaries such as attachments and elastics are mandatory in CAT (clear aligner orthodontic therapy) to achieve predictable results. Tooth shape has been shown to influence the efficiency of CAT [31–33], during correction of misalignment due to the geometric interaction between teeth and aligners. Rotation of round-shaped teeth remains one of the less predictable movements in CAT. According to the existing literature [34, 35], the least accurate movement during CAT is premolar rotation. The reduced control of orthodontic tooth movement could be related to the lack of interproximal undercuts between premolars, producing an incorrect force distribution. The biomechanical benefits of a TAD-based anchorage system such as the one used in this study can be utilized for correcting premolar rotations with aligner therapy too. A further study needs to be conducted, and more cases need to be published in orthodontic literature concerning TADs and aligners in conjunction, to understand the possibilities of widening the horizons of orthodontic treatment.

TADs may seem like an overkill to derotate severely rotated teeth, but in fact, they are the most fail-safe mechanics that can guarantee no deleterious effects on adjacent teeth, if used with proper training and understanding of orthodontic biomechanics.

9. Conclusion

Severely rotated teeth need a specifically designed treatment plan when using a fixed orthodontic appliance. Using TADs for correction, such rotated second premolars have a variety of benefits:

(1) Provide maximum anchorage without any effect on the adjacent teeth (zero anchorage loss)

(2) Help reduce the overall treatment time, as the derotations were being carried out simultaneously alongside leveling and alignment

(3) Use TADs as anchorage allowed for use of pure couple forces without any deleterious side effects

Consent

The patient's consent is not required as the patient's identity is not disclosed or compromised. But following usual protocol consent was taken and signed by the patient herself and her parents.

Acknowledgments

The authors wish to thank the patient for her constant support throughout the treatment period.

References

[1] W. Proffit, H. W. Fields, and D. M. Sarver, *Contemporary Orthodontics*, Oxford, UK, Elsevier Health Sciences, 4th edition, 2006.

[2] K. A. Russell and M. A. Folwarczna, "Mesiodens–diagnosis and management of a common supernumerary tooth," *Journal of the Canadian Dental Association*, vol. 69, no. 6, pp. 362–366, 2003.

[3] S. Sunda, P. Khanna, and V. Panghal, "Modified Nance Palatal Arch," *Journal of Medical Research and Health Education*, vol. 1, no. 2, p. 9, 2017.

[4] S. J. Littlewood, D. T. Millett, B. Doubleday, D. R. Bearn, and H. V. Worthington, "Retention procedures for stabilizing tooth position after treatment with orthodontic braces," *Cochrane Database of Systematic Reviews*, vol. 2016, no. 1, article CD002283, 2016.

[5] A. Abdulwhab, J. H. Ku, F. Alfawaz, J. H. Park, and Y. Kook, "Adjunctive surgery after total arch distalization to optimize esthetics," *APOS Trends Orthod*, vol. 10, no. 3, pp. 185–190, 2020.

[6] C. C. H. Chang, J. S. Y. Lin, and H. Y. Yeh, "Extra-alveolar bone screws for conservative correction of severe malocclusion without extractions or orthognathic surgery," *Current Osteoporosis Reports*, vol. 16, no. 4, pp. 387–394, 2018.

[7] M. R. Almeida, "Biomechanics of extra-alveolar mini-implants," *Dental Press Journal of Orthodontics*, vol. 24, no. 4, pp. 93–109, 2019.

[8] A. Carano, S. Velo, P. Leone, and G. Siciliani, "Clinical applications of the mini-screw anchorage system," *Journal of Clinical Orthodontics*, vol. 39, no. 1, pp. 9–24, 2005.

[9] H. S. Park, S. M. Bae, H. M. Kyung, and J. H. Sung, "Micro-implant anchorage for treatment of skeletal class I bialveolar protrusion," *Journal of Clinical Orthodontics*, vol. 35, no. 7, pp. 417–422, 2001.

[10] R. Kanomi, "Mini-implant for orthodontic anchorage," *Journal of Clinical Orthodontics*, vol. 31, no. 11, pp. 763–767, 1997.

[11] K. J. Lee, Y. C. Park, W. S. Hwang, and E. H. Seong, "Uprighting mandibular second molars with direct miniscrew anchorage," *Journal of Clinical Orthodontics*, vol. 41, no. 10, pp. 627–635, 2007.

[12] S. H. Kyung, J. H. Choi, and Y. C. Park, "Miniscrew anchorage used to protract lower second molars into first molar extraction sites," *Journal of Clinical Orthodontics*, vol. 37, no. 10, pp. 575–579, 2003.

[13] J. C. Lin, E. J. Liou, and C. L. Yeh, "Intrusion of overerupted maxillary molars with miniscrew anchorage," *Journal of Clinical Orthodontics*, vol. 40, no. 6, pp. 378–83; quiz 358, 2006.

[14] Y. J. Jeon, Y. H. Kim, W. S. Son, and M. G. Hans, "Correction of a canted occlusal plane with miniscrews in a patient with facial asymmetry," *American Journal of Orthodontics and Dentofacial Orthopedics*, vol. 130, no. 2, pp. 244–252, 2006.

[15] S. Weinstein, D. C. Haak, L. Morris, B. B. Snyder, and H. Y. Attaway, "On equilibrium theory of tooth position," *The Angle Orthodontist.*, vol. 33, pp. 1–26, 1963.

[16] J. J. Pilon, A. M. Kuijpers-Jagtman, and J. C. Maltha, "Magnitude of orthodontic forces and rate of bodily tooth movement. An experimental study," *American Journal of Orthodontics and Dentofacial Orthopedics*, vol. 110, no. 1, pp. 16–23, 1996.

[17] J. Daskalogiannakis, *Glossary of Orthodontic Terms*, Quintessence Books, Michigan, 2000.

[18] P. K. Turley, C. Kean, J. Schur et al., "Orthodontic force application to titanium endosseous implants," *The Angle Orthodontist*, vol. 58, no. 2, pp. 151–162, 1988.

[19] U. Madhur and R. Nanda, *Biomechanics Principles in Mini-Implant Driven Orthodontics*, Vasiliadis books, Greece, 2020.

[20] J. C. Maltha, V. Vandevska-Radunovic, and A. M. Kuijpers-Jagtman, "The biological background of relapse of orthodontic tooth movement," in *Biological mechanisms of tooth movement*, pp. 225–248, John Wiley & Sons, 2015.

[21] T. Lv, N. Kang, C. Wang, X. Han, Y. Chen, and D. Bai, "Biologic response of rapid tooth movement with periodontal ligament distraction," *American Journal of Orthodontics and Dentofacial Orthopedics*, vol. 136, no. 3, pp. 401–411, 2009.

[22] R. Al-Jasser, M. Al-Subaie, N. Al-Jasser, and A. Al-Rasheed, "Rotational relapse of anterior teeth following orthodontic treatment and circumferential supracrestal fiberotomy," *Saudi Dent J.*, vol. 32, no. 6, pp. 293–299, 2020, Epub 2019 Oct 24.

[23] J. G. Edwards, "A study of the periodontium during orthodontic rotation of teeth," *American Journal of Orthodontics*, vol. 54, no. 6, pp. 441–461, 1968.

[24] W. Beertsen, "Remodelling of collagen fibers in the periodontal ligament and the supra-alveolar region," *The Angle Orthodontist*, vol. 49, no. 3, pp. 218–224, 1979.

[25] K. Reitan, "Tissue rearrangement during retention of orthodontically rotated teeth," *The Angle Orthodontist.*, vol. 29, no. 2, pp. 105–113, 1959.

[26] R. W. Block, D. G. Kerns, F. J. Regennitter, and L. L. Kerns, "The circumferential supracrestal fiberotomy," *General Dentistry*, vol. 46, no. 1, pp. 48–54, 1998.

[27] K. Dhingra, K. L. Vandana, P. V. Girish, and C. Cobb, "Effect of 980-nm diode laser-aided circumferential supracrestal fiberotomy on fluorosed root surfaces," *The Angle Orthodontist*, vol. 83, no. 3, pp. 425–430, 2013.

[28] S. J. Littlewood, D. T. Millett, B. Doubleday, D. R. Bearn, and H. V. Worthington, "Orthodontic retention: a systematic review," *Journal of Orthodontics*, vol. 33, no. 3, pp. 205–212, 2006.

[29] R. Al-Jasser, T. Al-Jewair, and A. Al-Rasheed, "One-year rotational relapse frequency following conventional circumferential supracrestal fiberotomy," *World Journal of Clinical Cases*, vol. 8, no. 2, pp. 284–293, 2020.

[30] S. Naraghi, A. Andrén, H. Kjellberg, and B. O. Mohlin, "Relapse tendency after orthodontic correction of upper front teeth retained with a bonded retainer," *The Angle Orthodontist.*, vol. 76, no. 4, pp. 570–576, 2006.

[31] S. Barone, A. Paoli, A. V. Razionale, and R. Savignano, "Computational design and engineering of polymeric orthodontic aligners," *Int J Numer Method Biomed Eng.*, vol. 33, no. 8, article e2839, 2017.

[32] W. Hahn, A. Zapf, H. Dathe et al., "Torquing an upper central incisor with aligners–acting forces and biomechanical principles," *European Journal of Orthodontics*, vol. 32, no. 6, pp. 607–613, 2010.

[33] F. Elkholy, B. Mikhaiel, F. Schmidt, and B. G. Lapatki, "Mechanical load exerted by PET-G aligners during mesial and distal derotation of a mandibular canine: an in vitro study," *Journal of Orofacial Orthopedics*, vol. 78, no. 5, pp. 361–370, 2017.

[34] N. D. Kravitz, B. Kusnoto, B. Agran, and G. Viana, "Influence of attachments and interproximal reduction on the accuracy of canine rotation with Invisalign. A prospective clinical study," *The Angle Orthodontist*, vol. 78, no. 4, pp. 682–687, 2008.

[35] A. Cortona, G. Rossini, S. Parrini, A. Deregibus, and T. Castroflorio, "Clear aligner orthodontic therapy of rotated mandibular round-shaped teeth: a finite element study," *The Angle Orthodontist*, vol. 90, no. 2, pp. 247–254, 2020.

18

Functional Band and Loop Space Maintainers in Children

V. Vinothini,[1] A. Sanguida,[2] A. Selvabalaji,[2] G. S. Prathima,[2] and M. Kavitha[2]

[1]*Vinu Dental Clinic, Erode 638 452, Gobichettipalayam, India*
[2]*Department of Paedodontics and Preventive Dentistry, Indira Gandhi Institute of Dental Sciences, Sri Balaji Vidyapeeth, Pillaiyarkuppam, Puducherry 607 402, India*

Correspondence should be addressed to V. Vinothini; drvinumds@gmail.com

Academic Editor: Michael W. Roberts

Premature loss of teeth in children leads to space loss and affects arch integrity. The band and loop space maintainer is used in majority of patients requiring single tooth space maintenance in both primary and mixed dentitions. It preserves the proximal dimensions, but it is nonfunctional. This paper describes a method to modify the conventional band and loop space maintainer into a functional one and reports its clinical application and follow-up in five children.

1. Introduction

A healthy primary dentition preserves space for permanent teeth and maintains arch integrity. Diverse dietary patterns make children more susceptible to dental caries and result in premature loss of primary teeth, thereby necessitating placement of space maintainers [1, 2]. Space maintainers guide the eruption of the permanent teeth and obviate the need for complex orthodontic treatment later. The most commonly used fixed space maintainer is the band and loop space maintainer. Although it is easier to construct, economical, and consumes less chair-side time, it fails to restore the occlusal function of the lost tooth. Hence, an attempt is made to modify the appliance so as to make it functional.

2. Technique of Fabrication of the Functional Band and Loop Space Maintainer

The first step is to construct a conventional band and loop space maintainer in the region of premature tooth loss. This is followed by the placement of an acrylic tooth in the edentulous area of the cast and stabilization with modeling wax. The occlusion is then checked with the cast of the opposing arch and adjusted. Cold cure acrylic is used to attach the pontic to the loop. The completed appliance is then finished and polished (Figure 1). Trial fit is done in patient's mouth, and the appliance is checked for the presence of soft tissue irritation or occlusal interferences and adjusted accordingly. The final cementation of the appliance is done.

3. Case 1

A 6-year-old female patient reported to the Department of Pedodontics with a chief complaint of pain in the upper right back tooth region. The right maxillary deciduous first molar was carious with the resorption of more than 2/3rd of its roots and hence had to be extracted. Model analysis was done followed by the placement of a fixed functional band and loop space maintainer (Figure 2).

4. Case 2

A 6-year-old boy had grossly decayed teeth 74, 75, 84, and 85. Radiograph of 74 showed poor prognosis and was extracted. Pulpectomy was done for the remaining teeth, and teeth were restored with stainless steel crowns. A functional band and loop space maintainer was cemented in relation to 74. Patient was recalled after three months, and it was found that there was no soft tissue irritation or dislodgement of the appliance (Figure 3).

5. Case 3

A 7-year-old female patient reported with the chief complaint of multiple decayed teeth and also with a history of

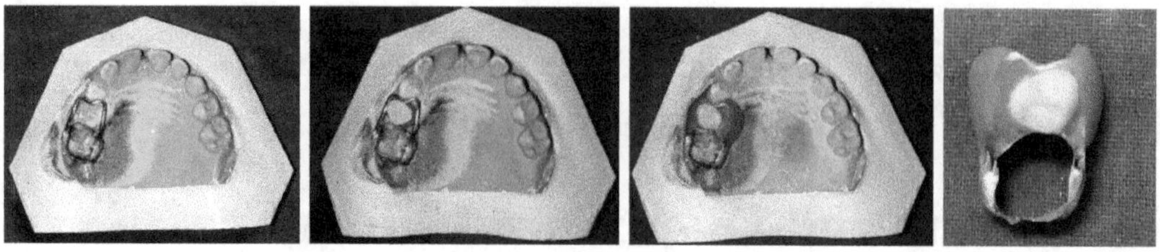

Figure 1: Steps in the construction of a functional band and loop space maintainer.

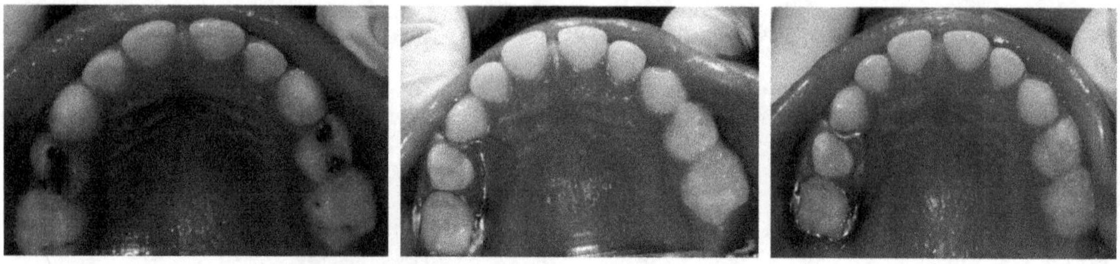

Figure 2: Preoperative, immediate postoperative, and one-year postoperative occlusal views of the maxillary arch with the functional band and loop space maintainer in the tooth 54 region.

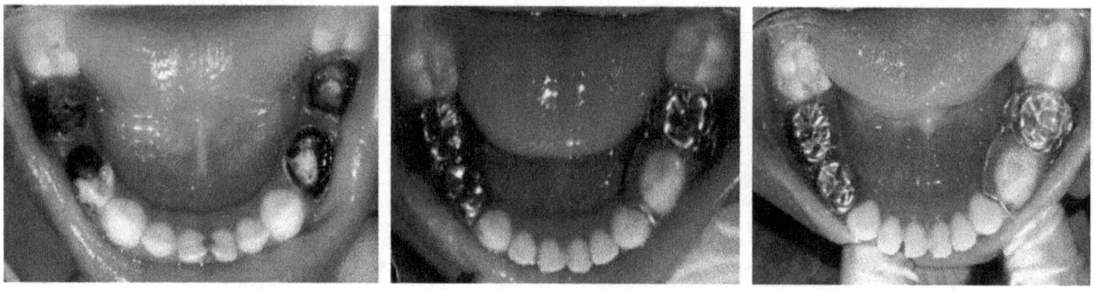

Figure 3: Preoperative, immediate postoperative, and one-year postoperative occlusal views of the mandibular arch with the functional band and loop space maintainer in the tooth 74 region.

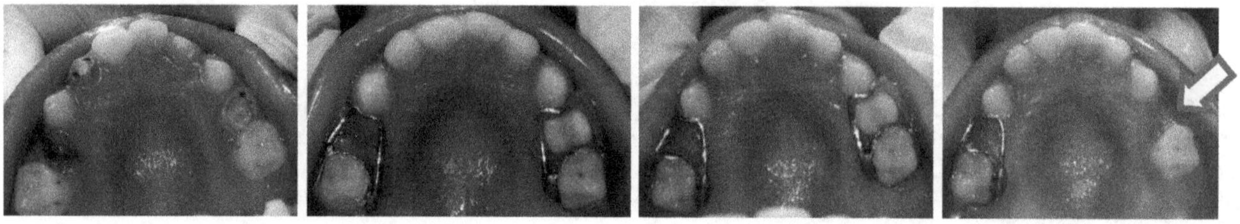

Figure 4: Preoperative, immediate postoperative, and one-year postoperative occlusal views of the maxillary arch with the conventional band and loop space maintainer in the tooth 54 region and functional band and loop space maintainer in the tooth 64 region. Note the absence of tissue changes (arrow).

extraction of the decayed right upper back tooth. Clinical examination revealed grossly decayed 53 and 64 and clinically missing 54. Radiograph of 64 revealed a poor prognosis and hence was extracted. Following model analysis, a conventional band and loop space maintainer in the 54 region and a functional band and loop space maintainer in the 64 region were cemented. Tooth 53 was endodontically treated and esthetically restored with composite resin (Figure 4). Patient was reviewed every three months, and she reported that the fixed functional band and loop space maintainer helped her to chew comfortably. There was no mucosal irritation in relation to the appliance.

6. Case 4

A 6-year-old female patient reported with clinically missing 74 and 84. Past dental records revealed the extraction of teeth 74 and 84 due to caries four months and two months earlier, respectively. History of difficulty in mastication was also reported. Model analysis was done. There was no space loss; hence, it was planned to maintain space with the functional band and loop space maintainer in relation to 84 and conventional one in relation to 74. Patient was recalled every three months for review, and she felt comfortable to chew on the right side (Figure 5).

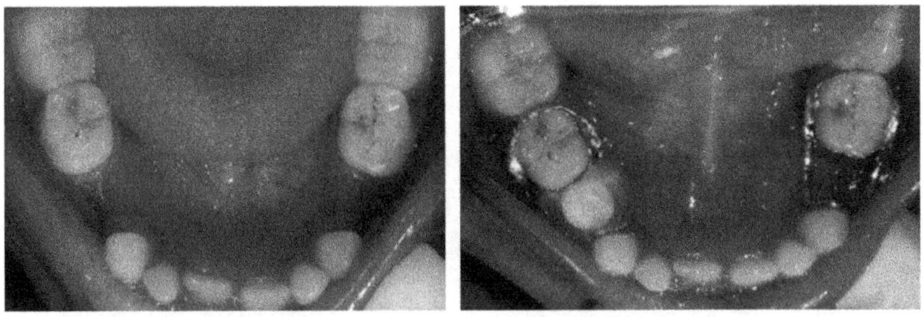

FIGURE 5: Preoperative and immediate postoperative views of the mandibular arch with the conventional band and loop space maintainer in the tooth 74 region and functional band and loop space maintainer in the tooth 84 region.

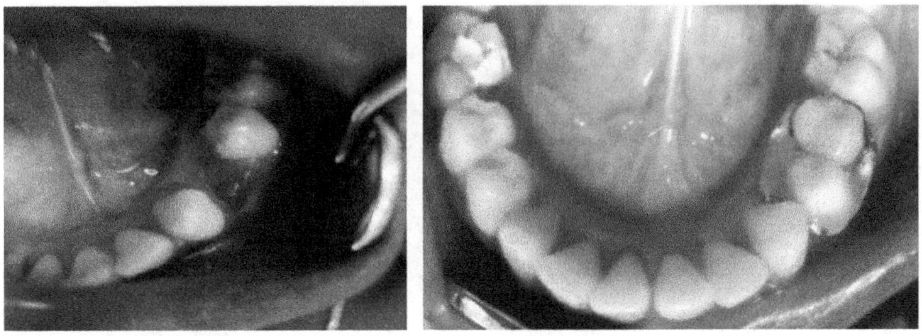

FIGURE 6: Preoperative and immediate postoperative occlusal views of the mandibular arch with the functional band and loop space maintainer in the tooth 34 region.

7. Case 5

A 13-year-old girl reported to the department with complaint of several broken teeth and one lost permanent tooth. Parents gave history of trauma to the chin region due to accidental fall from a tractor ten days before reporting. Her medical history was not remarkable. On intraoral examination, tooth numbers 15, 16, 25, 26, 35, 36, and 45 had sustained uncomplicated crown fractures. Tooth number 34 was clinically missing, and tooth number 46 showed a complicated crown fracture. Panoramic radiograph confirmed the avulsion of 34 and showed no evidence of fracture involving maxilla or mandible. It was planned to restore tooth numbers 15, 25, 35, and 45 with composite restorations, perform RCT in 46, and restore 16, 26, 36, and 46 with stainless steel crowns as they had extensive tooth structure loss due to the impact of trauma. A functional space maintainer (band and loop with acrylic pontic of tooth number 34) was planned as an interim prosthesis and a space maintainer in the tooth 34 region. As the tooth 35 had extensive tooth loss on lingual aspect, the band would also help in the retention of the composite restoration till future definitive restorative management (Figure 6).

TABLE 1

Advantages
(1) Aids in mastication.
(2) Prevents supraeruption of the opposing tooth.
(3) Distribution of occlusal forces on the pontic and hence less chance of loop distortion/slippage and impingement in gingiva.
(4) Prevents the development of abnormal tongue habits.
Limitations and possible solutions
(1) Direct visualization of the eruption of the successor is not possible.
(a) Hence, long-term and frequent follow-ups (preferably using radiographs—RVG) are required. Periodic removal and clinical inspection for signs of the eruption of the successor or tissue irritation followed by recementation should be performed as would be done for any traditional space maintainer.
(b) Parents should be informed that the pontic alone will be removed from the appliance when the child approaches the eruption age of the successor or if there is clinical or radiographic evidence of impending tooth emergence.
(2) Cement loss and solder failure can be possible reasons for failure of this appliance. Hence, quality designing of the appliance, close supervision, and frequent follow-ups at 2-4 month interval are imperative.

8. Discussion

Band and loop appliance is a versatile space maintainer for maintaining space due to premature loss of a single tooth [3]. It has shown good success rates [4–6]. However, the disadvantage is that it is not functional. Apart from maintaining the mesiodistal dimension of the space created by premature loss of a tooth, a space maintainer should aid in mastication and prevent overeruption of the opposing tooth or teeth. It should also be simple, not interfere with normal occlusal adjustments, or restrict normal growth and development [2]. However, no space maintainer fulfills all the ideal requirements. A new technique of the fabrication of a functional band and loop space maintainer was described in this report. Table 1 lists the pros and cons of the modified space maintainer compared to the traditional band and loop space maintainer.

In order to compare the acceptability of the modified band and loop space maintainer with that of the conventional one, two children were given both types. The two children reported satisfaction with the modified band and loop space maintainer and found that it is comfortable for eating.

All the children were recalled every three months. This appliance design did not interfere with oral hygiene maintenance nor did it causes soft tissue irritation, discomfort, or food lodgement. There were no reports of fracture of the appliance. However, it should be noted that the maximum follow-up period was only one year; hence, long-term follow-up is essential to evaluate the longevity of the appliance.

9. Conclusion

Managing space and at the same time improving the masticatory function and maintaining arch integrity in early loss of the primary teeth are challenging tasks. The functional band and loop space maintainer described in this report will be a good choice for use in premature loss of a single tooth in very young children.

References

[1] M. A. Qudeimat and S. A. Fayle, "The longevity of space maintainers: a retrospective study," *Pediatric Dentistry*, vol. 20, no. 4, pp. 267–272, 1998.

[2] J. R. Christensen and H. W. Fields Jr, "Space maintenance in the primary dentition," in *Pediatric Dentistry: Infancy Through Adolescence*, J. R. Pinkham, P. S. Casamassimo, H. W. Fields Jr, D. J. McTigue, and A. J. Nowak, Eds., pp. 419–448, Elsevier Saunders, Missouri, 2005.

[3] V. Setia, I. K. Pandit, N. Srivastava, N. Gugnani, and H. K. Sekhon, "Space maintainers in dentistry: past to present," *Journal Of Clinical And Diagnostic Research*, vol. 7, no. 10, pp. 2402–2405, 2013.

[4] C. Baroni, A. Franchini, and L. Rimondini, "Survival of different types of space maintainers," *Pediatric Dentistry*, vol. 16, no. 5, pp. 360-361, 1994.

[5] L. D. Rajab, "Clinical performance and survival of space maintainers: evaluation over a period of 5 years," *Journal of Dentistry for Children*, vol. 69, pp. 156–160, 2002.

[6] M. Fathian, D. B. Kennedy, and M. R. Nouri, "Laboratory-made space maintainers: a 7-year retrospective study from private pediatric dental practice," *Pediatric Dentistry*, vol. 29, no. 6, pp. 500–506, 2007.

19

Dental and Maxillofacial Manifestations of Axenfeld–Rieger Syndrome: Presentation of a Case in a 5-Year-Old Girl

Carlos-Martín Ardila and Efraín Álvarez-Martínez

Universidad de Antioquia, Medellín, Colombia

Correspondence should be addressed to Carlos-Martín Ardila; martin.ardila@udea.edu.co

Academic Editor: Maria Beatriz Duarte Gavião

In this case study, the dental and maxillofacial manifestations of a 5-year-old girl with Axenfeld–Rieger syndrome (ARS) are described. This syndrome is characterized by craniomaxillofacial, ocular, dental, and umbilical disorders. The patient presented ocular dyscoria and corectopia, iris abnormalities, midface hypoplasia with a thin upper lip, and a protruded lower lip. Hyperplastic maxillary labial frenulum, oligodontia, ghost teeth, bilateral Class III molar and canine relationship, and right posterior crossbite were also found. An everted umbilicus with redundant periumbilical skin was evident. Early diagnosis of ARS is essential to establishing preventive and corrective measures that provide a good quality of life for patients who suffer from this syndrome.

1. Introduction

Axenfeld–Rieger syndrome (ARS) is a rare autosomal dominant disorder with a worldwide incidence of 1 : 200,000. It encompasses a spectrum of genetically inherited disorders that are characterized by dental, ocular, craniofacial, and periumbilical abnormalities [1]. It is a hereditary disorder with almost complete penetrance and variable expression. Inheritance is autosomal dominant in 70% of cases [2]. In addition to its pathogenesis, there are no definitive data on its racial or gender prevalence. It is believed to arise as an ectodermal tissue defect caused by disorders of the neural crest. The differentiation and migration of the neural crest cells are responsible for (among other things) the induction of the enamel organ from the oral epithelium, and for the formation of normal ocular and craniofacial structures [3]. ARS has been associated with a wide variety of oral and dental abnormalities, including deciduous and permanent hypodontia (particularly maxillary anteriors), hyperplastic maxillary labial frenulum, microdontia, taurodontia, enamel hypoplasia, and peg-shaped teeth. Craniofacial features are dominated by midface hypoplasia due to maxillary hypoplasia, relative mandibular prognathism, and a broad, flat nasal root. Moreover, protruded lower lip or recessive upper lip and prominent supraorbital ridges are observed [2, 4].

Three types of ARS have been described. Type 1 is mainly characterized by dental abnormalities and midface hypoplasia secondary to underdeveloped maxillary sinuses. Type 2 includes hearing loss and heart defects, while Type 3 features ocular manifestations but lesser facial and dental abnormalities [5]. Recently, important innovations in the molecular genetics of ARS and associated phenotypes have been described. Three genetic loci have been recognized on chromosomes 4q25, 6p25, and 13q14. The genes at 4q25 and 6p25 have also been acknowledged and are termed "PITX2" and "FKHL7", respectively. The detection of these loci and genes has shed novel information on the interrelation of the Axenfeld–Rieger phenotypes. Therefore, all of these phenotypes may be considered together under the single heading of ARS, with the benefit of simplifying interaction between clinicians and scientists and remove subjective and unclear subclassification [6].

This article describes the maxillofacial and dental characteristics of one of the few cases worldwide of ARS that have been reported.

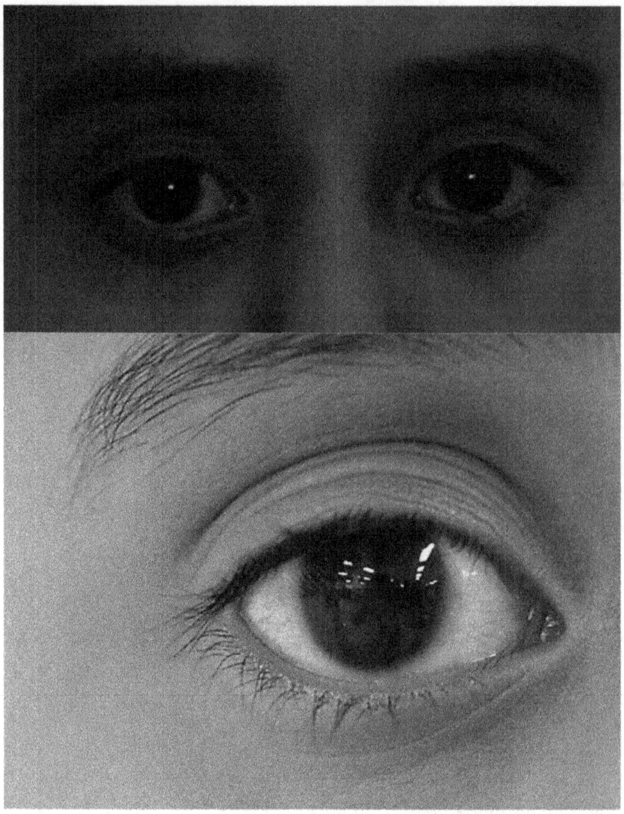

Figure 1: Evidence of pupillary dyscoria.

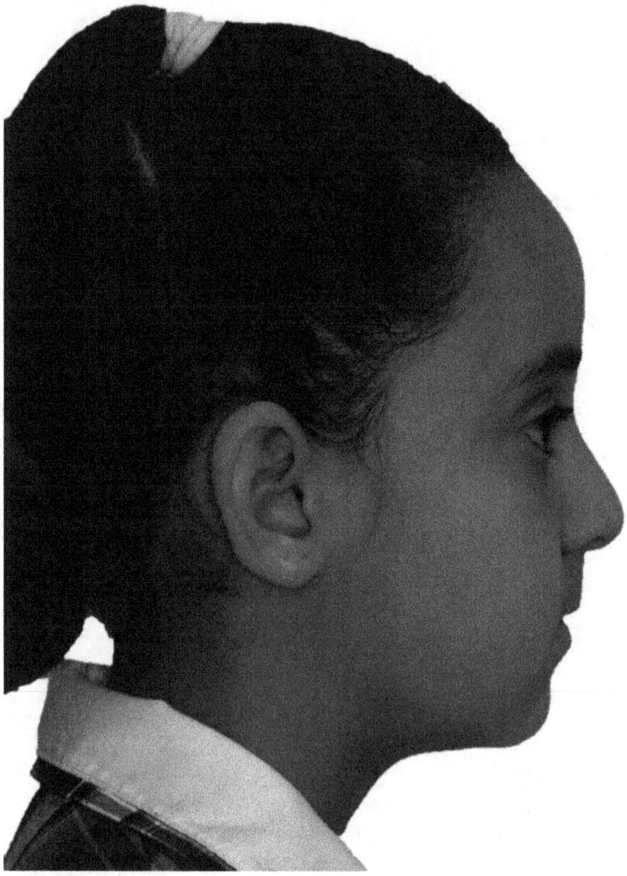

Figure 2: There is a greater predominance of the upper third of the face with respect to the middle and lower thirds. A slightly flattened mentolabial angle is observed.

2. Case Report

A 5-year-old girl, accompanied by her father, consulted for her daughter's dental alterations. The patient did not report any pain. The medical history revealed a consult for pupillary dyscoria, with no family history of craniofacial or dental anomalies. The patient's diagnosis of ARS was made during the first years of her life.

In the general examination, the patient had a good disposition, she was oriented in time, place, and person, and communicated easily.

Her extraoral characteristics included pupillary dyscoria (Figure 1), corectopia, blepharitis, abnormalities in the iris, and posterior embryotoxon. In profile analysis, there is a greater predominance of the upper third of the face with respect to the middle and lower thirds (Figure 2). Moreover, a slightly flattened infraorbital area, prominent cheekbones, straight nasolabial angle, superior retrochelia, resting labial seal, inferior normochelia, and slightly flattened mentolabial angle are observed (Figure 2).

In the lateral cephalic radiography, skeletal Class III due to mild maxillary macrognathism is shown. In addition, an increased lower facial third is observed (Figure 3).

The panoramic X-ray (Figure 4) shows a slightly narrower right nostril than the left. Early mixed maxillary dentition is observed where 16 and 26 are erupted. Teeth 17-11-21-23-24 and 27 are in intraosseous formation, in Nolla stage between 3 and 5; therefore, the formation of the other maxillary permanent teeth is not appreciated, indicating their agenesis (Figure 4). The patient presents mixed mandibular dentition (Figures 4 and 5); it is also observed that 36-31-41-46 erupted without apical closure (physiological phase), complete deciduous dentition, except 71 and 81 already exfoliated (Figure 4).

Intraorally, traction of the upper labial frenulum, associated with lack of vertical development of the superior alveolar process, is observed. Asymmetric oval arches and dental malocclusion Class III are shown (Figure 5).

Another prominent manifestation was the everted umbilicus with redundant periumbilical skin (Figure 6).

To ensure the preservation of the existing dentition, preventive dental measures were recommended, including oral hygiene instruction to the girl and her parents, as well as the sealing of pits and fissures of all molars. Trimestral check-ups with the dentist were also suggested. The orthodontist recommended a facial mask protocol with a Hyrax and a posteroinferior bite plane. The Hyrax was recommended to prevent cross-sectional discrepancy between the arches considering the Class III relationship and dental agenesis, in addition to disarticulating the circumpubertal sutures to perform the protraction of the maxilla. The posteroinferior bite plane was recommended to control verticality. The facial mask protracts the maxilla and contains mandibular growth.

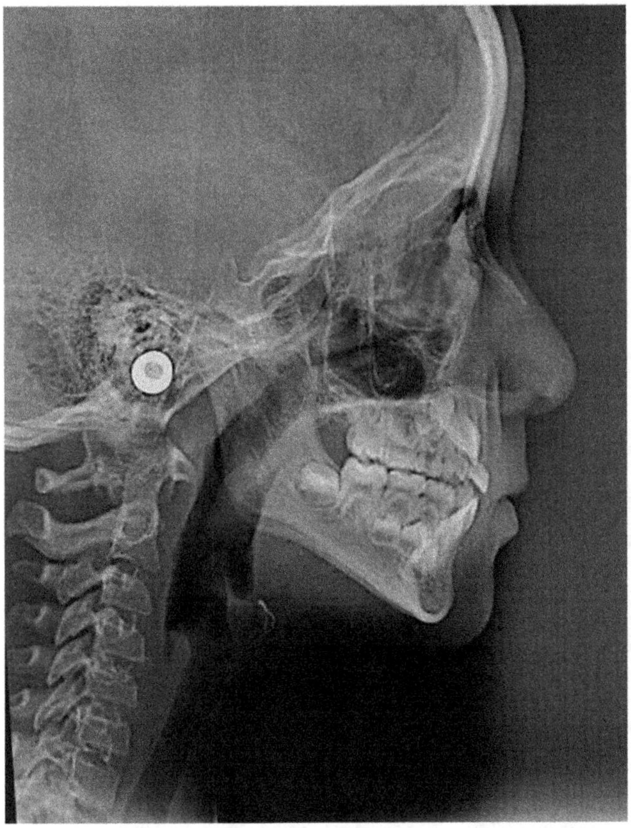

FIGURE 3: The lateral cephalic radiography shows skeletal Class III due to mild maxillary macrognathism.

3. Discussion

In this case, the dental and maxillofacial manifestations of a 5-year-old girl with ARS were described. To the authors' knowledge, this case represents the youngest patient with this syndrome, incorporating reportage of its dental and maxillofacial features. Early dental care of a patient with ARS allows establishing multidisciplinary prevention and treatment strategies that will improve the long-term prognosis of this complex condition. Early detection of ARS can also prevent serious ophthalmological problems.

The literature has extensively described the genetic etiology, ophthalmological and cardiac characteristics, and the treatment of ARS; however, the dental and facial characteristics and their management have been detailed to a lesser extent [7].

The craniomaxillofacial singularities found in ARS commonly include a broad forehead, sella turcica disorders, telecanthus, hypertelorism, dyscoria, disorders of the characteristics of the nose, hypoplasia of the midface, mandibular prognathism, an open-mouth appearance with a thin upper lip and retracted, and with a prominent lower lip [7]. However, some patients do not present any malformation of the craniofacial structures or skeletal bones, and are considered to have a variant of Rieger syndrome called ARS [8]. As in the case reported by Megighian et al. [8], in addition to the presence of dyscoria, the present case exhibits no major craniofacial bone changes, except for hypoplasia of the midface and a pseudoprognathism [5]. It has also been described that maxillary hypoplasia is found in around 90.5% of cases, with a skeletal Class III concave facial profile associated with a flat midface [7].

Oral manifestations include hyperplastic upper labial frenulum, enamel hypoplasia, hypodontia, oligodontia, microdontia, taurodontism, conical teeth, short roots, and delayed eruption [2, 4, 7, 9]. Some of these characteristics were evident in the present case, including that the upper anterior teeth are more frequently absent [8]. In this regard, it has been considered that the number of absent teeth has a specific role in the extent of maxillary hypoplasia due to the resulting alveolar hypoplasia [7, 9].

In this case, like that reported by Agarwal et al. [7], an everted umbilicus with redundant periumbilical skin was evidenced, mimicking an umbilical hernia [2].

Considering the characteristics of the present case, the multidisciplinary management includes the correction of maxillary hypoplasia using myofunctional orthopedic appliances, in addition to preserving the deciduous teeth as far as possible to maintain function and aesthetic appearance. Depending on the evolution of the dental eruption, the assisted eruption of the impacted teeth and the orthodontic correction of the preexisting dentition could be planned [10]. Oligodontia could be treated with prosthetic rehabilitation to restore form

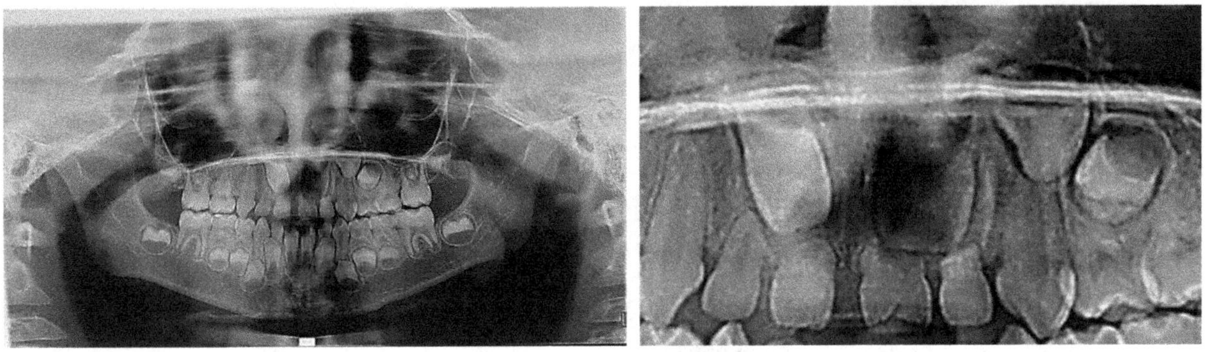

(a) (b)

FIGURE 4: Panoramic X-ray shows teeth 17-11-21-23-24 and 27 in intraosseous formation, in Nolla stage between 3 and 5. The formation of the other maxillary permanent teeth is not appreciated, indicating their agenesis (a and b). Panel (b) shows a close-up view of the anterosuperior area. The formation of teeth 12, 22, and 13 is not appreciated.

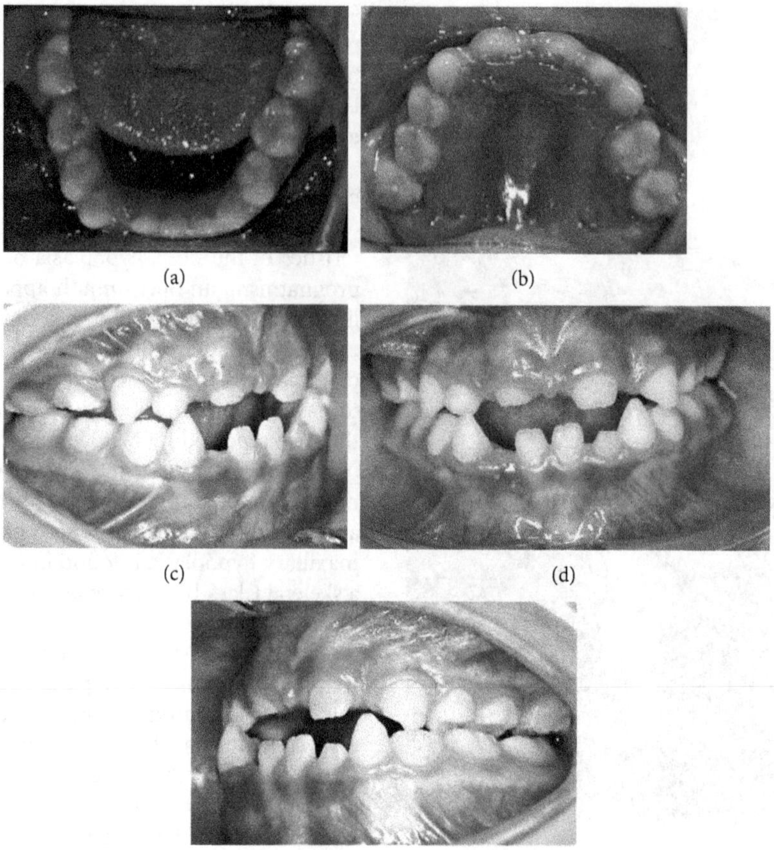

(a) (b) (c) (d) (e)

Figure 5: Asymmetrical oval arches and dental malocclusion Class III are shown (a and b). Traction upper labial frenulum associated with lack of vertical development of the superior alveolar process is observed (c, d, and e).

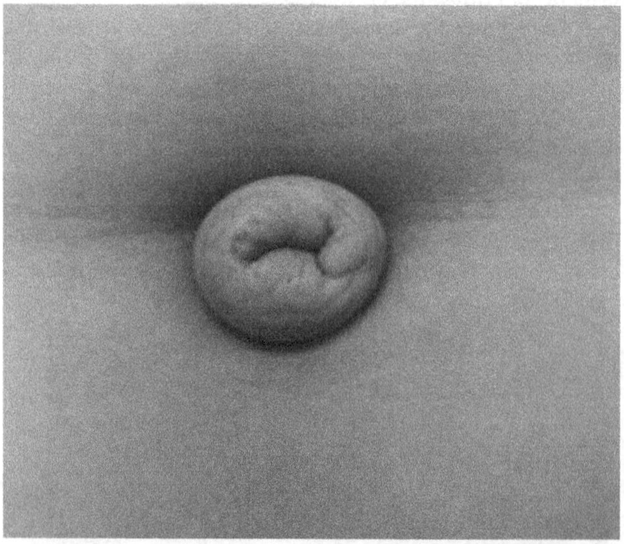

Figure 6: The existence of an everted umbilicus.

and function; dental implant restoration would be a feasible long-term treatment option. Consultation with ophthalmology is essential in order to control the evolution of vision.

Early diagnosis of ARS is essential to establish preventive and corrective measures that provide a good quality of life for patients who suffer from it.

Consent

The patient's father signed the informed consent related to hospital care and for academic purposes. Moreover, written consent to publish their clinical details and photographs was given by her father.

Acknowledgments

The authors acknowledge their employment relationship with the Universidad de Antioquia.

References

[1] F. Idrees, D. Vaideanu, S. G. Fraser, J. C. Sowden, and P. T. Khaw, "A review of anterior segment dysgeneses," *Survey of Ophthalmology*, vol. 51, no. 3, pp. 213–231, 2006.

[2] E. M. O'Dwyer and D. C. Jones, "Dental anomalies in Axenfeld-Rieger syndrome," *International Journal of Paediatric Dentistry*, vol. 15, no. 6, pp. 459–463, 2005.

[3] J. Dimitrakopoulos, N. Voyatzis, and T. Katopodi, "Rieger syndrome: a case report," *Journal of Oral and Maxillofacial Surgery*, vol. 55, no. 5, pp. 517–521, 1997.

[4] N. Fitch and M. Kaback, "The Axenfeld syndrome and the Rieger syndrome," *Journal of Medical Genetics*, vol. 15, no. 1, pp. 30–34, 1978.

[5] S. Singh, A. Narula, S. Chakarborty, and S. Chanana, "Axenfeld–Rieger syndrome: a rare developmental disorder," *Journal of Ophthalmology*, vol. 24, no. 4, 265 pages, 2014.

[6] W. L. Alward, "Axenfeld-Rieger syndrome in the age of molecular genetics," *American Journal of Ophthalmology*, vol. 130, no. 1, pp. 107–115, 2000.

[7] P. Agarwal, K. Jain, S. Sandesh, and S. Chopra, "Axenfeld-Rieger syndrome: rare case presentation and overview," *Journal of Oral and Maxillofacial Surgery*, vol. 19, no. 3, pp. 364–369, 2020.

[8] D. Megighian, M. Savastano, and P. Poli, "Rieger syndrome: case report," *The International Tinnitus Journal*, vol. 9, pp. 134–137, 2003.

[9] A. Villa, A. Albonico, and F. Villa, "Hypodontia and microdontia: clinical features of a rare syndrome," *Journal of the Canadian Dental Association*, vol. 77, article b115, 2011.

[10] C. A. Bender, M. J. Koudstaal, J. F. van Elswijk, C. Prahl, and E. B. Wolvius, "Two cases of Axenfeld-Rieger syndrome, report of the complex pathology and treatment," *The Cleft Palate-Craniofacial Journal*, vol. 51, no. 3, pp. 354–360, 2014.

20

Regenerative Endodontic Treatment of Maxillary Incisors with a History of Severe Traumatic Injury

Nazanin Chitsaz, Mehrfam Khoshkhounejad, Hadi Assadian, Behnam Bolhari, Mohammadreza Sharifian, and Zahra Mohammadi

Department of Endodontics, School of Dentistry, Tehran University of Medical Sciences (TUMS), Tehran, Iran

Correspondence should be addressed to Zahra Mohammadi; zahramohammadi704@gmail.com

Academic Editor: Hamdi Cem Gungor

The treatment objective for children with avulsed anterior teeth should concentrate on preserving the alveolar bone volume and contour. Posttraumatic external inflammatory root resorption (EIRR) is also a high-risk complication often observed in children. Regenerative endodontic procedure (REP) has been considered a successful treatment to arrest EIRR, especially in posttraumatic cases. This case report presents clinical outcomes of REP in two teeth of an 8-year-old systemically healthy patient with a history of severe dentoalveolar traumatic injury, one with a history of avulsion, and the other with an EIRR. The treatment consisted of REP on both teeth #8 and #9. The results showed some evidence of maturation in the apical third of tooth #9 and resolution of signs and symptoms on tooth #8.

1. Introduction

Dental trauma is a significant risk to dental health in young individuals. Dental trauma often occurs in children between 6 to 13 years of age, most commonly involving teeth with incomplete root formation. The most frequent dental injury at this age is crown fracture [1]. Avulsion of permanent teeth is the most severe dentoalveolar injury. It is relatively infrequent, ranging from 0.5% to 16% of traumatic injuries in the permanent dentition [2, 3]. In a literature review, Glendor concluded that one-fourth of all school children and one-third of adults suffered from traumatic dental injuries (TDIs) in permanent dentition [4]. Injuries include fracturing, displacing, or losing teeth, crushing and/or fracturing bone and soft tissue contusions, abrasions, and lacerations [5].

Tooth avulsion, which is also known as exarticulation or total luxation, is defined as complete displacement of the tooth out of its alveolar socket [6]. Loss of permanent teeth in growing children can result in severe atrophy of the residual ridge, which is difficult to restore with either implants or fixed partial dentures [5]. Therefore, preservation of the avulsed teeth is of utmost importance especially in anterior region for future reconstruction. Consequently, replantation is currently considered to be the treatment of choice for avulsed permanent teeth, and immediate replantation of the avulsed tooth is the best treatment at the place of the accident. However, common complications such as pulp necrosis and infection, ankylosis-related (replacement) resorption, and infection-related (inflammatory) resorption are frequently seen following replantation of avulsed permanent teeth [5–7]. The International Association for Dental Traumatology outlined guidelines advocating that replantation should be performed within 60 minutes after injury to have a better prognosis. Delayed replantation (>60 minutes) has been shown to have a poor long-term prognosis with eventual ankylosis and resorption [5, 8, 9]. Delayed replantation is preferred over not replanting in children with avulsed teeth because promotion of alveolar bone growth will be more predictable. In addition, replantation can provide improved esthetics, and function and psychological reasons are other benefits of replantation [10]. Following avulsion, the most desirable outcome can be met after a REP since the damaged tooth can pursue its maturation process [11].

It has been shown that delayed replantation of avulsed immature teeth provides a poor prognosis due to the sustained damages to the pulp and periodontal tissues which can impede further radicular development [6].

External root resorption (ERR) is considered a frequent consequence of severe dentoalveolar traumatic injury. EIRR which is a type of ERR is a pathologic process commonly seen after infection, pressure, trauma, or orthodontic tooth movement. In other words, EIRR occurs as a consequence inflammation and loss of radicular protective barriers following mechanical or chemical insults [12]. Posttraumatic EIRR is a considerable and common complication of dentoalveolar traumatic injuries in children [13]. Several treatment options have been proposed by authors to arrest EIRR with contradictory, uncertain, and unpredictable results [14–16]. Lately, Yoshpe et al. [14] described a case in which a regenerative endodontic procedure (REP) using PRF as a scaffold showed arrested EIRR of tooth #9, which had undergone trauma-induced EIRR.

This study is aimed at describing clinical outcomes of REPs in two teeth of a patient with a history of avulsion of tooth #8 and EIRR in tooth #9.

2. Case Report

An 8-year-old girl was referred to the Department of Endodontics at Tehran University of Medical Sciences (TUMS) School of Dentistry with a chief complaint of a sinus tract in the maxillary right central incisor (Figure 1(a)). She presented normal systemic health and corresponded to class I according to ASA health classification. Patient's dental history revealed a traumatic injury about one month before her referral that had caused avulsion of tooth #8 and complicated crown fracture of tooth #9. On the day of trauma, the patient had been referred to an emergency department of a hospital with a delay of 5 hours, and the tooth had been replanted. Patient's avulsed tooth had been kept in patient's mouth before replantation. Following replantation, a splint was established with sutures. Afterward, the patient was referred to the Department of Pediatric Dentistry the day after the injury for partial pulpotomy of tooth #9. Eventually, the patient was referred to the Department of Endodontics about one month later to evaluate and treat a sinus tract on tooth #8.

Tooth #8 did not respond to pulp sensibility tests. It had grade I mobility and was sensitive to percussion. The mucosal sinus tract was traced with a #30/.02 gutta-percha point, and a periapical radiograph was taken to ensure the origin of infection (Figure 2(a)). Tooth #8 had an open apex, short root, and thin root canal walls. Pulp revascularization treatment was considered regarding root development and apical maturation status. The patient was informed about the treatment process, and informed consent was taken. In the first session, buccal infiltration local anesthesia was administered using 2% lidocaine with 1 : 80,000 epinephrine. The access cavity was prepared under rubber dam isolation. The working length was determined using an electronic apex locator (Root ZX, J. Morita, Tokyo, Japan) and confirmed with a periapical radiograph. Then, chemical disinfection was carried out with use of 1.5% sodium hypochlorite as the irrigating solution with gentle mechanical instrumentation. Double antibiotic paste (DAP) was prepared using equal weight ratios of metronidazole and ciprofloxacin and placed within the prepared root canal after drying. The access cavity was sealed with reinforced zinc oxide eugenol cement (Zoliran, Golchai, Iran). Patient evaluation in the second treatment session, three weeks later, indicated complete resolution of the preexisting symptoms and healing of the sinus tract. In the second treatment session, after administering local anesthesia using infiltration of 3% mepivacaine without a vasoconstrictor, the tooth was isolated with a rubber dam. Intracanal medication was then removed with 20 mL of normal saline solution. Irrigation was carried out using 20 mL of 17% EDTA solution for 5 min. The root canal was then dried with sterile paper points. A blood sample was taken from the patient, and platelet-rich fibrin (PRF) was prepared using a duo centrifuge (Process for PRF, Nice, France). Afterward, bleeding was induced using a sterile #30 hand K-file (Mani, Japan) beyond the apex. The prepared PRF was placed within the coronal part of the root canal 3 mm apical to the cementoenamel junction (CEJ). Then, a light-cured dentin-bonding agent (Solobond Plus, DMG, Hamburg, Germany) was applied to the labial surface of the pulp chamber to seal off the dentinal tubules of the crown. Ortho-MTA (BioMTA, Daejon, Seoul, Korea) was used as the coronal barrier, and the access cavity was temporarily filled with reinforced zinc oxide eugenol cement (Zoliran, Golchai, Iran) after placing a moist cotton pellet on the coronal barrier.

The final setting of the OrthoMTA as the coronal barrier material was confirmed four days later, and the tooth was permanently restored using Filtek Z350 (3M ESPE) nanocomposite material after applying a thin layer of restorative light-cured glass-ionomer cement (GC Fuji II LC, GC, Tokyo, Japan) (Figure 2(b)). At 2-month (Figure 2(c)) and 4-month (Figures 1(b) and 2(d)) recall visits, tooth #8 showed no significant discoloration or mobility. The probing depths were within normal range, with no sensitivity to percussion or palpation. At the 2-month recall, tooth #9 responded positively to pulpal sensibility tests, but it was slightly sensitive to percussion. Probing depth and mobility were within the normal range. At the 4-month recall, it was sensitive to percussion and showed evidence of external root resorption. Therefore, a CBCT examination was ordered for a thorough three-dimensional evaluation of the resorptive defect.

According to CBCT (Figure 3) and evidence of external root resorption, a new treatment plan was scheduled for tooth #9. Since it had an open apex, short roots, and thin walls, pulp revascularization treatment was considered using the same procedure as described above for tooth #8.

At 14-month recall (Figures 1(c) and 2(e)) (10 months after initial regenerative endodontic treatment of tooth #9), teeth #8 and #9 were asymptomatic. They showed no sensitivity to percussion and palpation. Probing depth and mobility were within the normal range. External root resorption at tooth #9 was arrested. Both teeth showed evidence of tooth discoloration. Radiographic examination showed open apex in tooth #8 and little evidence of apical closure in tooth #9.

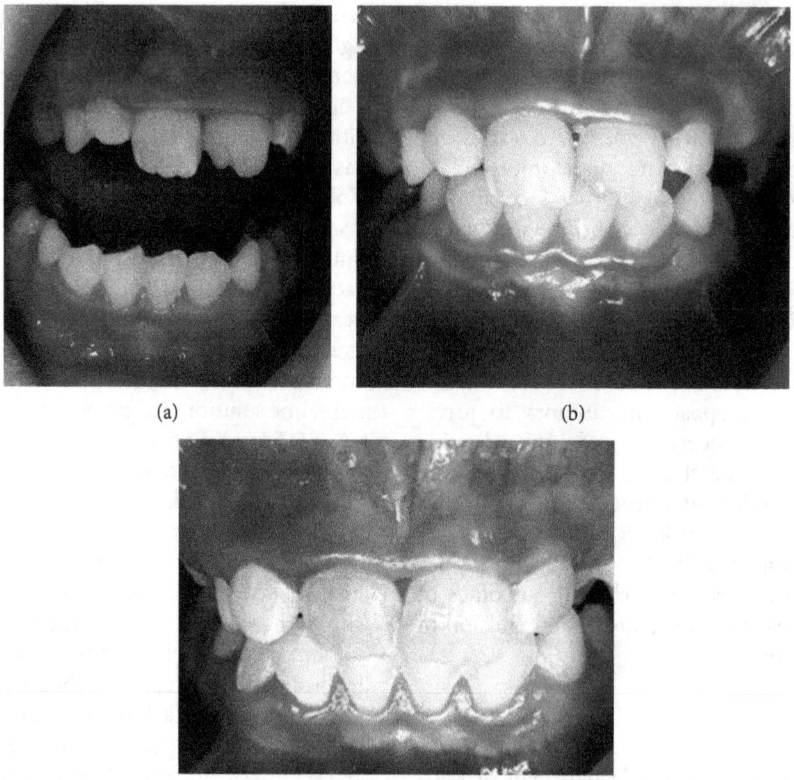

(a) (b) (c)

FIGURE 1: (a) Mucosal sinus tract on the maxillary right central incisor. (b) Four-month follow-up. (c) Fourteen-month follow-up.

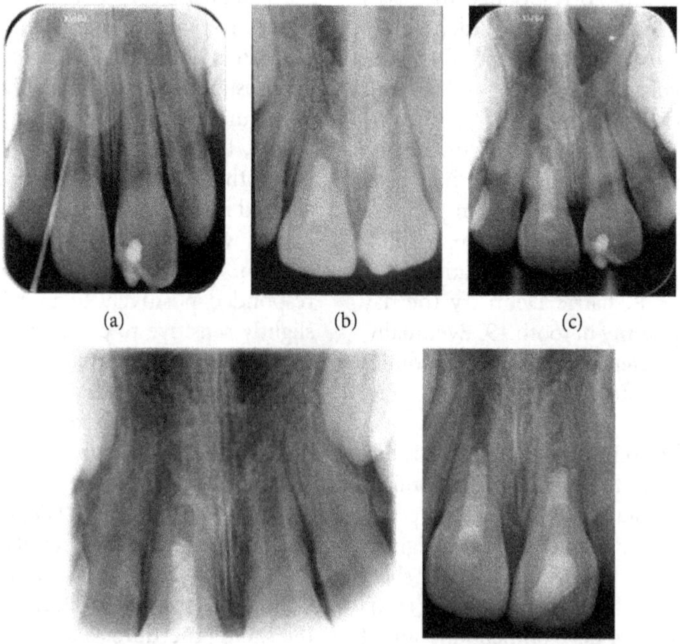

(a) (b) (c) (d) (e)

FIGURE 2: (a) Periapical radiograph of the maxillary right central incisor with traced mucosal sinus tract using a no. 30/0.02 gutta-percha point. (b) Immediate postoperative radiograph showing completion of RET. (c) Two-month follow-up. (d) Four-month follow-up. (e) Fourteen-month follow-up.

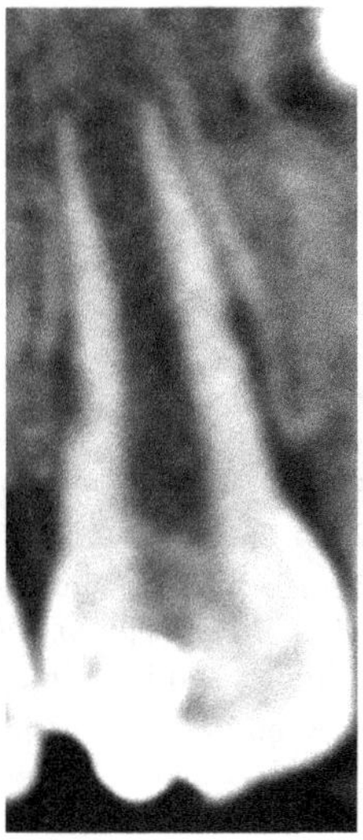

FIGURE 3: Coronally sectioned CBCT image indicating evidence for external root resorption.

3. Discussion

Traditionally, necrotic traumatized immature permanent teeth have been treated with either long-term calcium hydroxide or MTA apical plug; nevertheless, these methods have a number of disadvantages. One of the disadvantages of calcium hydroxide apexification is the possibility of higher tooth fragility due to long-term use of calcium hydroxide and long period of treatment. Disadvantages of MTA apical plugs include lack of root canal development and the possibility of further tooth fracture due to thin root walls. Another treatment option in these cases is regenerative endodontic procedures (REPs), with benefits such as the possibility of tooth root development and the possibility of increasing the thickness of the root canal walls [17, 18]. For the same benefits, REP was used in this case report of necrotic immature teeth of a patient with history of dental trauma (complicated crown fracture and avulsion).

A recent study revealed that the root development potential of immature necrotic teeth is related to the vitality of Hertwig's epithelial root sheath (HERS) [15]. Lack of continuous root development in the present case could be attributed to the damage to HERS during the traumatic injury. This case had a history of avulsion in tooth #8, considered the most severe dental injury with an unpredictable prognosis [16]. Therefore, we do not expect root development in tooth #8, while there is a higher probability of root development in tooth #9 with a history of complicated crown fracture trauma. In this case in tooth #8, no increase in root length or apex closure was observed in a 14-month follow-up, while tooth #9 with a history of complicated crown fracture showed evidence of apex closure on periapical radiography.

The long-term prognosis of replanted teeth is usually influenced by the extra-alveolar time of storage and the medium used, which are crucial in significantly increasing the viability of periodontal ligament cells and cementum [19, 20]. The International Association for Dental Traumatology (IADT) recommends that avulsed teeth be replanted immediately [5, 19].

There is a possibility of revascularization of permanent immature teeth in dry time less than an hour (IADT) [5]. In one study, it has been shown that replantation within 45 minutes increases the chance of revascularization [18].

Although it has been shown that saliva may not be the most suitable medium for long-time avulsed teeth, it can serve as a short-term storage medium for more than an hour for PDL cells. However, storage for 2 to 3 hours causes swelling and damage to the membrane of PDL cells and is also not desirable due to the presence of microorganisms in the saliva of the storage medium [21]. In this case, tooth #8 had been kept in patient's mouth for 5 hours before replantation. Therefore, prolonged extraoral time and inappropriate storage medium will be responsible for its compromised prognosis.

External root resorption (ERR) is often a consequence of a severe traumatic injury to dental structures. The presence of pulp necrosis combined with trauma to the tooth may have led to external inflammatory resorption of the root [22]. Long-term calcium hydroxide has been used for treatment of external root resorption. Calcium hydroxide can change the acidic environment of the resorbed root surface and prevent osteoclasts and odontoclasts from functioning. Calcium hydroxide may also be able to induce hard tissue. Recently, regenerative therapy has been used to manage the external root resorption of traumatized teeth. The resorption includes dentin and cementum, which is repaired by new cementum due to the presence of periodontal ligament stem cells, which, if properly signaled, can differentiate into cementoblast, not odontoblast, and repair the area with cementum [17].

In this case, tooth #9 showed external root resorption in the coronal third of the root, which was arrested after RET, and a normal periodontal ligament was seen around the area of arrested resorption at 10-month follow-up. However, longer follow-up is recommended. Likewise, Yoshpe et al. reported that REP is a promising treatment modality for arresting ERR [14]. Lu et al. showed that REP might be used to manage traumatized immature permanent teeth with necrotic pulp and apical periodontitis associated with severe external root resorption and root perforation. It was also shown that the resorptive area could be arrested and subsequently be repaired with hard tissue [17]. Dastpak et al. performed regenerative endodontic procedures for necrotic immature upper central incisor with external root resorption and chronic apical periodontitis in a patient with history of trauma. In a 12-month follow-up, the tooth was completely asymptomatic, and crown discoloration was observed. This case showed that REP can be effective in arresting ERR [23]. Giorgio et al. reported management of a case with external root resorption in an immature tooth #8 with a history of avulsion and presence of complicated crown fracture in a necrotic tooth #9. Apexification treatment by MTA apical plug was performed for both teeth. A 24-month follow-up revealed arresting root resorption in tooth #8, as well as ankylosis [24].

One serious complication after tooth avulsion and reimplantation is replacement root resorption (RRR) (ankylosis). The risk of ankylosis increases with prolonged period of dry time [24, 25, 5]. However, there is no definitive treatment for arresting RRR. According to Yoshpe et al., RET using PRF has the potential to arrest RRR [14]. Anyway, if ankylosis occurred, and there was evidence of intolerable infraocclusion from esthetic point of view that cannot be managed by restorative material, decoronation is needed [24]. Preservation of bone height and width following decoronation was observed [26].

Tooth discoloration is a common complication of RET [27]. This discoloration can be due to three reasons: intracanal drug, intracanal bleeding, and biomaterials. The intracanal medicament minocycline in triple antibiotics paste is responsible for discoloration [28], which, of course, was not used in this case, and DAP was used. Tripathi et al. reported that coronal tooth discoloration occurred after using white MTA as a coronal barrier in RET [29]. Additionally, in this case, teeth #8 and #9 showed minor discolorations at the 14-month follow-up, although the resolution of symptoms and restoration of dental functions happened following RET. Discoloration in the present case can be due to both bleeding and biomaterial. To prevent this, the use of bonding is recommended [30, 31].

American Association of Endodontics (AAE) [30] categorized success rates of RETs as primary, secondary, and tertiary goals, with elimination of symptoms and bone healing as primary, root maturation as secondary, and positive response to vitality testing as the tertiary goals. European Society of Endodontology (ESE) [31] describes success of regenerative endodontic procedure as lack of signs and symptoms, discoloration, and patient's acceptance and radiographic detection of new PDL along the inner wall of root canal.

From this point of view, tooth #8 belongs to "primary success" and tooth #9 belongs to "secondary success" according to AAE [30]. However, taking the ESE guidelines into consideration, the treatment was considered as "failed" due to the lack of root length increase and discoloration [31]. Therefore, AAE criteria for success in RETs seems to be a more comprehensive, more specifically in border line cases.

The current case report indicated that continued root development and increase in root canal wall thickness are not mere success criteria for RET. However, tooth functionality and esthetics, especially for young patients and supporting bone growth through the skeletal maturation period, should also be considered as further criteria for success. If the involved tooth becomes symptomatic in the future, other treatment options such as using dental implants in the defective site will be considered to restore patient's esthetics and function.

References

[1] J. O. Andreasen, F. M. Andreasen, and L. Andersson, *Textbook and Color Atlas of Traumatic Injuries to the Teeth*, John Wiley & Sons, 2018.

[2] B. J. Ö. R. N. Hedegård and I. N. G. E. B. O. R. G. Stålhane, "A study of traumatized permanent teeth in children 7-15 years. I," *Svensk tandlakare tidskrift. Swedish dental journal*, vol. 66, no. 5, pp. 431–452, 1973.

[3] J. J. Ravn, "Dental injuries in Copenhagen schoolchildren, school years 1967–1972," *Community Dentistry and Oral Epidemiology*, vol. 2, no. 5, pp. 231–245, 1974.

[4] A. Singla, S. Garg, A. Dhindsa, and S. K. Jindal, *Reimplantation: clinical implications and outcome of dry storage of avulsed teeth*, Journal of Clinical and Experimental Dentistry, 2010.

[5] A. F. Fouad, P. V. Abbott, G. Tsilingaridis et al., "International Association of Dental Traumatology guidelines for the management of traumatic dental injuries: 2. Avulsion of permanent teeth," *Dental traumatology*, vol. 36, no. 4, pp. 331–342, 2020.

[6] M. T. Flores, L. Andersson, J. O. Andreasen et al., "Guidelines for the management of traumatic dental injuries. II. Avulsion of permanent teeth," *Dental Traumatology*, vol. 23, no. 3, pp. 130–136, 2007.

[7] A. Filippi, Y. Pohl, and T. Von Arx, "Decoronation of an ankylosed tooth for preservation of alveolar bone prior to implant placement," *Dental Traumatology*, vol. 17, no. 2, pp. 93–95, 2001.

[8] S.-i. Iwaya, M. Ikawa, and M. Kubota, "Revascularization of an immature permanent tooth with apical periodontitis and sinus tract," *Dental Traumatology*, vol. 17, no. 4, pp. 185–187, 2001.

[9] Z. Fuss, I. Tsesis, and S. Lin, "Root resorption–diagnosis, classification and treatment choices based on stimulation factors," *Dental Traumatology*, vol. 19, no. 4, pp. 175–182, 2003.

[10] J. O. Andreasen and E. Hjorting-Hansen, "Replantation of teeth. I. Radiographic and clinical study of 110 human teeth replanted after accidental loss," *Acta Odontologica Scandinavica*, vol. 24, no. 3, pp. 263–286, 1966.

[11] G. Tsilingaridis, B. Malmgren, J. O. Andreasen, and O. Malmgren, "Intrusive luxation of 60 permanent incisors: a retrospective study of treatment and outcome," *Dental Traumatology*, vol. 28, no. 6, pp. 416–422, 2012.

[12] K. M. Campbell, M. J. Casas, and D. J. Kenny, "Ankylosis of traumatized permanent incisors: pathogenesis and current approaches to diagnosis and management," *Journal of the Canadian Dental Association*, vol. 71, pp. 763–768, 2005.

[13] S. Lin, M. Ashkenazi, M. Karawan, S. T. Teich, and Z. Gutmacher, "Management of ankylotic root resorption following dental trauma: a short review and proposal of a treatment protocol," *Oral Health & Preventive Dentistry*, vol. 15, no. 5, pp. 467–474, 2017.

[14] M. Yoshpe, S. Einy, N. Ruparel, S. Lin, and A. Y. Kaufman, "Regenerative endodontics: a potential solution for external root resorption (case series)," *Journal of Endodontics*, vol. 46, no. 2, pp. 192–199, 2020.

[15] M. Y.-H. Chen, K.-L. Chen, C.-A. Chen, F. Tayebaty, P. A. Rosenberg, and L. M. Lin, "Responses of immature permanent teeth with infected necrotic pulp tissue and apical

periodontitis/abscess to revascularization procedures," *International endodontic journal*, vol. 45, no. 3, pp. 294–305, 2012.

[16] D. D. Müller, R. Bissinger, M. Reymus, K. Bücher, R. Hickel, and J. Kühnisch, "Survival and complication analyses of avulsed and replanted permanent teeth," *Scientific reports*, vol. 10, no. 1, pp. 1–9, 2020.

[17] J. Lu, L. He, Z. Lu, B. Kahler, and L. M. Lin, "Regenerative endodontic procedures for traumatized immature permanent teeth with severe external root resorption and root perforation," *Journal of Endodontics*, vol. 46, no. 11, pp. 1610–1615, 2020.

[18] M. G. Al-shammari, "Regenerative endodontic procedure in immature permanent teeth," *Clinical Concepts and Practical Management Techniques in Dentistry*, 2021.

[19] M. V. D. P. Reis, C. J. Soares, P. B. F. Soares et al., "Replanted teeth stored in a newly developed powdered coconut water formula," *Dental Traumatology*, vol. 34, no. 2, pp. 114–119, 2018.

[20] B. Petrovic, D. Marković, T. Peric, and D. Blagojevic, "Factors related to treatment and outcomes of avulsed teeth," *Dental Traumatology*, vol. 26, no. 1, pp. 52–59, 2010.

[21] V. I. S. Khinda, G. Kaur, G. S. Brar, S. Kallar, and H. Khurana, "Clinical and practical implications of storage media used for tooth avulsion," *International journal of clinical pediatric dentistry*, vol. 10, no. 2, pp. 158–165, 2017.

[22] R. S. Cunha, F. C. Abe, R. A. Araujo, E. R. Fregnani, and C. E. Bueno, "Treatment of inflammatory external root resorption resulting from dental avulsion and pulp necrosis: clinical case report," *General Dentistry*, vol. 59, no. 3, 2011.

[23] M. Dastpak, H. Jafarzadeh, and E. Najafi, "Revascularization procedure in an open apex tooth with external root resorption: a case report," *Journal of Dental Materials and Techniques*, vol. 6, no. 2, pp. 79–82, 2017.

[24] G. Di Giorgio, A. Salucci, G. L. Sfasciotti, F. Iaculli, and M. Bossù, "External root resorption management of an avulsed and reimplanted central incisor: a case report," *Dentistry Journal*, vol. 9, no. 6, p. 72, 2021.

[25] E. Lauridsen, J. O. Andreasen, O. Bouaziz, and L. Andersson, "Risk of ankylosis of 400 avulsed and replanted human teeth in relation to length of dry storage: a re-evaluation of a long-term clinical study," *Dental Traumatology*, vol. 36, no. 2, pp. 108–116, 2020.

[26] J. V. N. Mohadeb, M. Somar, and H. He, "Effectiveness of decoronation technique in the treatment of ankylosis: a systematic review," *Dental Traumatology*, vol. 32, no. 4, pp. 255–263, 2016.

[27] A. Diogenes, M. A. Henry, F. B. Teixeira, and K. M. Hargreaves, "An update on clinical regenerative endodontics," *Endodontic Topics*, vol. 28, no. 1, pp. 2–23, 2013.

[28] W. Almutairi, G. H. Yassen, A. Aminoshariae, K. A. Williams, and A. Mickel, "Regenerative endodontics: a systematic analysis of the failed cases," *Journal of Endodontics*, vol. 45, no. 5, pp. 567–577, 2019.

[29] R. Tripathi, S. Cohen, and N. Khanduri, "<p>Coronal tooth discoloration after the use of white mineral trioxide Aggregate</p>," *Clinical, Cosmetic and Investigational Dentistry*, vol. - Volume 12, pp. 409–414, 2020.

[30] American Association of Endodontists, *AAE clinical considerations for a regenerative procedure*, 2016.

[31] K. M. Galler, G. Krastl, S. Simon et al., "European Society of Endodontology position statement: revitalization procedures," *International endodontic journal*, vol. 49, no. 8, pp. 717–723, 2016.

Infected Dentigerous Cyst of Maxillary Sinus Mimicking Intraoral Abscess in a Pediatric Patient: Management of Misdiagnosis and Inaccurate Treatment

Damian Chybicki, Alicja Popielarczyk, Wojciech Markowski, Gaja Torbicka, and Anna Janas-Naze

Department of Oral Surgery, Central Clinical Hospital, Medical University of Lodz, Poland

Correspondence should be addressed to Damian Chybicki; damian.chybicki@gmail.com

Academic Editor: Hamdi Cem Gungor

The article presents the case of a 12-year-old male patient who was suffering from exacerbated (infected) dentigerous cyst of maxillary sinus, associated with impacted canine whose symptoms were deceptively similar to intraoral abscess. The first-aid treatment performed by general dental practitioner consisted of intraoral incision and resulted in oroantral fistula formation. Eventually, the patient's ailments were not resolved, and we had to deal with serious local complications and difficulties. The treatment was performed under general anesthesia in one-day surgery system and included enucleation of the lesion, excision, and closure of oroantral fistula. Dislocated canine was not removed, and its subsequent eruption was observed.

1. Introduction

Many different types of inflammatory lesions can be seen in the oral cavity of pediatric patients. Odontogenic cysts represent the most common form of cystic lesions affecting the maxillofacial region [1]. Dentigerous cysts (also known as follicular cysts) are the second most common form of developmental odontogenic cysts that occur over a relatively broad age range, most frequently in the second to fourth decade of life. These lesions are the second most common odontogenic cysts (after radicular cysts) and account for almost 24% of all true cysts of the jaws [2, 3]. It is recognized that the formation of this type of cysts results from fluid accumulation between residual enamel epithelium, which is attached to cementoenamel junction, and the crown of an unerupted tooth (most frequently mandibular third molars, maxillary canines, and mandibular premolars) [2, 4].

Development of dentigerous cysts, just like many other cystic lesions, is slow and asymptomatic. They are usually discovered accidentally during routine radiographic examination performed for any other reason. However, the size of these lesions may lead to facial asymmetry or displacement of adjacent teeth, which makes them indirectly noticeable even during extraoral examination [4, 5]. It needs to be highlighted that cysts may also be affected by a bacterial infection, which results in pain, edema and pus accumulation. They can be misdiagnosed with abscesses in cases when radiographic examination was not performed or was misinterpreted. Effects of such circumstances are presented in this paper.

2. Case Report

A 12-year-old male patient with no general diseases presented to Department of Oral Surgery, Medical University of Lodz due to pain and edema of the right part of his face. The patient was referred to our Department by a general dental practitioner who diagnosed an abscess and performed intraoral incision to evacuate a pus discharge and prescribed antibiotic (amoxicillin 500 mg every 12 h) but symptoms did not decrease for the next three days.

During extraoral examination edema and redness of the skin of the right infraorbital and buccal area were noticed.

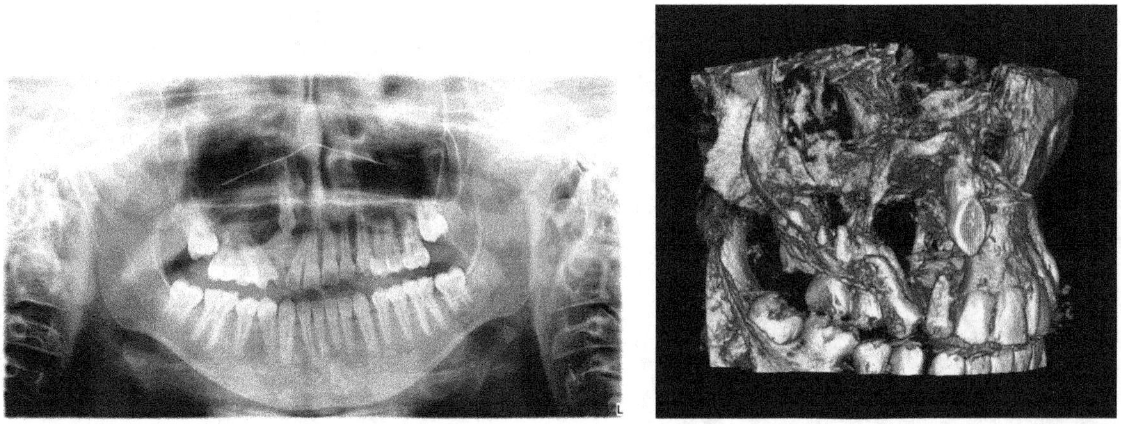

(a) (b)

FIGURE 1: OPG (a) and CBCT 3D scan (b). A considerable size of the lesion and translocation of tooth 13 are visible (arrow).

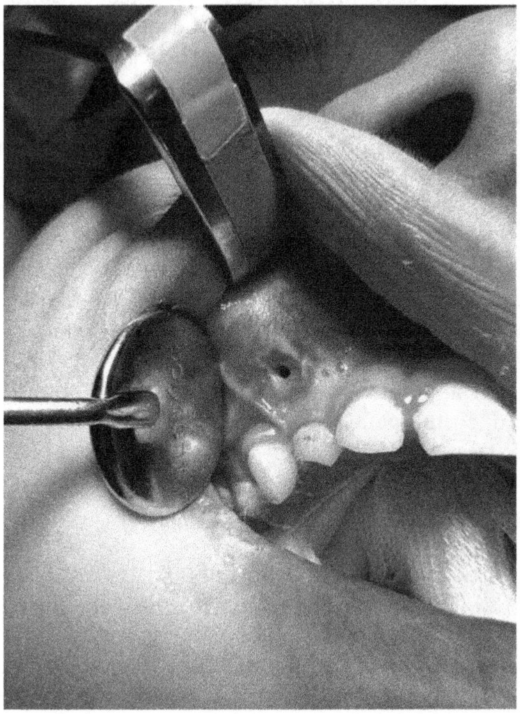

FIGURE 2: Intraoral view on operative region. Pus discharge is still present despite antimicrobial treatment.

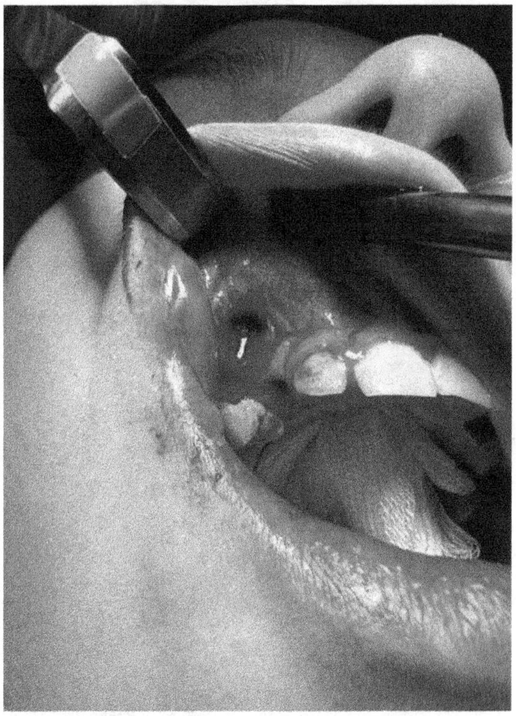

FIGURE 3: Tooth 53 is removed and oroantral fistula is excised.

Intraoral examination revealed a bulge in the area of teeth 54-52 and an opening after incision with pus discharge outflow.

Despite the patient's age, tooth 53 with slight mobility was still present in his oral cavity, so our diagnosis included a possible occurrence of infected dentigerous cyst. We performed an orthopantomogram (OPG) and CBCT (Cone-Beam Computed Tomography) which revealed a massive cyst-like lesion in the right maxillary sinus with translocation of tooth 13 (Figure 1) what confirmed our initial diagnosis. In the light of this evidence the previous dentist created an oroantral communication with his incision and after three days this opening became an oroantral fistula.

We established a treatment plan which included daily rinsing of the cyst and maxillary sinus with 0.02% chlorhexidine solution for the next 7 days through the fistula and continuation of the antibiotic (amoxicillin 500 mg every 12 h) to eliminate the acute inflammation symptoms and subsequently excision of the fistula, extraction of tooth 53, and enucleation of the cyst under general anesthesia. Decision whether to save tooth 13 or not was planned to be made intraoperatively, depending on its exact position and mobility after enucleation. We presented the treatment plan to patient's parents, collected all the necessary consents, and gave all of the recommendations that must be followed before surgery (e.g., laboratory blood tests, i.e., complete blood count and APTT). Despite the antimicrobial treatment, pus discharge was still present (Figure 2). In our

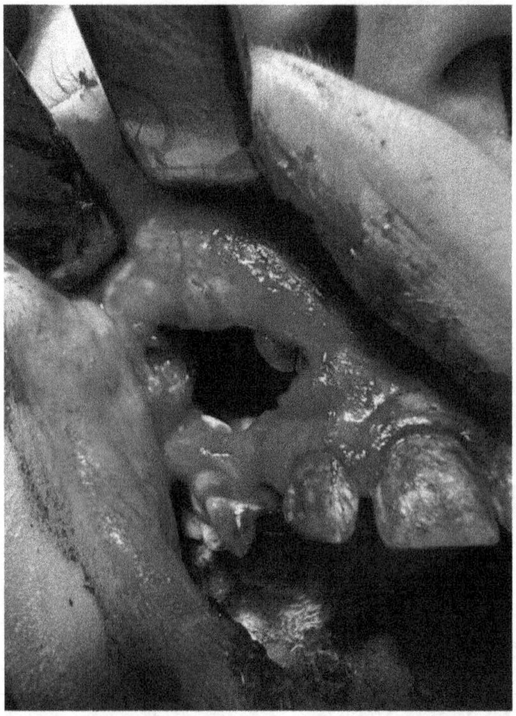

FIGURE 4: After incision and mucoperiosteal flap reflection, tooth 13 is visible. The anterior wall of maxillary sinus has been resorbed by the cyst.

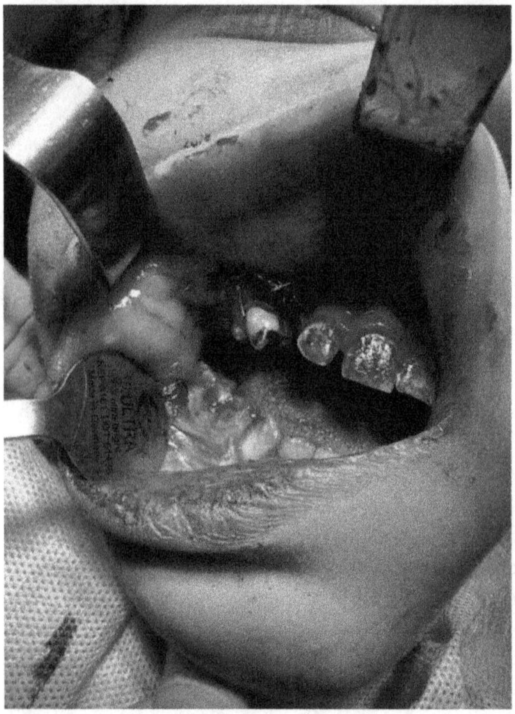

FIGURE 5: The wound closed with resorbable sutures. Depth of the vestibule is decreased due to the necessity of closing oroantral fistula.

opinion, tooth 53 extraction should have been applied as first aid, which would have resulted in outflow of the discharge from infected cyst, as well as alleviation of acute inflammation symptoms. Subsequently, a surgery should have been scheduled with the flap designed without any deficiency in soft tissues (because fistula has to be excised) and without shallowing the vestibule after suturing as its result.

Under general anesthesia (87.5 mg of propofol and 100 μg of phentanyl) with monitoring of oxygen saturation and heart rate (by pulse oximeter attached to patient's finger), tooth 53 was removed and the fistula was excised (Figure 3). A full-thickness mucoperiosteal flap was designed through the excised fistula. The flap was reflected with anterior part of the cyst attached to it as the anterior wall of maxillary sinus was completely resorbed and tooth 13 became visible immediately (Figure 4). The next steps included separation of the cyst from the flap and enucleation of the entire lesion. We decided that the stabilization and position of tooth 13 are favorable to be used effectively in orthodontic treatment. The flap was repositioned with two layers of resorbable sutures: the first layer consisted of continuous suture (Novosyn 4/0) and the second of single interrupted sutures (Novosyn 3/0) to achieve better adaptation. The wound after tooth 53 extraction was sutured with a horizontal mattress (Novosyn 2/0). (Figure 5).

The patient regained consciousness in the recovery room and was discharged home. Postoperative antibiotic (150 mg of clindamycin every 8 hours) and analgesic (200 mg of ibuprofen every 6 hours) were prescribed.

The follow-up appointments are as follows: first after 3 days, second after 2 weeks, and third after two months were scheduled. Proper healing of the wound and gradual reduction of the ailments were observed during first two visits. On the third appointment, the eruption of the tooth 13 was noticed, so the patient was referred for subsequent orthodontic treatment (Figure 6).

3. Discussion

Many articles describing dentigerous cysts have been published so far. The specific reason for this pathologic lesion remains unclear; however, numerous hypotheses are suggested. According to the "intrafollicular hypothesis," a dentigerous cyst is a result of liquid accumulation between the external and internal surfaces of the epithelium. This amassing happens during the development of the crown. There is also the "enamel hypoplasia hypothesis" which proposes the formation of the cyst resulting from stellate reticulum degeneration. On the other hand, "Main's hypothesis" suggests that the cyst growth is a consequence of the hydrostatic tension applied by the affected tooth on the follicle, whose effect is the division of the affected crown from the encompassing follicle [2, 6]. According to histological evaluation, a dentigerous cyst can be described as inflammatory or noninflammatory. The former results from inflammation in a nonvital deciduous tooth, while the latter appears because of the pressure applied by an erupting tooth on an impacted follicle [2, 7].

Although dentigerous cysts usually occur as single lesions, cases of their bilateral formation have also been described. Although such situations are extremely rare, they have been reported in patients suffering from

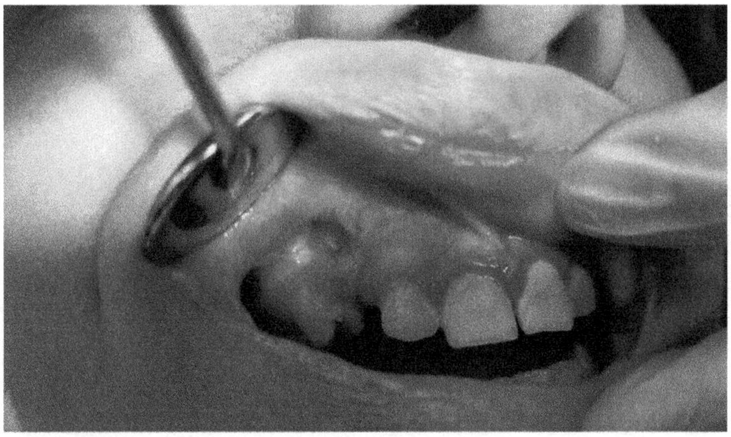

FIGURE 6: Intraoral view on operative area 2 months after surgery. Tooth 13 has started its eruption.

mucopolysaccharidosis, basal cell nevus syndrome (Gorlin syndrome), or cleidocranial dysplasia [8]. Among all the lesions that may be encountered in oral and facial areas, the following should be included in initial differential diagnosis due to their similar appearance in radiographic examination: radicular cyst, keratocystic and adenomatoid odontogenic tumors, unilocular ameloblastoma, and primordial cyst [3, 9, 10]. The three treatment methods of dentigerous cysts include enucleation, marsupialization, and decompression [1, 2, 4, 5, 11]. The decision which method should be used is based on the following criteria: cyst location and size, removal vs. preservation of unerupted tooth, pediatric patient's age and cooperation, and follow-up possibilities [2]. Marsupialization results in the formation of additional pocket in oral cavity from the cyst and is achieved by removal of its anterior wall. This method is considered conservative and is used when the preservation of the displaced teeth is desirable, especially in a young patient. It is also indicated in cases of huge cysts in mandible, whose enucleation could lead to bone fracture [12]. In the decompression method, a window in the cyst wall is created and a small acrylic device with a projectile is made to prevent the opening from closing. This results in a decrease of size of the cyst by internal pressure reduction and enables the enucleation to follow [13]. These two methods cannot be used in the area of maxillary sinuses for obvious reasons (e.g., chronic sinusitis).

In relation to cancer prevention, enucleation is the most favorable as the histopathological examination of the entire lesion can be performed and possible sites of neoplastic transformation can be detected. As an example, the following articles describe cancers arising from dentigerous cysts: intraosseous verrucous carcinoma [14] and primary intraosseous squamous cell carcinoma [15].

A method of treatment of massive dentigerous cysts involving the maxillary sinuses, not from the field of oral and maxillofacial surgery but otolaryngology, is the endoscopic-assisted transantral approach [16, 17]. The endonasal endoscopic approach by using various endoscopes and instruments is a minimally invasive surgery preserving physiological function while minimizing morbidity and preventing complications. Tooth and cyst that are close to the ostiomeatal complex can be managed through a fully endonasal endoscopic approach, preferably via a middle meatal antrostomy [17]. In our case, this method could not be used due to the lack of control over translocated canine and the presence of oroantral fistula.

4. Conclusions

Differentiation of infected cysts and intraoral abscesses still poses a serious problem for dentists who are not specialized in oral or maxillofacial surgery. Unfortunately, the inability to interpret radiographic examinations often results in misdiagnosis and inaccurate treatment. The necessity of more extensive education of dentists in the field of radiology should be emphasized.

Acknowledgments

The article was financed by Medical University of Lodz as a part of statutory activity no. 503/2-163-01/503/01.

References

[1] S. Kajjari, A. Gowtham, P. Meharwade, C. Uppin, S. M. Hugar, and C. Badakar, "Infected radicular cyst of deciduous second molar mimicking dentigerous cyst of second premolar in a young child: a rare entity," *International Journal of Clinical Pediatric Dentistry*, vol. 14, no. 3, pp. 434–437, 2021.

[2] E. G. Rajae and E. H. Karima, "Dentigerous cyst: enucleation or marsupialization? (a case report)," *The Pan African Medical Journal*, vol. 40, p. 149, 2021.

[3] N. R. Johnson, O. M. Gannon, N. W. Savage, and M. D. Batstone, "Frequency of odontogenic cysts and tumors: a systematic review," *Journal of Investigative and Clinical Dentistry*, vol. 5, no. 1, pp. 9–14, 2014.

[4] S. L. McKinney and S. M. Lukes, "Dentigerous cyst in a young child: a case report," *Canadian Journal of Dental Hygiene*, vol. 55, no. 3, pp. 177–181, 2021.

[5] A. S. Patil, P. N. Jathar, A. M. Panse, S. R. Bahutule, R. U. Patil, and M. Patil, "Infected dentigerous cyst and its conservative management: a report of two cases," *International Journal of Clinical Pediatric Dentistry*, vol. 12, no. 1, pp. 68–72, 2019.

[6] B. AlKhudair, A. AlKhatib, G. AlAzzeh, and A. AlMomen, "Bilateral dentigerous cysts and ectopic teeth in the maxillary sinuses: a case report and literature review," *International Journal of Surgery Case Reports*, vol. 55, pp. 117–120, 2019.

[7] E. Zerrin, D. K. Husniye, and C. Peruze, "Dentigerous cysts of the jaws: clinical and radiological findings of 18 cases," *Journal of Oral and Maxillofacial Radiology*, vol. 2, no. 3, pp. 77–81, 2014.

[8] L. Ghandour, H. F. Bahmad, and S. Bou-Assi, "Conservative treatment of dentigerous cyst by marsupialization in a young female patient: a case report and review of the literature," *Case Reports In Dentistry*, vol. 2018, 7621366 pages, 2018.

[9] R. Duhan, S. Tandon, S. Vasudeva, and M. Sharma, "Dentigerous cyst in maxillary sinus region: a rare case report and outline of clinical management for paediatric dentists," *IOSR J Dent Med Sci.*, vol. 14, no. 8, pp. 84–88, 2015.

[10] Z. Agani, V. Hamiti-Krasniqi, J. Recica, M. P. Loxha, F. Kurshumliu, and A. Rexhepi, "Maxillary unicystic ameloblastoma: a case report," *Bmc Research Notes*, vol. 9, no. 1, p. 469, 2016.

[11] F. Chouchene, W. B. Ameur, H. Hamdi et al., "Conservative approach of a dentigerous cyst," *Case Reports In Dentistry*, vol. 2021, 2021.

[12] R. V. Khandeparker, P. V. Khandeparker, A. Virginkar, and K. Savant, "Bilateral maxillary dentigerous cysts in a nonsyndromic child: a rare presentation and review of the literature," *Case Reports In Dentistry*, vol. 2018, 7583086 pages, 2018.

[13] S. Sevekar, H. N. Subhadra, and V. Das, "Radicular cyst associated with primary molar: surgical intervention and space management," *Indian Journal of Dental Research*, vol. 29, no. 6, pp. 836–839, 2018.

[14] C.-Y. Peng, Y.-F. Huang, M.-Y. Lu, Y.-H. Lee, and C.-H. Yu, "Intraosseous verrucous carcinoma arising from an infected dentigerous cyst—a case report," *Journal of the Formosan Medical Association*, vol. 114, no. 8, 2015.

[15] C. Gay-Escoda, O. Camps-Font, M. López-Ramírez, and A. Vidal-Bel, "Primary intraosseous squamous cell carcinoma arising in dentigerous cyst: report of 2 cases and review of the literature," *Journal Of Clinical And Experimental Dentistry*, vol. 7, no. 1, p. 5 e665-70, 2015.

[16] F. Y. Alhashim, F. S. Almarhoon, H. Y. Alhashim, and A. Moumen, "Endonasal endoscopic management of different cases of dentigerous cysts and ectopic teeth," *Journal of Surgical Case Reports*, vol. 2021, no. 4, p. rjab099, 2021.

[17] B. Sigdel, K. Sah, D. Kandel, M. Karn, A. Moran, and A. Panta, "Endoscopic-assisted transantral-endonasal approach to large dentigerous cyst of maxillary sinus," *Clinical Case Reports*, vol. 9, article e05027, p. 10, 2021.

22

Ameloblastic Fibroma of the Mandible Reconstructed with Autogenous Parietal Bone: Report of a Case and Literature Review

Conor Carroll,[1] **Mishaal Gill**,[1] **Eleanor Bowden**,[1] **John Ed O'Connell**,[1] **Rajeev Shukla**,[2] **and Chris Sweet**[1]

[1]*Department of Oral and Maxillofacial Surgery, Alder Hey Children's NHS Foundation Trust, East Prescot Road, Liverpool L14 5AB, UK*
[2]*Department of Pathology, Alder Hey Children's NHS Foundation Trust, East Prescot Road, Liverpool L14 5AB, UK*

Correspondence should be addressed to Conor Carroll; conorcarroll9@gmail.com

Academic Editor: Junichi Asaumi

Ameloblastic fibroma (AF) is a rare, slow-growing benign neoplasm, comprised of tissues of odontogenic origin. It constitutes 2% of odontogenic tumours, occurring at any age, but has a predilection to present in the first two decades of life. AF principally affects the posterior mandible. It is characterized by epithelial islands and cords immersed in ectomesenchyme that mimics the dental papilla and enamel organ but without actual hard tissue formation. Herein, we describe the case of a 6-year-old Caucasian male who presented to the Oral and Maxillofacial Department at Alder Hey Children's Hospital, Liverpool, UK, with a painless expansile mass in the left mandible which was diagnosed as a benign ameloblastic fibroma and subsequently enucleated and reconstructed with a parietal calvarial bone graft. A brief literature review and the issues surrounding diagnosis are discussed.

1. Introduction

Ameloblastic fibroma (AF) is a tumour, classified under the World Health Organization as "odontogenic epithelium with odontogenic ectomesenchyme, with or without hard tissue formation" [1]. They tend to develop "de novo," without an apparent aetiological factor. They are usually asymptomatic and may be identified incidentally as a radiographic finding during routine examination. They are benign in nature and share some clinical, radiographic, and histological features similar to other mixed odontogenic tumours, for example, ameloblastic fibro-odontoma (AFO), ameloblastic fibrodentinoma (AFD), complex and compound odontoma, odontoameloblastoma, and calcifying odontogenic cyst. These lesions can pose a diagnostic and therapeutic challenge.

We present a rare case of AF affecting the left body of mandible in a 6-year-old boy, which was surgically enucleated and reconstructed with a parietal calvarial bone graft (CBG).

2. Case Presentation

A 6-year-old boy was referred to the Oral and Maxillofacial Department at Alder Hey Children's Hospital, Liverpool, UK, with a painless left mandibular swelling. The mass had been present for two weeks and was gradually increasing in size. There was no complaint of difficulty in mastication, and there was no history of paraesthesia or discharge. The patient was systemically well and a full blood count was within normal limits. He had no relevant medical, drug, or familial history.

Clinical examination did not reveal any facial asymmetry or cervical lymphadenopathy. Intraorally, there was a localized swelling with expansion of the mandibular buccal plate extending from the left mandibular canine to the left first permanent molar (Figure 1). On palpation, the swelling was nontender with a hard consistency and was fixed to the deeper tissues. The overlying mucosa was within normal limits. All four first and second deciduous molars were

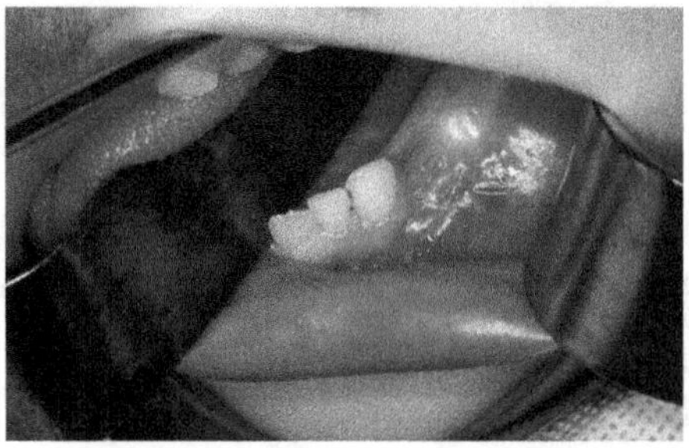

Figure 1: Intraoral view demonstrating swelling overlying the alveolar ridge with associated expansion of the left buccal plate. (Note that the lower left first and second deciduous molars were extracted previously at the incisional biopsy).

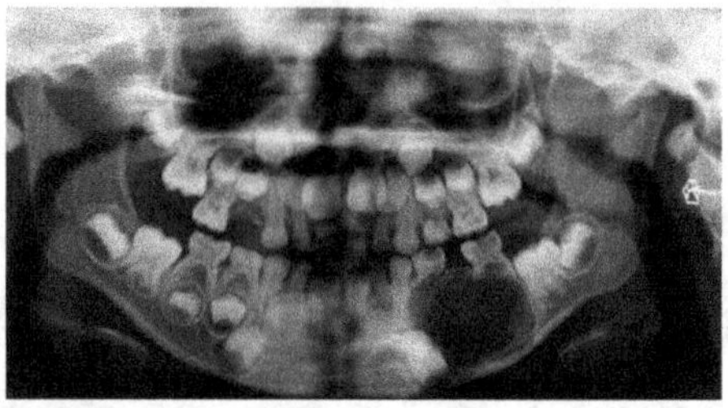

Figure 2: Orthopantomogram showing a well-defined multilocular radiolucent lesion with a sclerotic border in the left body of the mandible. The second deciduous molar has been displaced distally and is supraerupted.

carious, and the lower left first deciduous molar and lower left second deciduous molar were splayed due to the lesion.

Radiographically, an orthopantomogram (OPG) showed a multilocular, radiolucent lesion with scalloped margins affecting the left hemimandible (Figure 2). It extended anteroposteriorly from the distal aspect of the unerupted lower left canine to the mesial aspect of the lower left first permanent molar and approached the inferior border of mandible. The roots of the lower left first and second deciduous molars were resorbed, and the first and second premolar tooth germs were absent. A computed tomogram (CT) showed marked cortical thinning and some internal calcification but no evidence of internal septations. In some areas, the cortex appeared breached (Figures 3(a)–3(d) and 4).

An incisional biopsy and removal of all carious primary teeth under general anaesthesia was performed. The lesion was submitted for histopathological examination. Histological sections (Figures 5, 6(a), and 6(b)) showed a soft tissue specimen consisting of cellular/fibroblastic fibromyxoid stroma resembling primitive mesenchyme or developing dental papillae. The stromal fibroblasts had a diffuse or nodular arrangement. Towards the periphery of the fibroblastic stroma were various collections of "budding" cords and nests of odontogenic epithelium. Some islands of cells showed peripheral palisading and central squamatization and calcification. Several of the cords were rimmed by hyalinised material but not developed enough to qualify as dentine. Given that the lesion appeared uniformly radiolucent on imaging and did not include aberrant tooth germ-like structures, the features were consistent with a diagnosis of an AF.

The case was discussed at a craniofacial multidisciplinary team meeting. The proposed treatment involved enucleation of the tumour and reconstruction of the defect with a full-thickness parietal calvarial bone graft. The lesion was exposed via a transoral mucoperiosteal flap which extended from the lower left central incisor to the lower left wisdom tooth. While the lesion was successfully enucleated (Figure 7), it was found to have perforated both the buccal and lingual (posterosuperiorly adjacent to the molar teeth) cortices. In addition, it was found to be enveloping the mental nerve via the foramen and therefore the nerve was sacrificed.

The parietal bone graft was harvested via a full-thickness parietal scalp incision. The outer and inner tables were harvested as a single block, then separated on a "back-table," with the inner table replaced over the dura and secured via titanium miniplates. The outer cortex and underlying cancellous bone were then cut into several small pieces (cortic-cancellous) facilitating placement into the mandibular defect.

The surgical specimen was then sent for formal histopathological examination. Gross pathological analysis showed an irregular mass of white rubbery tissue measuring 30 × 25 × 15 mm (Figure 8). The cut surface was yellowish/white in colour with a rubbery consistency and clearly extended to the resection margin of the enucleation. Histological sections showed small islands and strands of basophilic ameloblastic epithelium in a background of abundant stroma with bland oval to spindle cells. No necrosis, atypia, or mitoses were present. There was focal inflammation and collection of macrophages. Further soft tissue specimens from the superior, inferior, and posterior-lingual margins did not show any tumour invasion. Overall, the histological features were considered to be characteristic of a conventional ameloblastic fibroma, neither the granular nor cystic variant.

The postoperative period was uneventful, and the patient was discharged two days following surgery. He is currently under regular clinical and radiographic follow-up. An OPG taken 10 months post-surgery shows good bone formation with no signs of tumour recurrence (Figure 9).

3. Discussion

An electronic literature search was conducted using the PubMed, Embase, and CINAHL applications. The general search criteria were (Ameloblastic)*, (Fibroma)*, (Ameloblastic Fibroma)*, and (Odontogenic Tumor)*. In the second phase of the review, terms related to the initial keywords used above were enabled to allow for a broader search criteria of the topic. This allowed for wider search terms across all databases to include all articles which may be relevant. The literature review yielded 604 papers; duplicates were then removed to provide 334 papers.

Evidence of greatest hierarchical value was a systematic review on AF by Chrcanovic et al., 2017; the most common publications that are related to AF and ameloblastic fibrosarcoma (AFS) were case reports and literature reviews descriptive in nature.

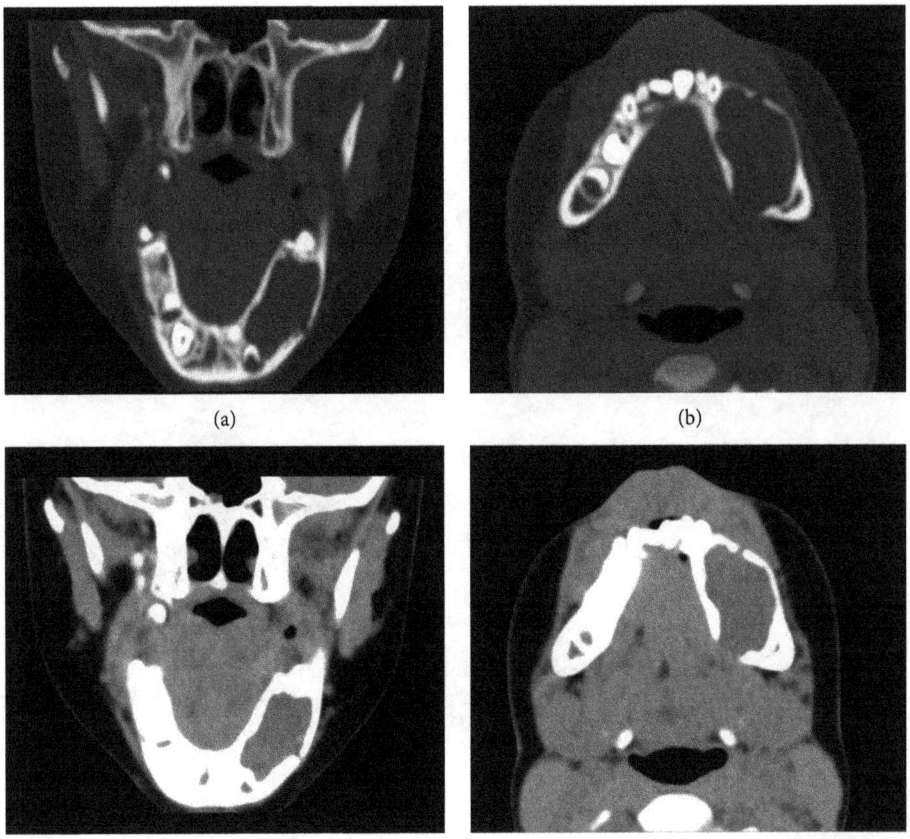

(a) (b) (c) (d)

FIGURE 3: (a–d) Computed tomogram demonstrates an expansile mass to the left mandible with small buccal and lingual perforation of the cortices.

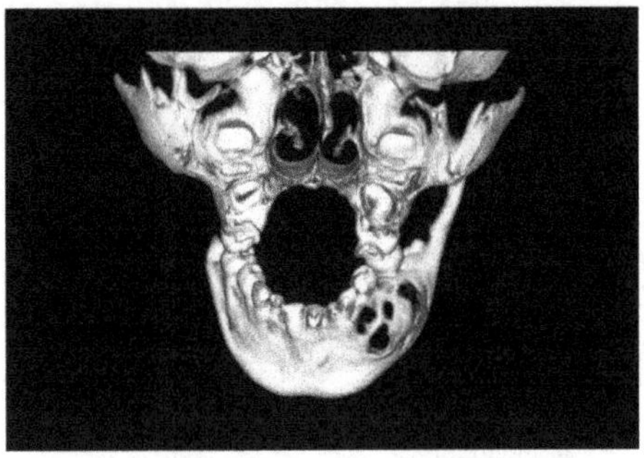

FIGURE 4: Three-dimensional tomographic reconstruction illustrating bony destruction with fenestration.

The first publication of AF was by Kruse in 1891 [2]. It is considered to be the least differentiated of the group of mixed odontogenic tumours as the neoplastic cells do not produce calcified tooth tissue, i.e., enamel and dentine [3]. AF is a true mixed odontogenic tumour as both the epithelial and ectomesenchymal tissues are neoplastic [4].

It is reported that AF has a propensity to affect males more than females in a ratio of 1.4:1 [4]. It has a predilection to occur in the first and second decades of life [5], although cases have been reported in middle-aged groups, for example, that of an extensive AF in a 45-year-old male [6]. The most commonly affected site is the posterior mandible [7]. There have been reported cases arising in the maxillary sinus [8].

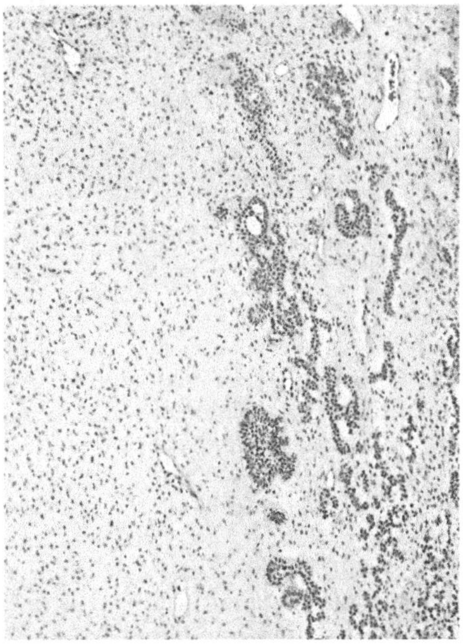

FIGURE 5: H&E (×100) biphasic lesion with dominant stromal and smaller epithelial component.

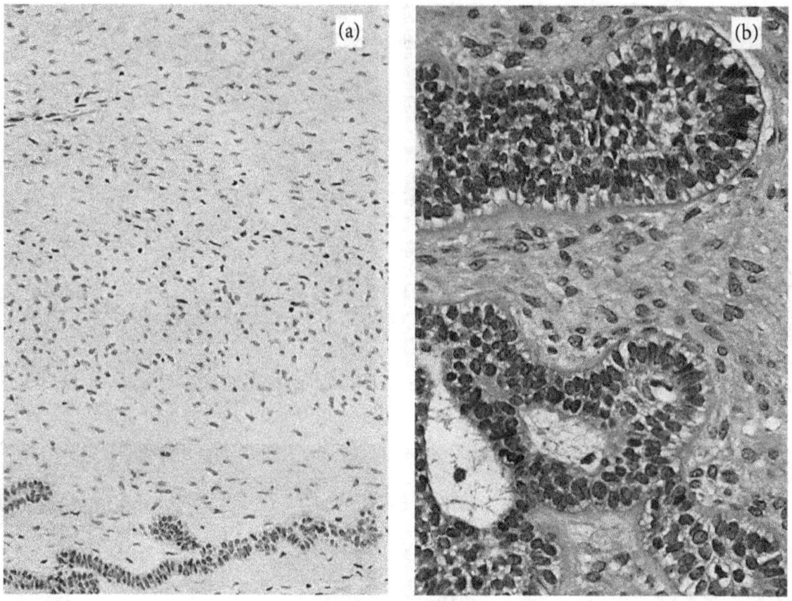

(a) (b)

Figure 6: (a) H&E (×200) stromal element is composed of bland spindle cells with no cellular atypia or mitosis; small islands and cords of markedly attenuated ameloblastic epithelium are seen at the bottom of the field. (b) H&E (×400) epithelial element with peripheral palisading and reverse polarization away from basement membrane (Vickers-Gorlin change).

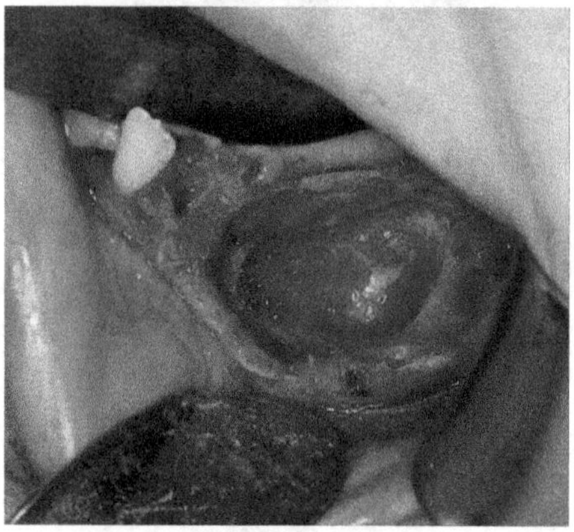

Figure 7: The tumour cavity in body of mandible following enucleation and curettage.

The most likely presentation is that of a unilateral painless swelling [4, 5]. Associated characteristics are mobility of teeth, root resorption, expansion of buccal and lingual cortices, pathological fracture, and paraesthesia [9, 10]. The lesion may be mistaken to be a dentigerous cyst as it can be associated with delayed/failure of tooth eruption [4, 11–13].

The radiographic features are variable, ranging from a well-circumscribed small lucent unilocular lesion to a more expansile multiloculated appearance seen in larger tumours [14]. The borders of the lesion are well-defined with sclerotic margins [7]. There may be cortical expansion in a buccolingual plane but this may be misinterpreted on a 2D image and therefore, we advocate the use of computed tomography to assess tumour extent and invasion. Furthermore, in cases where soft tissue invasion is suspected, magnetic resonance imaging should be considered.

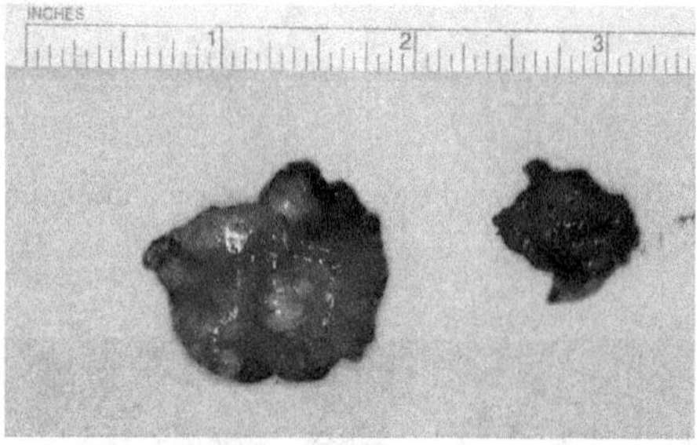

Figure 8: Gross pathological specimen.

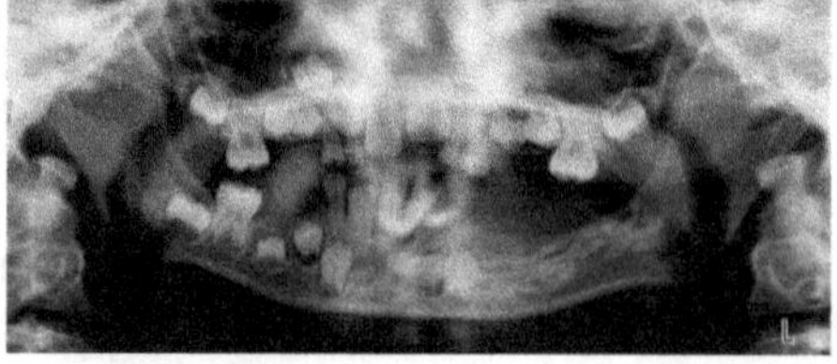

Figure 9: Postoperative OPG demonstrating satisfactory healing in the left body of the mandible with no evidence of recurrence.

Histologically, AF is a biphasic tumour made up of odontogenic ectomesenchyme resembling tooth-related structures such as dental papilla and epithelial strands and nests similar to the dental lamina and enamel organ, but without dental hard tissues [15]. The stromal component features spindled and angular cells with little collagen, imparting a myxomatous appearance. The epithelial component is made up of thin cords or small nests of odontogenic epithelium with little cytoplasm and basophilic nuclei.

Histological differential diagnosis of AF includes its malignant counterpart AFS and ACS and other mixed odontogenic tumours. AF along with AFD and AFO histologically resemble various stages of odontogenesis. AF lacks significant dental hard tissue formation such as dentin or enamel. If there is dentin or enamel present, the lesion is classified as AFD or AFO, respectively [16]. AFS is a neoplasm with a similar architecture to AF, but it is composed of a benign epithelium and malignant mesenchymal tissue typically comprising marked cellularity, nuclear pleomorphism, and a moderate-to-high number of mitotic figures in the mesodermal component. These characteristic histological findings were absent in this case which supports the diagnosis of AF.

In general terms, AF is primarily diagnosed morphologically, with immunohistochemistry having a limited diagnostic role. Ki-67, p53, and proliferating cell nuclear antigen (PCNA) are useful biomarkers of malignant transformation of AF into AFS in borderline cases, as AFS shows higher positivity of these markers [17, 18].

Immunohistochemistry has been applied to understand histogenesis. AF express CK7, CK13, and CK14, similar to the immunophenotype of the dental lamina [19]. A recent study assessed the immunohistochemical expression of odontogenic ameloblast-associated proteins; amelotin, ameloblastin, and amelogenin in diverse odontogenic tumours, including AF. Among these four proteins, AF was positive only for amelogenin. This further supports that the tumour cells of AF recapitulate dental lamina cells [20].

The management of AF can be a challenge, and there is no clear consensus regarding the optimal approach. In our opinion, a "case-specific" approach is appropriate. The aims of treatment are to remove the tumour and decrease the chances of recurrence while preserving adjacent vital structures. Management is dictated by patient age, extent and spread of the lesion, and histopathological findings.

In young patients, an AF could represent the primitive stages of a developing complex odontoma [4, 21]. Currently, we are unable to differentiate a hamartomatous lesion from a neoplasm merely on histological grounds; thus, age of the patient should be a significant factor when choosing therapeutic management.

Philipsen et al. [22] proposed that the innocuous behaviour of the lesion does not justify aggressive initial treatment but rather meticulous surgical enucleation with close clinical follow-up.

This is especially pertinent in a young patient where the emphasis is to preserve masticatory function and maintain dentofacial growth.

A more radical approach of marginal or segmental resection is suggested by some authors because of the possibility of malignant transformation of an ameloblastic fibroma [23, 24]. It is thought that around one-third of ameloblastic fibrosarcomas develop as a result of the malignant transformation of an ameloblastic fibroma [25]. Most papers included in our literature review agree a conservative surgical approach initially, followed by further aggressive excision for recurrent lesions, very large tumours, or those involving the maxilla.

In a large review of 123 cases of AF by Chen et al. [26], univariate analysis of malignant transformation-free survival indicated that, among all the analysed clinical variables, only the age of patients at the first presentation was significantly related to malignant transformation of AF. Patients younger than 22 years were unlikely to develop malignant transformation (3.3%) in comparison to patients older than 22 years (26.1%).

There is conflicting data in the literature on the recurrence rate of AF. Furthermore, not all reported cases have long-term follow-up, and so it is difficult to determine the prognosis of AF. Dallera et al. [21] reported no recurrences for 5 cases treated with enucleation and curettage with an average follow-up period of 15 years. A similar review of 9 AF cases by Gorlin et al. [8] indicated that there was no recurrence subsequent to conservative therapy. However, in a review of the literature on recurrences of AF, Zallen et al. [27] found a cumulative recurrence rate of 18.3%. The reason for the discrepancy in recurrence rates is uncertain and suggests that the cause of recurrence is due to incomplete removal and presence of satellite tumours at the edge of the lesion [6].

Long-term follow-up is recommended [28]. It is our intention to review our patient (clinically and radiographically) at 3 monthly intervals, for 6 months, followed by 6 monthly intervals for 2 years, and yearly thereafter for a prolonged period of time, likely in the region of 10-15 years given that malignant transformation can occur years after initial diagnosis.

In our opinion, reconstructive options should be case and defect-specific and depend on a number of factors including site and extent of defect, patient age, and associated medical comorbities. Autogenous bone grafts are considered to be the gold standard for maxillofacial reconstruction [29]. In this particular case, the use of a parietal calvarial bone graft to reconstruct the mandibular defect was utilised. We chose to reconstruct immediately given the distinct histological findings from the initial biopsy and to avoid exposing the patient to a repeat general anaesthetic. Given the extent of the defect and loss of integrity of the buccal and lingual cortical plates, reconstruction with autogenous parietal bone provided structural stability to the mandible and aided against pathological fracture. Furthermore, osteogenesis will facilitate adequate bone formation to assist oral rehabilitation with strategic placement of dental implants when the patient is older [30, 31].

Calvarial bone grafts are considered to be a safe and effective source of bone due to their low donor and recipient site complications [32]. This is because of the greater potential for osteointegration and revascularization as the cortical bone can act as a rigid platform for the regeneration of new tissue. The volume of bone harvested to reconstruct a large defect may be a limiting factor to this technique. However, in this case, given the size of the mandibular defect to be restored, this was not significant. The possible complications which may be encountered when harvesting a calvarial bone graft include dural tear, intracerebral haematoma, cerebrospinal fluid leaks, meningitis, and aesthetic defects to the skull. In a study of fifty consecutive patients treated with a

CBG for maxillofacial reconstruction, a low donor and recipient site complication rate of 4 and 4.8%, respectively, was found [33].

The CBG is considered a viable alternative to the anterior iliac crest graft [32]. However, given that our patient was six years of age, this donor site was not chosen for mandibular reconstruction because of: incomplete ossification of the growth plates; to avoid damage to the lateral cutaneous nerve and; to avoid disturbance to iliac wing growth [34]. Major complications of iliac crest bone grafting can also include chronic pain, arterial injury, arteriovenous fistula formation, abdominal organ herniation, and pelvic instability [34].

In extensive cases partial mandibular resection may be indicated involving reconstruction with rigid fixation or a composite vascularised free-flap.

4. Conclusion

This case demonstrates that ameloblastic fibroma can be managed with enucleation and immediate reconstruction with autogenous parietal bone. Patients with AF, however, must be followed up for a long period because of AF's ability to transform into its malignant counterpart, ameloblastic fibrosarcoma. Heretofore, there has been no clinical or radiographic evidence for recurrence 2 years postoperatively, and the patient has made a successful return to function.

Abbreviations

AF: Ameloblastic fibroma
AFS: Ameloblastic fibrosarcoma
AFD: Ameloblastic fibrodentinoma
AFO: Ameloblastic fibro-odontoma
ACS: Ameloblastic carcinosarcoma
CBG: Calvarial bone graft.

Consent

The authors can confirm that written and signed parental consent was obtained on behalf of the patient for the publication of this case report.

Authors' Contributions

All the authors contributed to the work-up of this case report, and the manuscript has been reviewed and approved by all the authors.

References

[1] S. Muller and M. Vered, "Ameloblastic fibroma," in *WHO Classification of Head and Neck Tumours*, A. K. El-Naggar, J. K. C. Chan, J. R. Grandis, T. Takata, and P. J. Slootweg, Eds., pp. 222-223, IARC, Lyon, 4th edition, 2017.

[2] A. Kruse, "Ueber die Entwickelung cystischer Geschwülste im Unterkiefer," *Archiv für pathologische Anatomie und Physiologie und für klinische Medicin*, vol. 124, no. 1, pp. 137–148, 1891.

[3] C. Jindal and R. Bhola, "Ameloblastic fibroma in six-year-old male: hamartoma or a true neoplasm," *Journal of Oral and Maxillofacial Pathology*, vol. 15, no. 3, pp. 303–305, 2011.

[4] D. Cohen and I. Bhattacharyya, "Ameloblastic fibroma, ameloblastic fibro-odontoma, and odontoma," *Oral and Maxillofacial Surgery Clinics of North America*, vol. 16, no. 3, pp. 375–384, 2004.

[5] P. Slootweg, "An analysis of the interrelationship of the mixed odontogenic tumors—ameloblastic fibroma, ameloblastic fibro-odontoma, and the odontomas," *Oral Surgery, Oral Medicine, and Oral Pathology*, vol. 51, no. 3, pp. 266–276, 1981.

[6] B. C. Vasconcelos, E. S. Andrade, N. S. Rocha, H. H. Morais, and R. W. Carvalho, "Treatment of large ameloblastic fibroma: a case report," *Journal of Oral Science*, vol. 51, no. 2, pp. 293–296, 2009.

[7] A. Buchner and M. Vered, "Ameloblastic fibroma: a stage in the development of a hamartomatous odontoma or a true neoplasm? Critical analysis of 162 previously reported cases plus 10 new cases," *Oral Surgery, Oral Medicine, Oral Pathology, Oral Radiology*, vol. 116, no. 5, pp. 598–606, 2013.

[8] R. Gorlin, A. Chaudhry, and J. Pindborg, "Odontogenic tumors. *Classification, histopathology, and clinical behavior in man and domesticated animals*," *Cancer*, vol. 14, no. 1, pp. 73–101, 1961.

[9] R. Gorlin, L. Meskin, and R. Brodey, "Odontogenic tumors in man and animals: pathologic classification and clinical behavior—a review," *Annals of the New York Academy of Sciences*, vol. 108, no. 3, pp. 722–771, 1963.

[10] B. W. Neville, D. D. Damm, C. M. Allen, and J. R. Bouquot, *Oral and Maxillofacial Pathology*, Saunders, Philadelphia, PA, USA, 1995.

[11] B. Nelson and G. Folk, "Ameloblastic fibroma," *Head and Neck Pathology*, vol. 3, no. 1, pp. 51–53, 2008.

[12] C. E. Tomich, "Benign mixed odontogenic tumors," *Seminars in Diagnostic Pathology*, vol. 16, no. 4, pp. 308–316, 1999.

[13] L. S. Hansen and G. Ficarra, "Mixed odontogenic tumors: an analysis of 23 new cases," *Head & Neck Surgery*, vol. 10, no. 5, pp. 330–343, 1988.

[14] L. R. Cahn and T. Blum, "Ameloblastic odontoma: case report critically analyzed," *Journal of Oral Surgery*, vol. 10, pp. 169-170, 1952.

[15] P. J. Slootweg, "Odontogenic tumors," in *World Health Organization Classification of Tumours. Pathology and Genetics of Head and Neck Tumours*, L. Barnes, J. Eveson, P. Reichart, and D. Sidransky, Eds., p. 308, IARC Press, Lyon, 2005.

[16] V. F. Bernardes, C. C. Gomes, and R. S. Gomez, "Molecular investigation of ameloblastic fibroma: how far have we gone?," *Head & Neck Oncology*, vol. 4, no. 2, p. 45, 2012.

[17] H. Pontes, F. Pontes, B. de Freitas Silva et al., "Immunoexpression of Ki67, proliferative cell nuclear antigen, and Bcl-2 proteins in a case of ameloblastic fibrosarcoma," *Annals of Diagnostic Pathology*, vol. 14, no. 6, pp. 447–452, 2010.

[18] A. Batista de Paula, J. da Costa Neto, E. da Silva Gusmão, F. Guimarães Santos, and R. Gomez, "Immunolocalization of the p53 protein in a case of ameloblastic fibrosarcoma,"

Journal of Oral and Maxillofacial Surgery, vol. 61, no. 2, pp. 256–258, 2003.

[19] M. Crivelini, V. de Araujo, S. de Sousa, and N. de Araujo, "Cytokeratins in epithelia of odontogenic neoplasms," *Oral Diseases*, vol. 9, no. 1, pp. 1–6, 2003.

[20] M. Crivelini, R. Felipini, G. Miyahara, and S. de Sousa, "Expression of odontogenic ameloblast-associated protein, amelotin, ameloblastin, and amelogenin in odontogenic tumors: immunohistochemical analysis and pathogenetic considerations," *Journal of Oral Pathology & Medicine*, vol. 41, no. 3, pp. 272–280, 2011.

[21] P. Dallera, F. Bertoni, C. Warchetti, P. Bacchini, and A. Campobassi, "Ameloblastic fibroma: a follow-up of six cases," *International Journal of Oral and Maxillofacial Surgery*, vol. 25, no. 3, pp. 199–202, 1996.

[22] H. P. Philipsen, R. P. Reichart, and F. Pratorius, "Mixed odontogenic tumours and odontomas. Considerations on interrelationship. Review of the literature and presentation of 134 new cases of odontomas," *Oral Oncology*, vol. 33, no. 2, pp. 86–99, 1997.

[23] S. Muller, D. C. Parker, S. B. Kapadia, S. D. Budnick, and E. L. Barnes, "Ameloblastic fibrosarcoma of the jaws. A clinicopathologic and DNA analysis of five cases and review of the literature with discussion of its relationship to ameloblastic fibroma," *Oral Surgery, Oral Medicine, Oral Pathology, Oral Radiology, and Endodontology*, vol. 79, no. 4, pp. 469–477, 1995.

[24] Y. Takeda, R. Kaneko, and A. Suzuki, "Ameloblastic fibrosarcoma in the maxilla, malignant transformation of ameloblastic fibroma," *Virchows Archiv. A, Pathological Anatomy and Histopathology*, vol. 404, no. 3, pp. 253–263, 1984.

[25] A. Kousar, M. Hosein, Z. Ahmed, and K. Minhas, "Rapid sarcomatous transformation of an ameloblastic fibroma of the mandible: case report and literature review," *Oral Surgery, Oral Medicine, Oral Pathology, Oral Radiology, and Endodontics*, vol. 108, no. 3, pp. e80–e85, 2009.

[26] Y. Chen, J. Wang, and T. Li, "Ameloblastic fibroma: a review of published studies with special reference to its nature and biological behavior," *Oral Oncology*, vol. 43, no. 10, pp. 960–969, 2007.

[27] R. Zallen, M. Preskar, and S. McClary, "Ameloblastic fibroma," *Journal of Oral and Maxillofacial Surgery*, vol. 40, no. 8, pp. 513–517, 1982.

[28] D. O. Costa, A. T. Alves, M. D. Calasans-Maia, R. L. Cruz, and S. Q. Lourenço, "Maxillary ameloblastic fibroma: a case report," *Brazilian Dental Journal*, vol. 22, no. 2, pp. 171–174, 2011.

[29] W. Smolka, N. Eggensperger, A. Kollar, and T. Iizuka, "Midfacial reconstruction using calvarial split bone grafts," *Archives of Otolaryngology - Head & Neck Surgery*, vol. 131, no. 2, pp. 131–136, 2005.

[30] A. Oppenheimer, J. Mesa, and S. Buchman, "Current and emerging basic science concepts in bone biology," *Journal of Craniofacial Surgery*, vol. 23, no. 1, pp. 30–36, 2012.

[31] J. Fearon, I. Munro, and D. Bruce, "Observations on the use of rigid fixation for craniofacial deformities in infants and young children," *Plastic and Reconstructive Surgery*, vol. 95, no. 4, pp. 634–637, 1995.

[32] L. De Luca, R. Raszewski, N. Tresser, and B. Guyuron, "The fate of preserved autogenous bone graft," *Plastic and Reconstructive Surgery*, vol. 99, no. 5, pp. 1324–1328, 1997.

[33] R. Movahed, L. Pinto, C. Morales-Ryan, W. Allen, and L. Wolford, "Application of cranial bone grafts for reconstruction of maxillofacial deformities," *Baylor University Medical Center Proceedings*, vol. 26, no. 3, pp. 252–255, 2013.

[34] R. Rossillon, D. Desmette, and J. J. Rombouts, "Growth disturbance of the ilium after splitting the iliac apophysis and iliac crest bone harvesting in children: a retrospective study at the end of growth following unilateral Salter innominate osteotomy in 21 children," *Acta Orthopaedica Belgica*, vol. 65, no. 3, pp. 295–301, 1999.

23

A Pragmatic Approach to the Management of Severe Awake Bruxism in an Adolescent with Cerebral Palsy and Global Developmental Delay

N. Ismail, [1,2] S. H. Hamzah, [1] and I. Wan Mokhtar [1,3]

[1] *Centre for Paediatric Dentistry & Orthodontics Studies, Faculty of Dentistry, Universiti Teknologi MARA, Sungai Buloh Campus, Jalan Hospital, 47000 Sungai Buloh, Selangor, Malaysia*
[2] *Ministry of Health, Malaysia*
[3] *Centre for Comprehensive Care Studies, Faculty of Dentistry, Universiti Teknologi MARA. Sungai Buloh Campus, Jalan Hospital, 47000 Sungai Buloh, Selangor, Malaysia*

Correspondence should be addressed to I. Wan Mokhtar; ilham@uitm.edu.my

Academic Editor: Leandro Napier de Souza

Cerebral palsy is a neurological and motor condition characterised by muscle balance and posture impairments. Bruxism and malocclusion were frequently observed in patients with cerebral palsy, in contrast to other oral anomalies. The report outlines how severe awake bruxism is managed in a 16-year-old Korean boy who has nonverbal spastic cerebral palsy and global developmental delay. The treatment protocol involved the fabrication of soft occlusal splints of three and four millimetres in thickness, followed by the placement of stainless-steel crowns on all first permanent molars whilst video recording and a bruxism diary was kept. Fixed restorations demonstrate increased endurance in withstanding bruxism force in persons who are dependent on their caretaker.

1. Introduction

Cerebral palsy (CP) is a neurological disorder characterised by disturbances in muscular control that occur during pregnancy, perinatal life, or postnatal life [1]. The Surveillance of Cerebral Palsy in Europe (SCPE) has agreed to define CP as a group of permanent, but not irreversible, disorders of movement and posture, as well as motor function, caused by a nonprogressive interference, lesion, or abnormality of the developing/immature brain [2]. The prevalence of this clinical condition has been estimated to be two children per 1,000 births with a preference for males and African American populations [3]. Cerebral palsy is classified based on the nature of the motor symptoms (spastic, dyskinetic, or ataxic) and the degree of impairment (hemiplegia, diplegia, or tetraplegia).

When the masticatory muscles are harmed, oral health may be compromised as a result of altered orofacial structure, the development of parafunctional behaviours, nutritional problems, and difficulties with oral hygiene care [4]. Individuals with CP have a greater proclivity for delayed permanent molar eruption, Angle's Class II malocclusion [5, 6], dental trauma [7], and bruxism [8].

Bruxism is an affliction of a repetitive jaw-muscle activity characterised by tooth clenching or grinding and mandible bracing or thrusting. Bruxism manifests itself in two distinct circadian patterns: during sleep (referred to as sleep bruxism) or during wakefulness (referred to as awake bruxism) [9]. This repetitive grinding and gnashing can result in masseter muscle hypertrophy, headaches, temporomandibular disorder (TMD), and tooth abrasion [10]. Instrumental and noninstrumental approaches can be used to assess bruxism [11]. Instrumental approaches include the use of polysomnography (PSG) with audiovisual (AV) recording or a portable electromyograph (EMG) device to monitor the patient's masticatory muscle activity [12]. Noninstrumental approaches, on the other hand, were based on self-report (clinical history or questionnaires) and clinical

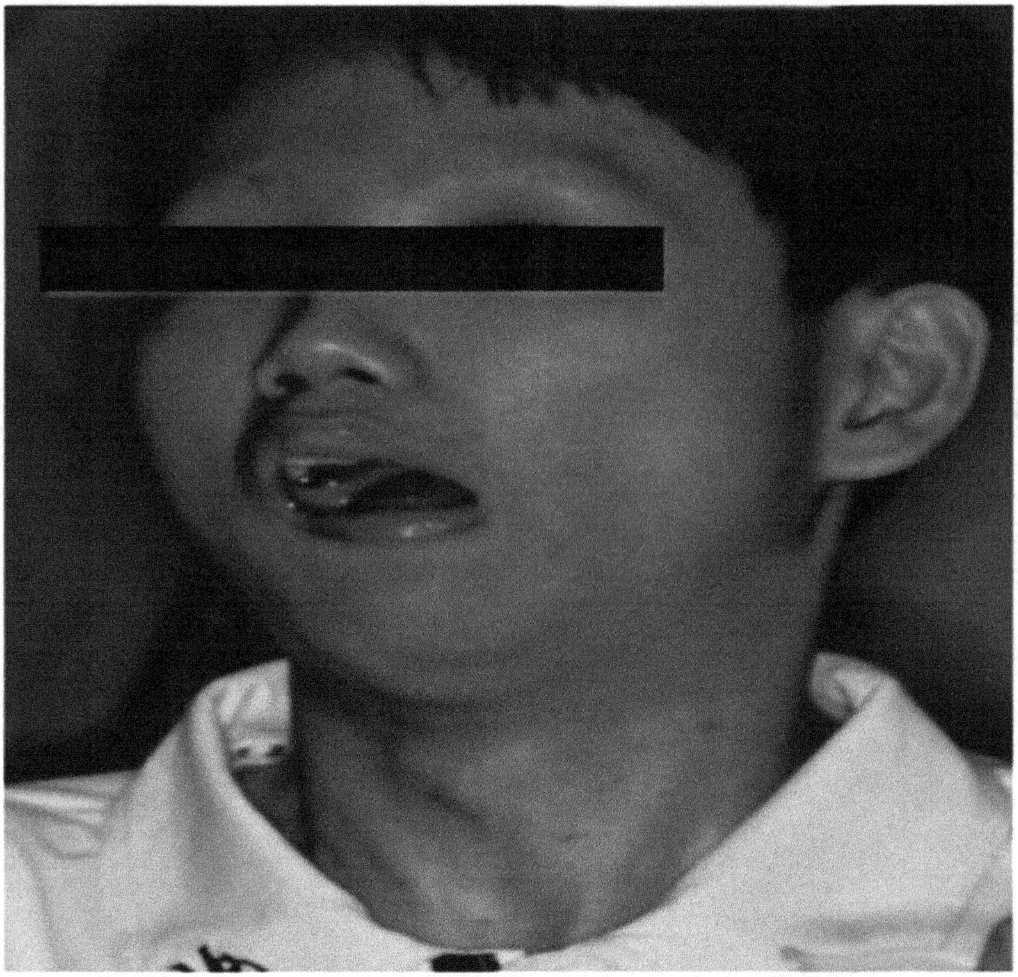

FIGURE 1: Extraoral photo of the patient.

examination, such as multifacet tooth wear [12]. Prevalence of bruxism in children with cerebral palsy ranges from 25.0% to 69.4% [8].

Additionally, dental attrition/erosion, a possible consequence of spasticity/bruxism, is significantly greater in subjects with CP than in age-matched controls [13]. Reduced and altered saliva production, as well as frequent gastroesophageal reflux, also contribute to dental attrition/erosion [14, 15]. The following case study and discussion detail the treatment given to a teenager with CP and global developmental delay (GDD) who suffered from severe awake bruxism.

2. Case Report

A sixteen-year-old Korean boy presented to the Special Care Dentistry Clinic (for children), with spastic cerebral palsy (type quadriplegia) and global developmental delay diagnosed at the age of three months. He arrived with his mother in a wheelchair and was nonverbal. The mother concerned of his continuous grinding and clenching behaviours especially when he is stressful, which causing attrition and wear tooth facets generally on his dentition and generalised staining on the permanent tooth. The anamnesis reveals that the pregnancy and delivery were both normal, and he was born at full term. There was no family history of cerebral palsy or other hereditary disorders.

He had previously experienced multiple convulsive crises triggered by a high fever and flashing lights during his five years of life and was previously prescribed with an anticonvulsant medication (Carbamazepine) only during that period. He is closely monitored by a multidisciplinary team comprised of a paediatrician, physiotherapist, psychologist, and neurologist. Physical examination revealed a weight of 47 kilogrammes and a height of 160 centimetres. He had a combination of movement impairments caused by abnormal reflexes, limb and trunk rigidity, abnormal posture, involuntary movements, and unsteady walking, which necessitated his reliance on a wheelchair for mobility. On a dietary note, he ate mostly semiblended or pureed foods.

Extraoral palpation reveals hypertrophy of the masseter muscle on a class II skeletal pattern. Facial and hypoglossal nerve dysfunction were apparent, which exacerbates salivary drooling symptoms and poor in swallowing (Figure 1). The intraoral examination reveals a permanent dentition stage with optimal oral hygiene, visible generalised chromogenic bacteria with a blackish stain on the posterior tooth (Figure 2(a)). The blunt cusps on the first permanent molar

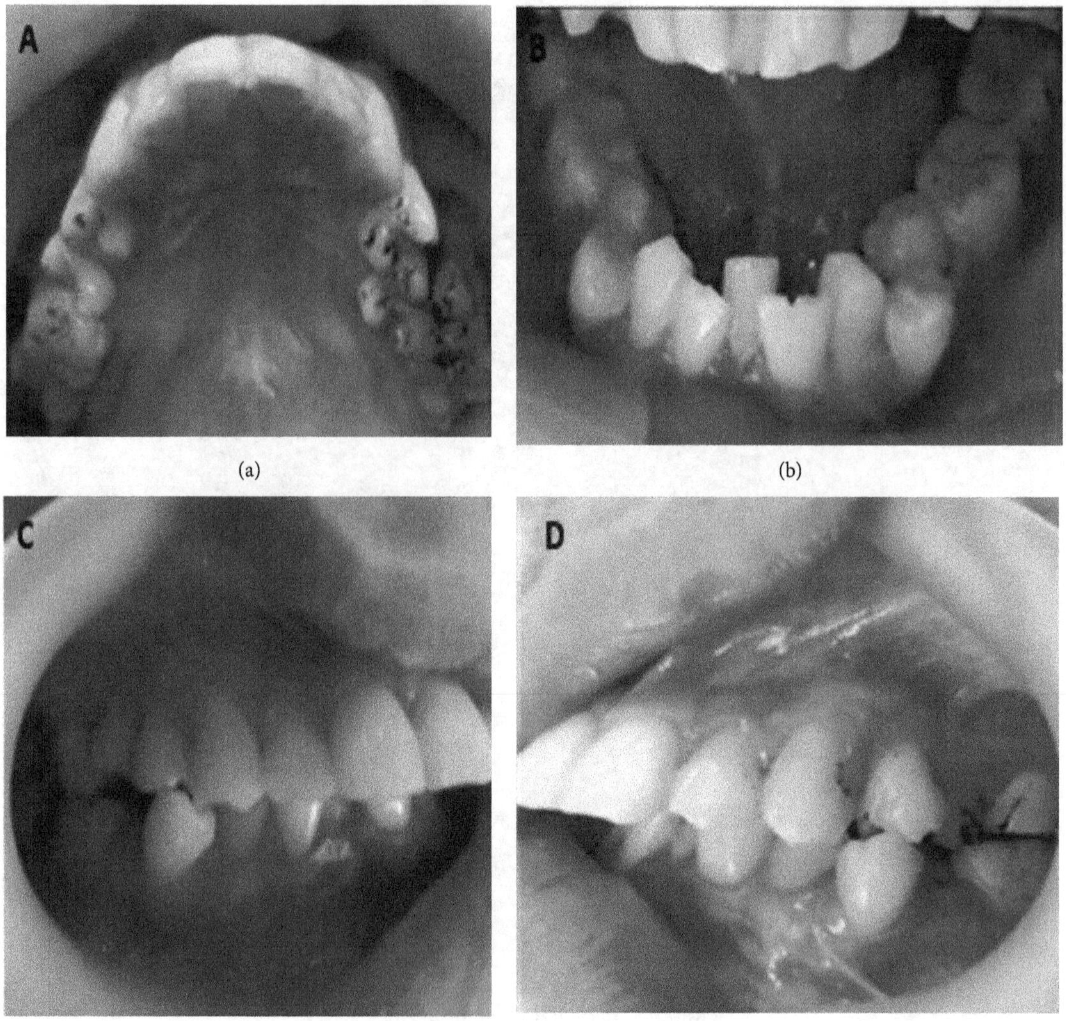

(a) (b) (c) (d)

Figure 2: (a) Intraoral photograph of upper occlusal view showing generalised blackish staining on posterior teeth. (b) Intraoral photograph of lower occlusal view showing severe crowding complicated with a fusion of tooth 31 and tooth 32. (c) Intraoral photograph (right buccal view) showing buccally placed tooth 44, severely attritted incisal tip of 13. (d) Intraoral photograph (left buccal view) showing scissor bite between upper and lower first premolar and severe incisor overjet.

and canine were evident. An incidental discovery of fusion tooth anomalies is observed on lower left incisors, teeth 31 and 32 (Figure 2(b)). Additionally, he had a Class II div I malocclusion, which included a deep overbite (lower incisors impinging on the anterior palate), bilateral posterior cross-bite associated with a buccally displaced first lower premolar, and severe crowding on the lower anterior segment (Figures 2(c) and 2(d)). Radiographic examination was not possible due to the patient's unwillingness to cooperate during the acquisition.

3. Clinical Management

The treatment management started with a 3 mm thick oral protective appliance (occlusal soft splint) fabrication. Impressions with alginate material were taken using a passive immobilisation technique. The splint issued within 2 weeks, with reassurance on the importance of proper oral hygiene. Unfortunately, patient returned within a month with a fractured split. Henceforth, a millimetre thicker (4 mm) splint is fabricated. Two splints were provided for daytime (Figure 3(a)) and another for sleep-time (Figure 3(b)).

The patient was followed up on a regular basis to remove and clean the appliances, apply topical fluoride, and be reminded to practise good oral hygiene. After a year of observation, the bruxism behaviour decreased, but the intensity is somewhat unchanged. It is noticed that the bruxism is more intense during daytime comparing to the nighttime as the daytime splint exhibits more wear off surfaces. As a result, a decision was made to increase the vertical height of the first permanent molars and thus reduce premature contacts. This is to achieve by placing stainless-steel crown (SSC) on the permanent molars.

Due to his unfavourable behaviour, the procedures were scheduled under general anaesthesia (GA). To engage the optimal occlusal force, a thorough occlusal analysis was

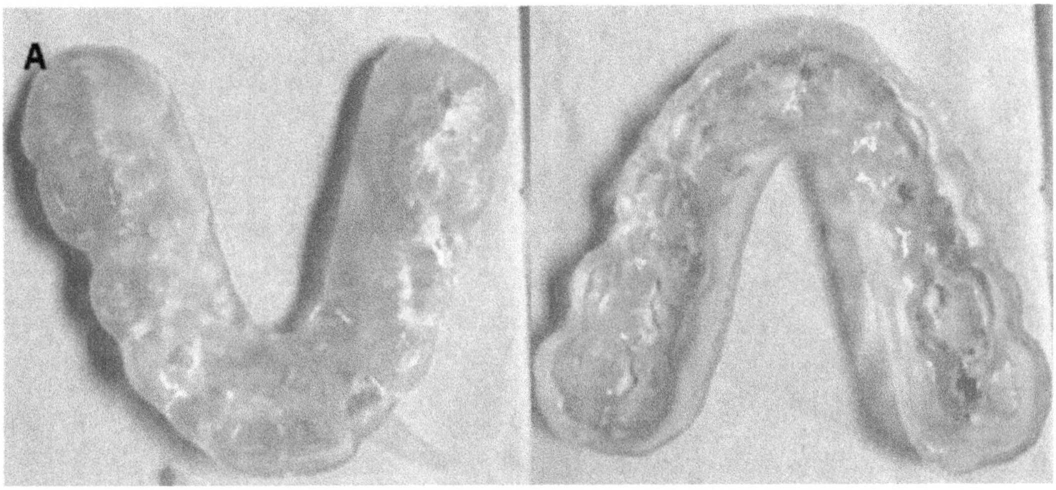

(a)

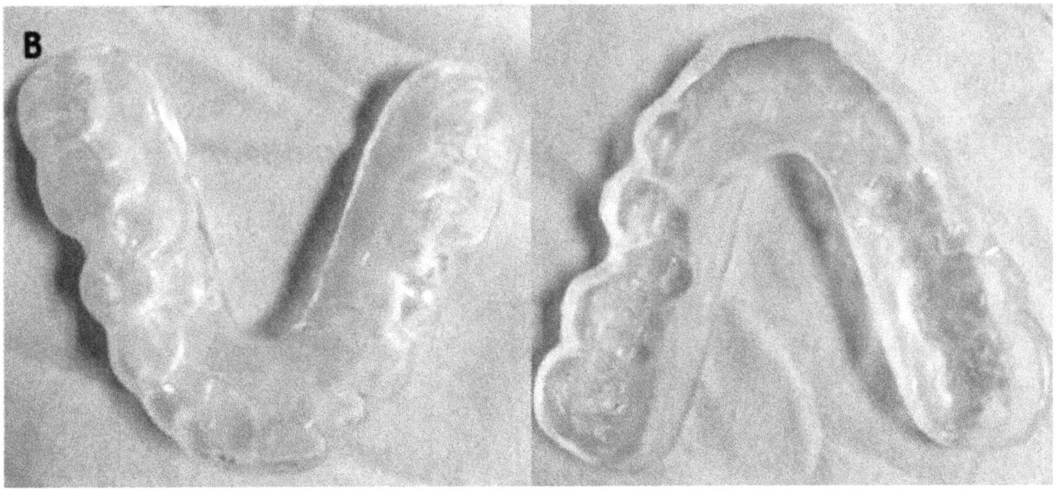

(b)

FIGURE 3: (a) Upper and lower soft occlusal splint wore during daytime. (b) Upper and lower soft occlusal splint wore at sleep-time.

performed prior in the dental office and repeated under the influence of GA. The distal cusps of the second permanent molars are submerged; thus, the crown is placed only on the first permanent molars. The crowded lower anterior segment, which contributed to the premature contact, was relieved by extracting both lower right and left first permanent premolars that were buccally displaced. Additionally, the tooth appears to complicate oral hygiene measures, justifying its extraction. The incisal third of the fusion tooth's indentation was restored using composite resin as a preventive resin restoration (Figures 4(a) and 4(b)).

4. Review and Maintenance

Postoperatively, the patient was on close monitoring regime; First visit after 1 month, 2nd to 4th visit in every 3 months, followed by 5th visit after 6 month until the condition deemed nonaggressively progressive. Within the first seven-month review visit, the mother reported that his son continued to have bruxism, but only when he was stressed or bored. Intraoral examination revealed that only the palatal cusp of SSC placed on the upper left first permanent molar tooth (26) attritted, exposing the underlying GIC cement (Figures 4(c) and 4(d)). The progression of attrition was monitored until there is need for replacement. Both parents and clinician decided on starting on a bruxism diary to engage with the habit intensity and timing. The mother agreed and advised on video recording with written log capturing the timing, frequency, and severity of the habit. The records would aid in identifying the specific stressors that contribute to the parafunctional habits, allowing for a better understanding and intervention to the habit.

5. Discussion

Various modalities of treatment for the management of bruxism have been investigated such as occlusal intervention (either by occlusal appliance or "Nociceptive Trigeminal Inhibition (NTI) Clenching Suppression System"—a small anterior splint). Biofeedback therapy is based on the principle that bruxers can "unlearn" their behaviour when a stimulus makes them aware of their adverse jaw muscle

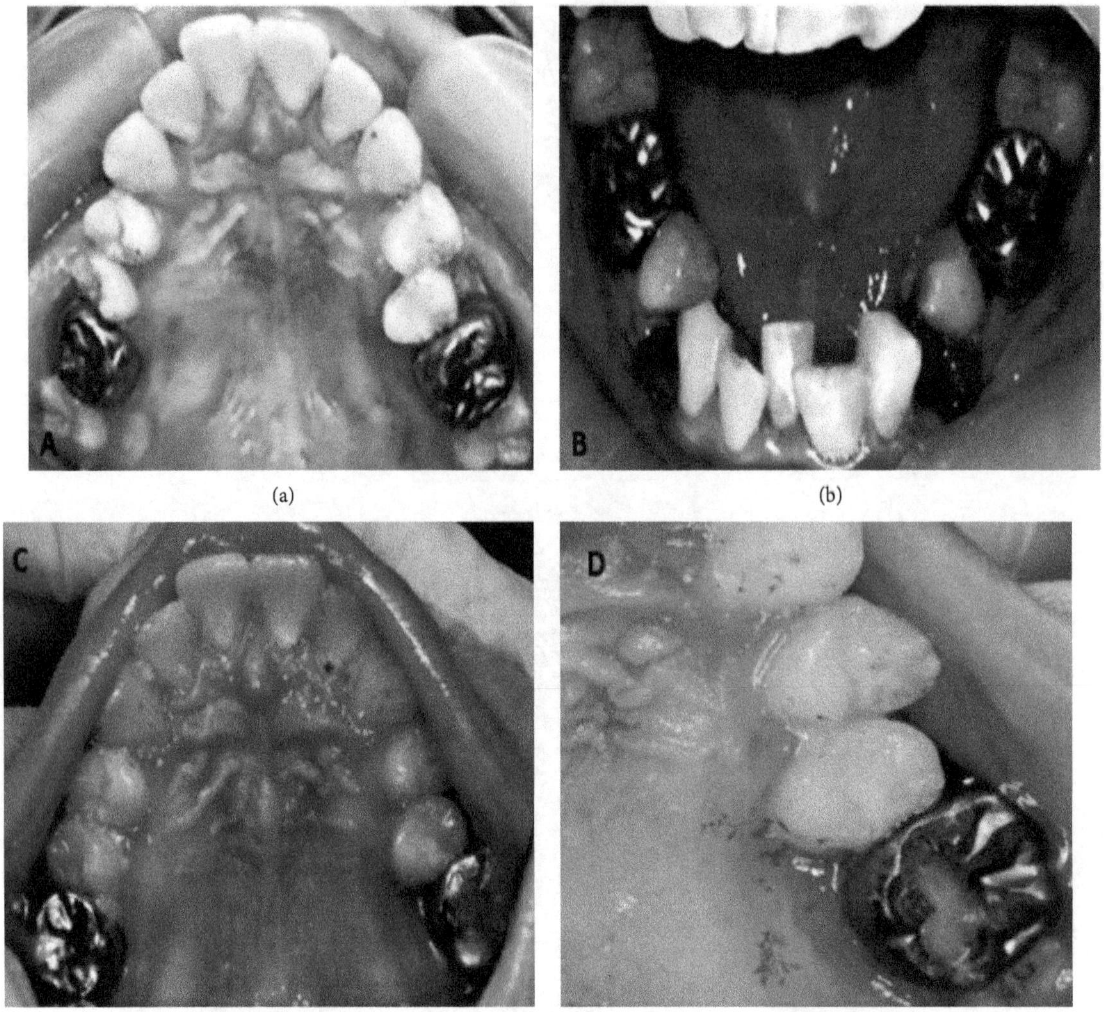

(a) (b)

(c) (d)

Figure 4: (a) Intraoperative upper occlusal views of cemented of stainless-steel crown on tooth 16 and tooth 26. (b) Intraoperative lower occlusal view showing mandibular first premolars were extracted and indentation on incisal edge of fusion teeth 31 and 32 was restored with composite resin. (c) Upper occlusal view after 7-month follow-up showing intact stainless-steel crowns (SSCs) on tooth 16 and tooth 26 with evidence of attritted crown on 26. (d) Intraoral pictures focusing on tooth 26 revealed that palatal cusp of tooth 26 is severely attritted and exposing the cement of the crown after 7-month follow-up.

activities ("aversive conditioning") and pharmacological approach like antidepressant drugs (benzodiazepine or L-dopa) or drugs that have paralytic effect on the muscle through an inhibition of acetylcholine release at the neuromuscular junction (botulinum toxin) which decreases bruxism activity [16].

Bruxism was diagnosed in this patient using noninstrumental methods, where self-reported signs and symptoms by mother as well as clinical evidence of generalised attrition. Despite the low concordance with instrumental assessment, particularly in assessing sleep bruxism [17], self-reported assessment may be entirely valid for a particular application and remains the primary tool in research and clinical practise [12]. After the treatment with soft splint, the study learned that his awake bruxism is more intense comparing to the sleep bruxism. This is concluded based on the attrition evidence difference between both splints as suggested by Koyano et al. [18].

A systematic review by Canales et al. [19] showed that most studies using botulinum toxin injection focused on sleep bruxism, whilst awake bruxism has been addressed only with single case reports. Botulinum toxin injection may influence only the last phase of a sleep bruxism episode, by reducing the intensity of the contraction, whilst it cannot have any effects on its genesis [19]. It should also be noted that, despite awake bruxism is mainly related to anxiety or daily stress [20], some case reports showed that botulinum toxin injection in patients with severe awake bruxism episodes may be an alternative option to wearing oral appliances [21]. Despite botulinum toxin has been increasingly diffused in dentistry over recent years particularly for pain management in patient with bruxism, nonetheless, there is no consensus about its effects in this disorder as lack of clinical protocols, standardization of dosage, and different dilution of preparations between the various commercial brands may contribute to explain the incomplete knowledge on the topic [22].

Dental treatment of bruxism with an interocclusal appliance (splint) is based on Glaros and Melamed's local or mechanical theories [23]. This theory postulated that bruxism may be caused by tooth failing to achieve optimal intercuspal position or retruded cuspal position. Deviation from the ideal structure impairs the nervous feedback system and proprioceptive receptors in the mandible, lowering the irritability threshold, and bruxism occurs as a teleological response to restore ideal occlusion. Interocclusal appliances have been shown to reduce bruxing activity by decreasing bruxing frequency but not duration or amplitude [24].

In the initial treatment, the patient is prescribed with soft split (silicone type) to cover both maxillary and mandibular teeth, providing a cushion effect during intercuspation and preventing them from contacting one another, thereby preventing damage caused by the grinding habit and reducing masticatory activity [25]. We decided to use silicon-type material which is based on the study by Seifeldin and Elhayes that shows the use of soft occlusal splint exhibits superior and earlier improvement of some temporomandibular joint disorder (TMD) [26]. It was demonstrated that 3 mm splints can be used effectively in the treatment of bruxism as it is superior in comfort and has remarkable result for TMD compared to 5 mm and 6 mm splints [27, 28]. However, over the time, the soft splint became worn out and the second devices were constructed from the same material with increased occlusal height of 4 millimetres. Hegab et al. found that 4 mm splint therapy has as nearly as effectiveness like 3 mm splint therapy [29].

The consideration for a reversible and conservative treatment is crucial to avoid unnecessary treatment. However, the therapeutic effect appears to be limited to the duration of the device's ability to maintain the bruxism habit's frequency and usually recommended for short-term use because degradation can occur rapidly [30]. Due to the guarded changes in the grinding frequency, the treatment switched to a stainless-steel crown (SSC). SSC is shown to be less technique sensitive and can reduce chairside time which is an important consideration in managing patient with disability [31].

According to a previous study, the increased prevalence of Angle's Class II is due to an imbalance between the perioral and intraoral muscles, as evidenced by unusual tongue movement or positioning [6]. Bilateral extraction of buccally located lower first premolars was performed in this patient to alleviate lower anterior crowding and improve oral hygiene.

Numerous studies have attempted to establish a link between stress and bruxism. Children who brux experienced a greater level of stress than children who did not brux and bruxers were significantly more likely to experience increased levels of anxiety [32]. Vanderas et al. [33] discovered that children with significantly elevated stress levels had significantly higher catecholamine levels in their urine and a higher prevalence of bruxism [33]. The children's bruxism diary suggested to identify risk factors for bruxism. Aspects of behaviour such as anxiety management and occupying the patient's time with something interesting may aid in the treatment of this condition [34].

6. Conclusion

In conclusion, the occlusal splint is a reversible intervention that acts as a provisional treatment for tooth grinding and tooth wear control. We foresee that by placing stainless-steel crown on first permanent molar once it is fully erupted may be a promising prophylactic measure in patient with cerebral palsy (CP) and global developmental delay (GDD).

Consent

The case report obtained consent form provided by the parent.

Acknowledgments

The study is supported by Dana Universiti Cawangan Selangor (DUCS) research grant with reference number 600-UiTMSEL (PI. 5/4). The authors would like to express deepest gratitude to patient and his parent for their cooperation. The author would also like to thank the research assistant Zawani Nazura Zainuren as well as the clinical supporting staffs of Faculty of Dentistry and Faculty of Medicine Universiti Teknologi MARA (UiTM).

References

[1] W. Osler, *The Cerebral Palsies of Children*, Cambridge University Press, England, 1989.

[2] C. Cans, H. Dolk, M. J. Platt, and A. Colver, "Recommendations from the SCPE collaborative group for defining and classifying cerebral palsy," *Developmental Medicine and Child Neurology*, vol. 49, no. 49, pp. 35–38, 2007.

[3] K. Himmelmann and P. Uvebrant, "The panorama of cerebral palsy in Sweden. XI. Changing patterns in the birth-year period 2003–2006," *Acta Paediatrica*, vol. 103, no. 6, pp. 618–624, 2014.

[4] B. Rodrigues, M. T. dos Santos, D. Masiero, N. F. Novo, and M. R. Simionato, "Oral conditions in children with cerebral palsy," *Journal of Dentistry for children.*, vol. 70, no. 1, pp. 40–46, 2003.

[5] M. T. dos Santos, D. Masiero, and M. R. Simionato, "Risk factors for dental caries in children with cerebral palsy," *Special Care in Dentistry.*, vol. 22, no. 3, pp. 103–107, 2002.

[6] D. Bakarcić, V. Lajnert, B. M. Maricić et al., "The comparison of malocclusion prevalence between children with cerebral palsy and Healthy children," *Collegium Antropologicum*, vol. 39, no. 3, pp. 663–666, 2015.

[7] C. B. Miamoto, M. L. Ramos-Jorge, M. C. Ferreira, M. Oliveira, R. G. Vieira-Andrade, and L. S. Marques, "Dental trauma in individuals with severe cerebral palsy: prevalence and associated factors," *Brazilian Oral Research*, vol. 25, no. 4, pp. 319-323, 2011.

[8] A. C. Peres, M. O. Ribeiro, Y. Juliano, M. F. César, and R. C.

Santos, "Occurrence of bruxism in a sample of Brazilian children with cerebral palsy," *Special Care in Dentistry.*, vol. 27, no. 2, pp. 73–76, 2007.

[9] F. Lobbezoo, J. Ahlberg, A. G. Glaros et al., "Bruxism defined and graded: an international consensus," *Journal of Oral Rehabilitation*, vol. 40, no. 1, pp. 2–4, 2013.

[10] D. Manfredini and F. Lobbezoo, "Relationship between bruxism and temporomandibular disorders: a systematic review of literature from 1998 to 2008," *Oral Surgery, Oral Medi-cine, Oral Pathology, Oral Radiology, and Endodontology.*, vol. 109, no. 6, pp. e26–e50, 2010.

[11] F. Lobbezoo, K. Koyano, D. A. Paesani, and D. Manfredini, "Sleep Bruxism: Diagnostic Considerations," in *Principles and Practice of Sleep Medicine*, M. H. Kryger, T. Roth, and W. C. Dement, Eds., pp. 1427–1434, Elsevier, Philadelphia, PA, 6th edition, 2016.

[12] P. Svensson, T. Arima, G. Lavigne, and E. Castrillon, "Sleep Bruxism: Definition, Prevalence, Classification, Etiology and Consequences," in *Principles and Practice of Sleep Medicine*, M. H. Kryger, T. Roth, and W. C. Dement, Eds., pp. 1423–1426, Elsevier, Philadelphia, PA, 6th edition, 2016.

[13] G. K. Goncalves, F. G. Carmagnani, M. S. Correa, D. A. Duarte, and M. T. Santos, "Dental erosion in cerebral palsy patients," *Journal of Dentistry for Children*, vol. 75, no. 2, pp. 117–120, 2008.

[14] R. O. Guaré, M. C. Ferreira, M. F. Leite, J. A. Rodrigues, A. Lussi, and M. T. Santos, "Dental erosion and salivary flow rate in cerebral palsy individuals with gastroesophageal reflux," *Journal of Oral Pathology & Medicine*, vol. 41, no. 5, pp. 367–371, 2012.

[15] M. T. Rodrigues Santos, W. L. Siqueira, and J. Nicolau, "Amylase and peroxidase activities and sialic acid concentration in saliva of adolescents with cerebral palsy," *Quintessence International*, vol. 38, no. 6, pp. 467–472, 2007.

[16] S. Shetty, V. Pitti, C. S. Babu, G. S. Kumar, and B. C. Deepthi, "Bruxism: a literature review," *The Journal of Indian Prosthodontic Society*, vol. 10, no. 3, pp. 141–148, 2010.

[17] K. G. Raphael, M. N. Janal, D. A. Sirois et al., "Validity of self-reported sleep bruxism among myofascial temporomandibular disorder patients and controls," *J Oral Rehabil*, vol. 42, no. 10, pp. 751–758, 2015.

[18] K. Koyano, Y. Tsukiyama, R. Ichiki, and T. Kuwata, "Assessment of bruxism in the clinic," *Journal of Oral Rehabilitation*, vol. 35, no. 7, pp. 495–508, 2008.

[19] G. de la Torre Canales, M. B. Câmara-Souza, C. F. do Amaral, R. C. Garcia, and D. Manfredini, "Is there enough evidence to use botulinum toxin injections for bruxism management? A systematic literature review," *Clinical Oral Investigations*, vol. 21, no. 3, pp. 727–734, 2017.

[20] D. Manfredini and F. Lobbezoo, "Role of psychosocial factors in the etiology of bruxism," *Journal of Orofacial Pain*, vol. 23, no. 2, pp. 153–166, 2009.

[21] E. K. Tan and J. Jankovic, "Treating severe bruxism with botulinum toxin," *Journal of the American Dental Association (1939)*, vol. 131, no. 2, pp. 211–216, 2000.

[22] J. Ramirez-Castaneda, J. Jankovic, C. Comella, K. Dashtipour, H. H. Fernandez, and Z. Mari, "Diffusion, spread and migration of botulinum toxin," *Movement Disorders*, vol. 28, no. 13, pp. 1775–1783, 2013.

[23] A. G. Glaros and B. G. Melamed, "Bruxism in children: etiology and treatment," *Applied and Preventive Psychology*, vol. 1, no. 4, pp. 191–199, 1992.

[24] K. Holmgren, A. Sheikholeslam, and C. Riise, "Effect of a full-arch maxillary occlusal splint on parafunctional activity during sleep in patients with nocturnal bruxism and signs and symptoms of craniomandibular disorders," *The Journal of Prosthetic Dentistry*, vol. 69, no. 3, pp. 293–297, 1993.

[25] S. C. Shan and W. H. Yun, "Influence of an occlusal splint on integrated electromyography of the masseter muscles," *Journal of Oral Rehabilitation*, vol. 18, no. 3, pp. 253–256, 1991.

[26] S. A. Seifeldin and K. A. Elhayes, "Soft versus hard occlusal splint therapy in the management of temporomandibular disorders (TMDs)," *The Saudi Dental Journal*, vol. 27, no. 4, pp. 208–214, 2015.

[27] H. Abekura, M. Yokomura, S. Sadamori, and T. Hamada, "The initial effects of occlusal splint vertical thickness on the nocturnal EMG activities of masticatory muscles in subjects with a bruxism habit," *The International Journal of Prosthodontics*, vol. 21, no. 2, pp. 116–120, 2008.

[28] N. Akbulut, A. Altan, S. Akbulut, and C. Atakan, "Evaluation of the 3 mm thickness splint therapy on temporomandibular joint disorders (TMDs)," *Pain Research & Management*, vol. 2018, article 3756587, pp. 1–7, 2018.

[29] A. F. Hegab, A. H. Youssef, H. Hameed, and K. S. Karam, "MRI-based determination of occlusal splint thickness for temporomandibular joint disk derangement: a randomized controlled clinical trial," *Oral Surgery, Oral Medicine, Oral Pathology, Oral Radiology*, vol. 125, no. 1, pp. 74–87, 2018.

[30] G. Lavigne, C. Manzini, and N. T. Hyunth, *'Sleep Bruxism' in Principles and Practice of Sleep Medicine*, W.B. Saunders, 5th edition, 2011.

[31] R. C. Randall, "Preformed metal crowns for primary and permanent molar teeth: review of the literature," *Pediatric Dentistry*, vol. 24, no. 5, pp. 489–500, 2002.

[32] A. T. Cheifetz, S. K. Osganian, E. N. Allred, and H. L. Needleman, "Prevalence of bruxism and associated correlates in children as reported by parents," *Journal of Dentistry for Children*, vol. 72, no. 2, pp. 67–73, 2005.

[33] A. P. Vanderas, M. Menenakou, T. Kouimtzis, and L. Papagiannoulis, "Urinary catecholamine levels and bruxism in children," *Journal of Oral Rehabilitation*, vol. 26, no. 2, pp. 103–110, 1999.

[34] J. M. Serra-Negra, S. M. Paiva, C. E. Flores-Mendoza, M. L. Ramos-Jorge, and I. A. Pordeus, "Association among stress, personality traits, and sleep bruxism in children," *Pediatric Dentistry*, vol. 34, no. 2, pp. 30E–34E, 2012.

Management of a Hypomineralisation of the Enamel by Applying a Remineraliser Based on Zinc Hydroxyapatite (microRepair)

G. Solinas,[1] V. Grabesu,[2] M. Lattari,[3] R. Strinna,[1] N. Arnould,[4] and A. A. Amodeo[5,6]

[1]*RDH, Independent Researcher in Sassari, Italy*
[2]*DDS and SLP, Independent Researcher in Sassari, Italy*
[3]*RDH, Independent Researcher in Pavia, Italy*
[4]*DDS, Independent Researcher in Sassari, Italy*
[5]*RDH DHA, Adjunct Professor Degree Course Dental Hygiene University of Milan Department of Biomedical, Surgical and Dental Sciences, Italy*
[6]*RDH DHA, Foundation IRCCS Ca' Granda Ospedale Maggiore Policlinico, Italy*

Correspondence should be addressed to A. A. Amodeo; alessio.amodeo@unimi.it

Academic Editor: Andrea Scribante

According to our experience, the treatment with remineralising mousse based on biomimetic nanohydroxyapatite has the advantage of being easily implemented by all patients as it is economical and absolutely noninvasive. The following case report reports the results obtained from the use of a mousse based on biomimetic nanohydroxyapatite for the treatment of incisor and molar hypomineralisation. This case report illustrates the case of a 4-year-old patient who was diagnosed with MIH and was subjected to remineralising treatments at home for six months, at alternating periods. Throughout the observation period, the painful perception of the lesions was detected through an assessment scale, and the clinical appearance was documented photographically. One year after the diagnosis, all the elements involved no longer showed any symptoms.

1. Introduction

Incisor and molar hypomineralisation (MIH) is characterised by a defect in enamel development of systemic origin and affects at least one permanent first molar, often associated with enamel defects of the incisors [1].

MIH has a reported overall prevalence of 12.9% (11.7-14.3%) [2]. To date, the aetiology of this disease remains unclear. Several theories have developed over the years, including prenatal theories such as cigarette smoking or maternal infections, perinatal theories such as premature births, caesarean sections and complications during delivery, and postnatal theories such as breastfeeding, poor nutrition, childhood illnesses, and drug intake. None of these factors can be considered causal [3–5].

MIH elements show macroscopic clinical differences. Histologically, they show malposition of enamel crystals. Mechanically, they are more fragile and have reduced elasticity. Enamel is characterised by an increased amount of type I collagen, a1-antitrypsin, and antithrombin III, all of which inhibit the growth of hydroxyapatite crystals during enamel maturation.

Compared to healthy teeth, teeth affected by enamel defects show a less distinct histologically prism sheath, with a lack of hydroxyapatite crystals: the hypomineralised enamel has lower mechanical properties, such as hardness and elasticity, which have lower values than a normal enamel. In addition, the enamel affected by these pathologies shows a greater amount of proteins such as serum albumin, type I collagen, ameloblastin, a1-antitrypsin, and antitrobin III, which inhibit the growth of the hydroxyapatite crystals, resulting in the reduction of the enamel minerals [6].

The features for the diagnosis of MIH are shown in Table 1.

Recently, research is moving towards the introduction of remineralising material alternative to fluorine and based on the integration of calcium and phosphates at the level of demineralised dental surfaces [7].

Table 1: Features for the diagnosis of MIH.

Key features	Description
Bounded opacity	(i) Delimited opacity (ii) Variability of colour and size (iii) Defects of less than 1 mm
Loss of posteructive enamel	(i) Surface defect after tooth eruption (ii) Loss of enamel from a surface initially formed after tooth eruption (iii) Frequently associated with a preexisting demarcated opacity
Atypical restorations	(i) Size and shape of restorations not in accordance with carious images (ii) Frequent extensions to buccal and palatal/lingual surfaces (iii) Frequently associated with opacity at the margin of the restoration (iv) For the incisors, buccal restoration not related to trauma can be seen
Molar extraction due to MIH	(i) The absence of a permanent first molar should be related to the other teeth (ii) Opacities and atypical restorations in other permanent first molars combined with the lack of a permanent first molar (iii) Absence of the first permanent molars in an otherwise healthy dentition in combination with demarcated opacities on the incisors
Failure of a molar or incisor to erupt	(i) The permanent first molar or incisor to be examined has not yet been erupted

Biomimetic effect of the nanohydroxyapatite is based on its interaction with biological tissues and on its ability to mimic biogenic materials in their functionalities. Chemical composition is similar to enamel and dentin, with intermediate characteristics. Gradual action of biomimetic nanohydroxyapatite crystals allows the linkage to dentinal and enamel tooth surfaces due to bioreabsorption properties under physiological conditions. This property can be modulated by ion substitution, and crystallinity degree achieved implementing innovative synthesis with nanosized crystal control [7, 8].

2. Differential Diagnosis

Particular emphasis should be placed on differential diagnosis with other abnormalities of the enamel structure. The correct diagnosis will result in a structured protocol for resolving the case. Specifically, we need to differentiate MIH from the following:

(i) Amelogenesis imperfecta: amelogenesis imperfecta is a genetic defect in enamel development and presents itself as hypoplastic, hypomatous or hypomineralised enamel depending on the stage of enamel formation affected by the congenital defect [9]. Depending on the type, it is complicated to distinguish it from a case of MIH. The family medical history and the involvement of the deciduous dentition should undoubtedly be taken into account [10]

(ii) *Enamel hypoplasia:* this is characterised by a defect in the amount of enamel and presents itself with reduced enamel thickness, including cavities or irregular areas. Enamel loss is localised [11]. The differentiation from MIH should be based on the characteristics of the lesion edges, which are smoother and more regular in hypoplasia and more irregular and deeper in cases of MIH [10]

(iii) *Fluorosis:* fluorosis is characterised by excessive fluoride absorption during the mineralisation phase of teeth [12]. The elements present with white, yellow or brown opacities but without a clear border with the enamel [9]. It is precisely the distinction of the lesions that is the decisive aspect in the differential diagnosis. The patient's medical history will provide additional help in making the diagnosis [10]

(iv) *White spot lesions:* these are the first signs of carious lesions. They are caused by a prolonged accumulation of bacterial plaque on the tooth surface. The position of these lesions leads to differentiation from MIH, as they are most often found on cervical areas of the elements [10–13]

3. Materials and Methods

3.1. Timeline. Figure 1 shows the timeline of the interventions. The timing of each intervention was agreed upon.

3.2. Patient Information. The female patient was 4 years old when she came to our attention. She was brought to the practice by her parents because she complained of hypersensitivity to heat and cold, even during normal breathing. The patient had never undergone a dental examination or treatment.

3.3. Objective Examination. During the examination, the patient presented hypomineralisation of the enamel on 11, 21, 31, 41, and 36. The appearance varies from one element to another. All the lesions on the incisors had well-defined borders and a white-yellow colour. 36 show areas of hypomineralisation at the occlusal and vestibular levels. The enamel is smooth on the incisors and broken on 36.

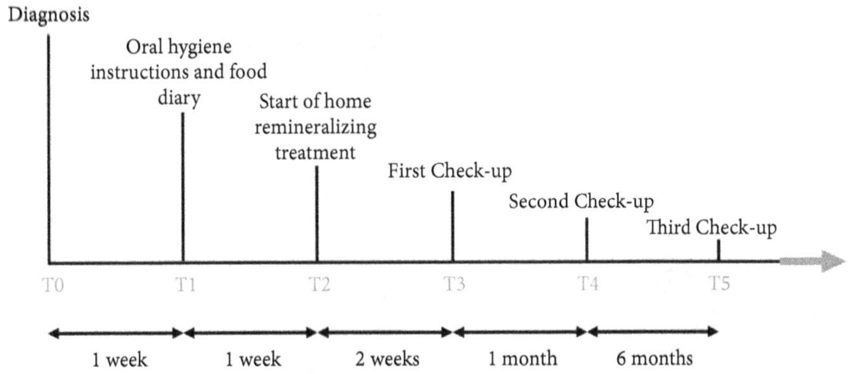

Figure 1: Timeline of interventions.

Table 2: MIH treatment need index (MIH-THI).

Grade	Description
Grade 0	No MIH
Grade 1	MIH without hypersensitivity, without defect
Grade 2	MIH without hypersensitivity, with defect
2a	<1/3 of the area involved
2b	>1/3 of the area involved
2c	>2/3 of the involved surface and/or defect close to the pulp or atypical extraction or restoration
Grade 3	MIH with hypersensitivity, without defect
Grade 4	MIH with hypersensitivity, with defect
4a	<1/3 of the area involved
4b	>1/3 < 2/3 of the surface involved
4c	>2/3 of the involved surface and/or defect close to the pulp or atypical extraction or restoration

Table 3: Subdivision into sextants.

Sextant 1	Sextant 2	Sextant 3
Right maxilla distal to/with 14 (54).	Anterior maxilla with 13-23 (53-63).	Left maxilla distal to/with 24 (64).
Sextant 6	Sextant 5	Sextant 4
Right mandible distal to/with 44 (84).	Anterior mandible with 33-43 (73-83).	Left mandible distal to/with 34 (74).

3.4. Diagnostic Evaluation. After careful assessment of the lesions during clinical follow-up, the diagnosis of MIH was made, evaluating the patient's medical history and creating a differential diagnosis with other enamel lesions.

There are currently several approaches to classifying the severity of MIH. In most cases, the pathology is subdivided and classified as mild or severe. The teeth show demarcated enamel opacities in mild cases without enamel breakdown and rarely hypersensitivity to external stimuli. In more severe cases, the enamel appears with demarcated opacities, enamel breakdown, and spontaneous hypersensitivity.

A new index, the MIH treatment need index (MIH-TNI), has recently been introduced (Table 2).

It is designed to classify MIH according to its severity based on two key symptoms that are clinically considered the most important: hypersensitivity and enamel breakdown [14–16].

For the diagnosis of our patient's MIH, we used the subdivision into sextants as proposed by the authors of the MIH-TNI [15]. The subdivision into sextants is shown in Table 3.

Table 4: Clinical case classification.

Sextant 1	Sextant 2	Sextant 3
0	2a	0
Sextant 6	Sextant 5	Sextant 4
0	4b	4b

This clinical case was classified as shown in Table 4.

3.5. Interventions. Treatment options for MIH tooth range from prevention to extraction are shown. To make the right choice, several factors need to be taken into account:

(i) The severity of the condition

(ii) Presence of symptoms

(iii) Age of the patient

(iv) Patient and parental compliance

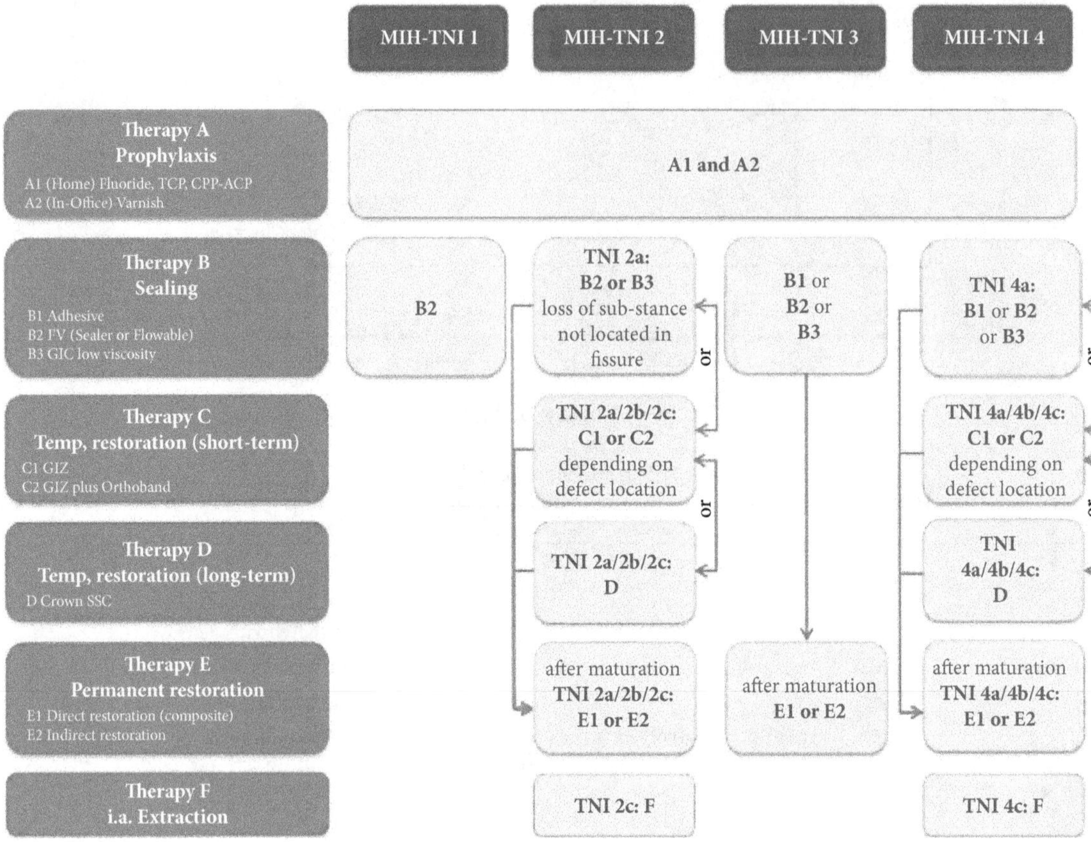

Figure 2: Therapy plan based on the MIH-TNI in patients with low caries risk.

(v) Patient and parental expectations [17]

The study by Williams et al. from 2006 [18] shows an initial clinical approach with six-step management:

(1) Risk identification

(2) Early diagnosis

(3) Remineralisation and desensitisation

(4) Prevention of tooth decay and enamel breakdown

(5) Restorations or extractions

(6) Maintenance

Also, in 2006, Mathu-Muju published another decision tree in the treatment of MIH [19], and Wright divided the injuries according to their severity (mild, moderate, and severe). Following this work, Lygidakis et al. published a practical guide in 2010 proposing various approaches depending on the severity and age of the patient [17].

By combining these guidelines and cross-referencing the data collected with the MIH-TNI table, taking the symptoms as a fixed point, therapeutic approaches ranging from prophylaxis to extraction have been developed [16] (Figures 2 and 3).

In this case report, we decided, in agreement with the patient's parents, to start with the least invasive treatment and then proceed gradually with increasingly invasive treatments in case of failure. Our treatment plan was exposed to the University's Internal Review Board which, with protocol 0077/2020, expressed a positive opinion.

In this case, the first step ($T0$) was to confirm the diagnosis, collect the clinical data, and photographically document the initial stage (Figure 4). During the first appointment, informed consent was given and explained to the patient's parents.

Before drawing up the treatment plan, we had to classify the patient's perception of pain on each element that presented hypoplasia.

The cause of this hypersensitivity would appear to be chronic inflammation of the pulp. The hypomineralised enamel and dentine layers do not sufficiently protect the pulp tissue of the dental elements from chemical and physical stimuli and thermal stimuli in the oral cavity. Although a large part of the literature [1] states that hypersensitivity occurs almost exclusively on the first molars, we will see how the patient in question also reported an increased pain perception on other elements.

Given the patient's age, who was 4 years old at $T0$, we used the Wong-Baker face (Figure 5).

For a more reliable figure, considering the patient's age, we repeated the test three times at a distance of one week. The results are superimposable and specifically are as follows:

(i) Element 11 (perceived value 0): (no pain)

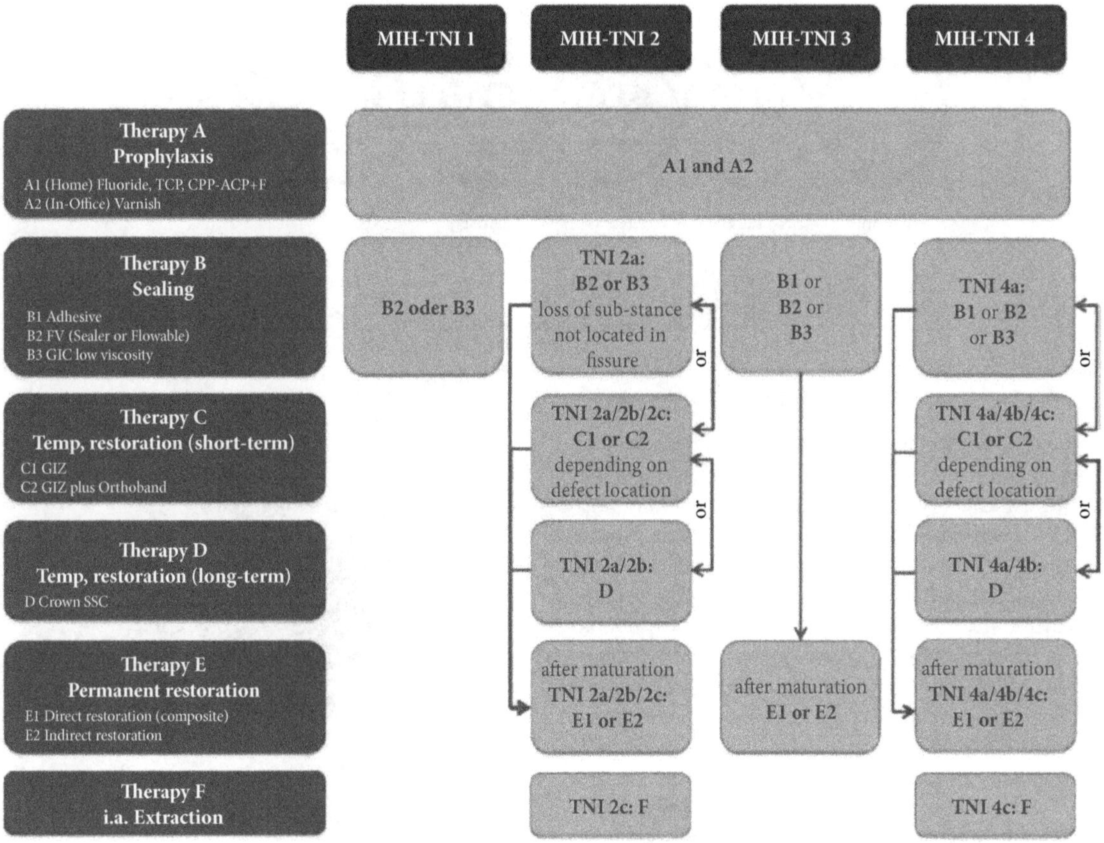

FIGURE 3: Therapy plan based on the MIH-TNI in patients with high caries risk.

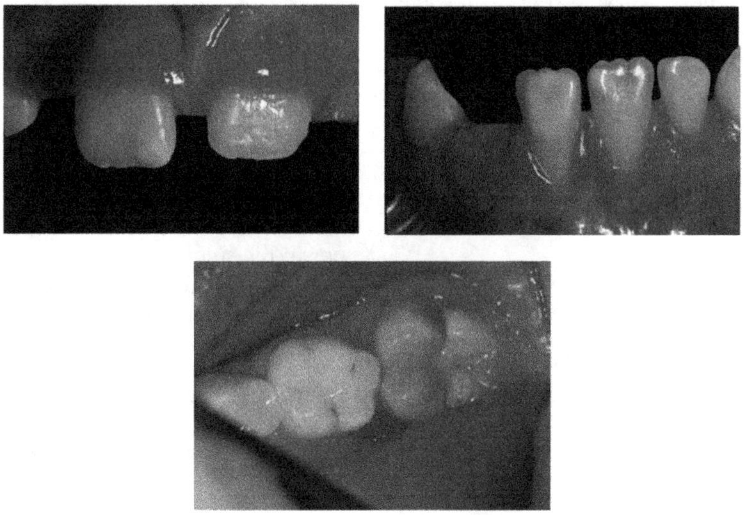

FIGURE 4: Photo of the patient at $T0$, i.e., at the time of diagnosis.

(ii) Element 21 (perceived value 0): (no pain)

(iii) Element 36 (perceived value 8): (very strong pain)

(iv) Element 41 (perceived value 8): (very strong pain)

The possibility of a potential enamel fracture on 36 was then considered very remote, and for this reason, it was decided, at least in this first phase, not to subject the element to restorative treatment.

The next appointment ($T1$) served to instruct and motivate both the patient and the parent to maintain proper, almost obsessive, oral hygiene at home. We provided the necessary tools (electric toothbrush and plaque detector tablets).

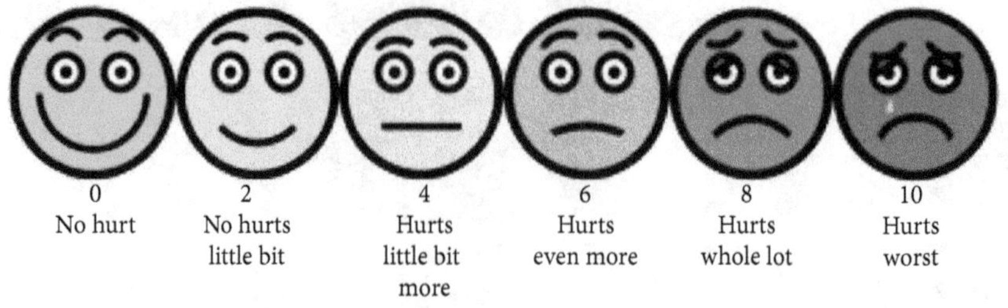

Figure 5: Wong-Baker face pain rating scale.

At the next appointment ($T2$), one week later, we proceeded to start the home remineralisation therapy with the application of a paste with zinc hydroxyapatite (Biorepair® Repair Shock Treatment, Coswell, S.p.A., Funo, Italy; ingredients: aqua, zinc hydroxyapatite 30%, hydrated silica, silica, sodium myristoyl sarcosinate, sodium methyl cocoyl taurate, sodium bicarbonate, aroma, sodium saccharin, phenoxyethanol, benzyl alcohol, sodium benzoate, citric acid, and menthol) once a day for 5 minutes, using a small disposable tray for topical fluoroprophylaxis (Figure 6) Furthermore, for the patient's daily oral hygiene, it was required to use a specific toothpaste containing zinc hydroxyapatite (Biorepair Kids 0/6 years, Coswell, S.p.A., Funo, Italy; ingredients: aqua, glycerin, zinc hydroxyapatite*, sorbitol, PEG-32, silica, cellulose gum, aroma, sodium myristoyl sarcosinate, sodium methyl cocoyl taurate, Fragaria vesca juice, Mentha piperita oil, sodium saccharin, citric acid, sodium benzoate, potassium sorbate, phenoxyethanol, benzyl alcohol, anethole, and menthol) under the supervision of the parents.

The toothpaste was used in a "pea size" dose, 2 minutes twice a day.

The parents were asked to check with the plaque detector once a week and take a photograph with their mobile phone. The pictures were sent to the practice to monitor the situation weekly without having to examine the patient so frequently.

The patient's food diary was collected and analysed, and there were no abnormalities in the weekly diet.

At time $T3$ (two weeks after the start of treatment), a clinical check-up was carried out with detection of pain perception:

(i) Element 11 (perceived value 0): (no pain)

(ii) Element 21 (perceived value 0): (no pain)

(iii) Element 36 (perceived value 8): (extreme pain)

(iv) Element 41 (perceived value 8): (extreme pain)

The data collected showed no change from $T0$.

After one month ($T4$), a further clinical check-up was carried out with data collection and photo documentation:

(i) Element 11 (perceived value 0): (no pain)

(ii) Element 21 (perceived value 0): (no pain)

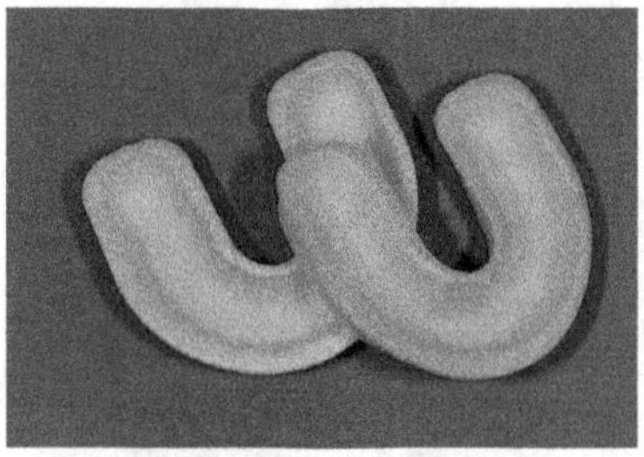

Figure 6: Disposable small fluoride trays.

(iii) Element 36 (perceived value 5): (mild pain)

(iv) Element 41 (perceived value 4): (mild pain)

(v) Element 32 (perceived value 9): (very strong pain)

(vi) Element 42 (perceived value 2): (very slight pain)

Given the excellent compliance achieved by both patient and mother, the absence of side effects of the treatment and pain perception at time $T4$ showed a reduction in pain; we decided to extend the therapy for another 6 months.

This choice was also dictated by the fact that other elements, such as 32 and 42, started erupting and had enamel defects referable to MIH.

At this point, we started scheduling bimonthly checkups in the studio.

We collected sensitivity data and documented the case photographically (Figure 7) and clinically.

The results of the test at time T5 were as follows:

(i) Element 11 (perceived value 0): (no pain)

(ii) Element 21 (perceived value 0): (no pain)

(iii) Element 36 (perceived value 0): (no pain)

(iv) Element 41 (perceived value 0): (no pain)

(v) Element 32 (perceived value 6): (mild pain)

(vi) Element 42 (perceived value 0): (no pain)

At 12 months after diagnosis ($T6$), we decided to safeguard the seal of the molars with the placement of glass ionomer cement (triage) as remineralisation of the elements after one year of treatment could guarantee stable adhesion of the product (Figure 8).

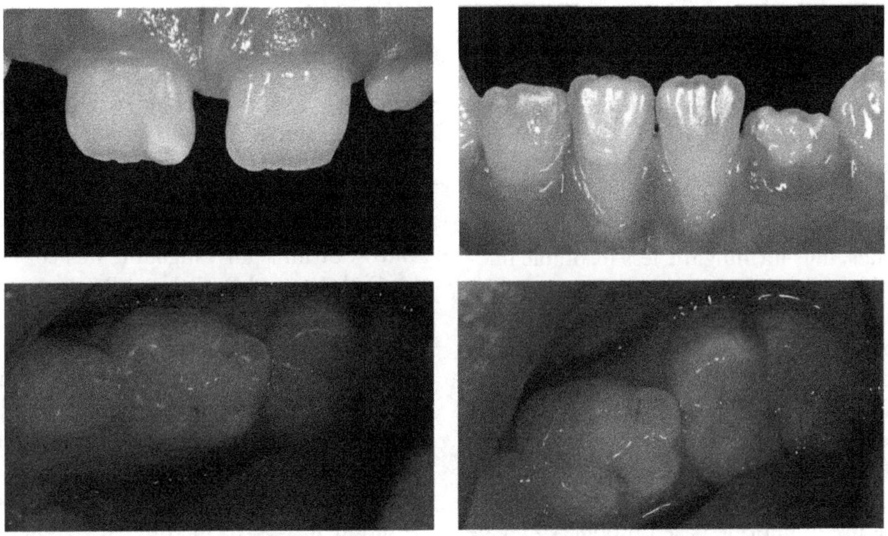

FIGURE 7: $T5$ photos (photos six months after the start of treatment).

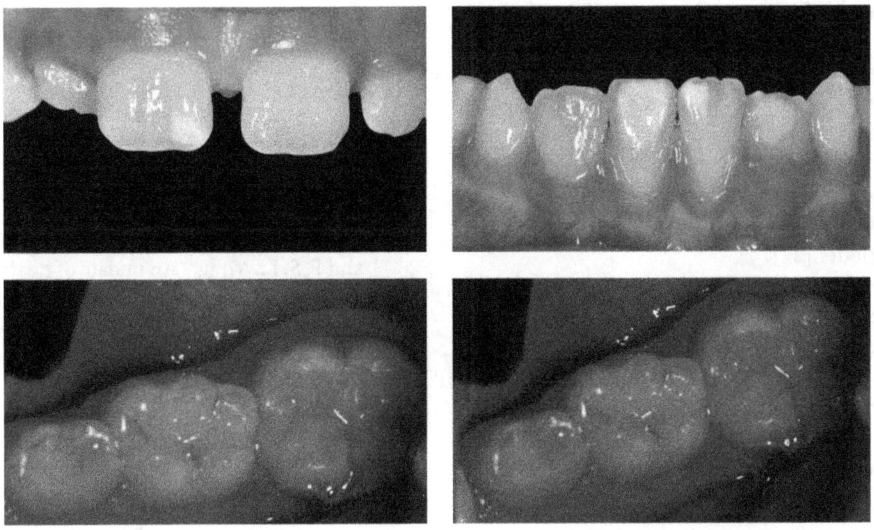

FIGURE 8: Photos at $T6$ (photos one year after the start of treatment before triage placement).

4. Discussion

This case report presents the results of home remineralisation treatment in a patient with MIH.

Incisor and molar hypomineralisation (MIH) can be defined as a delimited qualitative developmental defect of systemic origin in enamel involving the incisors and first permanent molars.

This condition leads to several dental complications, including hypersensitive teeth, increased susceptibility to tooth decay, impaired chewing due to rapid tooth loss, and aesthetic repercussions. These issues may affect patients' quality of life from an early age, so it is essential to diagnose these lesions early and set up treatment plans to preserve the teeth as much as possible. However, deciding on the most appropriate approach is complex. The main factors that need to be taken into account are patient compliance, stage of dental development, and severity of the defect; in addition, patient and parental preferences, other anomalies, and the psychosocial impact of treatment on the patient need to be considered [1].

In this case report, given the very young age of the patient and her compliance, a minimally invasive and as conservative as possible treatment was opted for.

One of the probable keys to our success was the patient's absolute cooperation. The remineralising paste was used for 5 minutes a day with a small disposable tray for topical fluoroprophylaxis; therefore, it was absolutely comfortable and atraumatic.

Several clinical trials [20–23] have investigated the benefits of using remineralising agents such as fluoride in its various formulations, casein-based mousses and amorphous calcium phosphate (CPP-ACP), and hydroxyapatite. Increasing the mineral component in teeth affected by MIH can improve the physical structure of the enamel, an improvement in symptoms and specifically in hypersensitivity, and an improvement in the aesthetic appearance of the teeth involved.

An important consideration which deserves to be done is the comparison of biomimetic hydroxyapatite with respect to fluoride.

Mouthwashes and toothpastes containing fluoride ions are among the most popular products for oral hygiene. Fluoride ions have the capability of interacting with dental hydroxyapatite crystals, thus forming the less insoluble fluoridated hydroxyapatite or fluorapatite, which are more resistant to the acid attack [24]. However, the efficacy of fluoride toothpastes is limited to a partial substitution of the hydroxyl groups with fluoride ions in natural hydroxyapatite, with no deposition of an additional mineral content.

Conversely, several studies [25] have shown that biomimetic hydroxyapatite even leads to a mineral deposition, thus forming a real coating on enamel and dental surfaces [26].

Additionally, the use of fluoride-based products may be linked to a risk of toxicity in the case of high dosage intake, respectively, consisting of fluorosis in children and bone diseases in the elderly.

The European Food Safety Authority (EFSA) suggests that the maximum level of fluoride content for oral care products, including toothpastes, is 1500 mg/kg. Also, the maximum fluoride intake should be 0.1 mg fluoride/kg/day in children aged 1–8 years [24].

Based on this consideration, in addition to the different remineralising effects, to lower the risk of toxicity linked to fluoride might suggest the safer use of biomimetic hydroxyapatite in young patients [27].

In our case report, one year after starting treatment with a hydroxyapatite paste, we can see that the probable increase in the mineral component has led to the almost complete resolution of hypersensitivity and improved aesthetic appearance of both the upper and lower central incisors. This encourages us to continue along this path in the hope that it will not be necessary to intervene in a more invasive manner in the future.

5. Conclusions

According to the latest scientific literature, MIH can significantly negatively impact children's lives, with hypersensitivity, increased susceptibility to caries, and repercussions on dental aesthetics among the most common symptoms.

Therefore, it is essential to know and distinguish MIH from other enamel lesions to intervene early and with a minimally invasive approach.

This case report reports our positive experience with treating a 4-year-old patient with stage 4b MIH using a hydroxyapatite-based cream (microRepair®). Within one year, the hypersensitivity was almost entirely resolved, and the aesthetics of the teeth improved.

Consent

Informed consent was obtained from all subjects involved in the study. Written informed consent has been obtained from the patient to publish this paper.

Authors' Contributions

Conceptualisation was done by G. Solinas, V. Grabesu, and A.A. Amodeo. Methodology was done by G. Solinas, V. Grabesu, and A.A. Amodeo. Software was acquired by V. Grabesu, M. Lattari, and R. Strinna. Validation was performed by G. Solinas, V. Grabesu, and A.A. Amodeo. Formal analysis was conducted by G. Solinas, M. Lattari, and R. Strinna. Investigation was conducted by G. Solinas, V. Grabesu, and R. Strinna. Resources were acquired by G. Solinas, M. Lattari, and R. Strinna. Data curation was performed by G. Solinas, M. Lattari, and R. Strinna. Writing and original draft preparation were done by G. Solinas, M. Lattari, and A.A. Amodeo. Writing and review and editing were done by N. Arnould and A.A. Amodeo. Visualisation was conducted by G. Solinas and V. Grabesu. Supervision was done by N. Arnould and A.A. Amodeo. Project administration was performed by N. Arnould and A.A. Amodeo. All authors have read and agreed to the published version of the manuscript.

References

[1] K. L. Weerheijm, B. Jalevik, and S. Alaluusua, "Molar-incisor hypomineralisation," *Caries Research*, vol. 35, no. 5, pp. 390-391, 2001.

[2] C. Somani, G. D. Taylor, E. Garot, P. Rouas, N. A. Lygidakis, and F. S. L. Wong, "An update of treatment modalities in children and adolescents with teeth affected by molar incisor hypomineralisation (MIH): a systematic review," *European Archives of Paediatric Dentistry*, pp. 1–26, 2021.

[3] A. Leppäniemi, P. L. Lukinmaa, and S. Alaluusua, "Nonfluoride hypomineralisation in the permanent first molars," *European Journal of Paediatric Dentistry*, vol. 3, p. 128, 2000.

[4] B. Jälevik, G. Klingberg, J. G. Norén, and L. Barregård, "Epidemiological study of idiopathic enamel hypomineralisation in permanent first molars," *European Journal of Paediatric Dentistry*, vol. 3, p. 128, 2000.

[5] V. E. V. M. Beentjes, K. L. Weerheijm, and H. J. Groen, "A match-control study into the aetiology of hypomineralized first permanent molars," *European Journal of Paediatric Dentistry*, vol. 3, p. 123, 2000.

[6] A. Butera, C. Maiorani, A. Morandini et al., "Assessment of genetical, pre, peri and post natal risk factors of deciduous molar hypomineralization (DMH), hypomineralized second primary molar (HSPM) and molar incisor hypomineralization (MIH): a narrative review," *Children*, vol. 8, p. 432, 2021.

[7] A. Scribante, M. R. Dermenaki Farahani, G. Marino et al., "Biomimetic effect of nano-hydroxyapatite in demineralized enamel before orthodontic bonding of brackets and attachments: visual, adhesion strength, and hardness in in vitro tests," *BioMed Research International*, vol. 2020, Article ID 6747498, 9 pages, 2020.

[8] M. Memarpour, F. Shafiei, A. Rafiee, M. Soltani, and M. H. Dashti, "Effect of hydroxyapatite nanoparticles on enamel remineralization and estimation of fissure sealant bond

strength to remineralized tooth surfaces: an in vitro study," *BMC Oral Health*, vol. 19, no. 1, p. 92, 2019.

[9] P. J. Crawford, M. Aldred, and A. Bloch-Zupan, "Amelogenesis imperfecta," *Orphanet Journal of Rare Diseases*, vol. 2, no. 1, p. 17, 2007.

[10] A. Ghanim, M. J. Silva, M. E. C. Elfrink et al., "Molar incisor hypomineralisation (MIH) training manual for clinical field surveys and practice," *European Archives of Paediatric Dentistry*, vol. 18, no. 4, pp. 225–242, 2017.

[11] Commission on Oral Health RE, "A review of the developmental defects of the enamel index (DDE index). Commission on oral health, research & epidemiology. Report of an FDI working group," *International Dental Journal*, vol. 42, no. 6, pp. 411–426, 1992.

[12] P. Denbesten and W. Li, "Chronic fluoride toxicity: dental fluorosis," *Monographs in Oral Science*, vol. 22, pp. 81–96, 2011.

[13] G. Solinas, G. Stellino, M. Lattari, A. A. Amodeo, and A. B. Giannì, "Case report: combined treatment with home bleaching and resin infiltration in treating two non-cavited carious lesions," *Acta Scientific Dental Sciences*, vol. 5, no. 8, pp. 59–64, 2021.

[14] R. Steffen, N. Kramer, and K. Bekes, "The Würzburg MIH concept: the MIH treatment need index (MIH TNI)," *European Archives of Paediatric Dentistry*, vol. 18, no. 5, pp. 355–361, 2017.

[15] K. Bekes and R. Steffen, "The Wuerzburg MIH concept: part 1. The MIH treatment need index (MIH TNI). A new index to assess and plan the treatment in patients with molar incisor hypomineralization (MIH)," *Oralprophylaxe & Kinderzahnheilkunde*, vol. 38, no. 4, pp. 165–170, 2016.

[16] K. Bekes, N. Krämer, H. van Waes, and R. Steffen, "The Wuerzburg MIH concept: part 2," *The treatment plan. Oralprophylaxe & Kinderzahnheilkunde*, vol. 38, no. 4, pp. 171–175, 2016.

[17] N. A. Lygidakis, F. Wong, B. Jalevik, A. M. Vierrou, S. Alaluusua, and I. Espelid, "Best clinical practice guidance for clinicians dealing with children presenting with molar-incisor-hypomineralisation (MIH)," *European Archives of Paediatric Dentistry*, vol. 11, no. 2, pp. 75–81, 2010.

[18] V. William, L. B. Messer, and M. F. Burrow, "Molar incisor hypomineralisation: review and recommendations for clinical management," *Pediatric Dentistry*, vol. 28, no. 3, pp. 224–232, 2006.

[19] K. Mathu-Muju and J. T. Wright, "Diagnosis and treatment of molar incisor hypomineralisation," *The Compendium of Continuing Education in Dentistry*, vol. 27, no. 11, pp. 604–610, 2006.

[20] M. Bakkal, Z. Abbasoglu, and B. Kargul, "The effect of casein phosphopeptide-amorphous calcium phosphate on molar-incisor hypomineralisation: a pilot study," *Oral Health & Preventive Dentistry*, vol. 15, no. 2, pp. 163–167, 2017.

[21] C. Baroni and S. Marchionni, "MIH supplementation Strategies," *Journal of Dental Research*, vol. 90, no. 3, pp. 371–376, 2011.

[22] A. M. Biondi, S. G. Cortese, L. Babino, and D. E. Fridman, "Comparison of mineral density in molar incisor hypomineralization applying fluoride varnishes and casein phosphopeptide-amorphous calcium phosphate," *Acta Odontológica Latinoamericana*, vol. 30, no. 3, pp. 118–123, 2017.

[23] M. Restrepo, F. Jeremias, L. Santos-Pinto, R. Cordeiro, and A. Zuanon, "Effect of fluoride varnish on enamel Remineralization in anterior teeth with molar incisor Hypomineralization," *The Journal of Clinical Pediatric Dentistry*, vol. 40, no. 3, pp. 207–210, 2016.

[24] M. Lelli, O. Marchisio, I. Foltran et al., "Different corrosive effects on hydroxyapatite nanocrystals and amine fluoride-based mouthwashes on dental titanium brackets: a comparative in vitro study," *International Journal of Nanomedicine*, vol. 8, pp. 307–314, 2013.

[25] A. Butera, M. Pascadopoli, S. Gallo et al., "SEM/EDS evaluation of the mineral deposition on a polymeric composite resin of a toothpaste containing biomimetic Zn-carbonate hydroxyapatite (microRepair®) in oral environment: a randomized clinical trial," *Polymers*, vol. 13, no. 16, p. 2740, 2021.

[26] M. Lelli, A. Putignano, M. Marchetti et al., "Remineralization and repair of enamel surface by biomimetic Zn-carbonate hydroxyapatite containing toothpaste: a comparative in vivo study," *Frontiers in Physiology*, vol. 5, p. 333, 2014.

[27] M. Bossù, M. Saccucci, A. Salucci et al., "Enamel remineralization and repair results of biomimetic hydroxyapatite toothpaste on deciduous teeth: an effective option to fluoride toothpaste," *Journal of Nanbiotechnology*, vol. 17, no. 1, p. 17, 2019.

25

Use of a Modified Nance Appliance for Esthetic Rehabilitation of a Child Patient with Rare Nonfamilial and Nonsyndromic Oligodontia

Abbas O. Al-Ahmadi,[1] Ali A. Assiry,[2] Siraj D. A. A. Khan,[2] Anand Marya,[3,4] Adith Venugopal,[4] and Mohmed Isaqali Karobari[5]

[1]*Specialized Dental Centre, King Fahad Hospital, Medina, Saudi Arabia*
[2]*Pediatric Dentistry, Faculty of Dentistry, Najran University, Saudi Arabia*
[3]*Department of Orthodontics, Faculty of Dentistry, University of Puthisastra, Phnom Penh, Cambodia*
[4]*Department of Orthodontics, Saveetha Dental College, Saveetha Institute of Medical and Technical Sciences, Saveetha University, Chennai, India*
[5]*Conservative Unit, School of Dental Sciences, Universiti Sains Malaysia, Health Campus, Kubang Kerian, 16150 Kota Bharu, Kelantan, Malaysia*

Correspondence should be addressed to Anand Marya; amarya@puthisastra.edu.kh

Academic Editor: Husamettin Oktay

Congenital absence of more than 6 teeth except the third molar is known as oligodontia. It can affect both primary and permanent dentitions. The affected individuals usually demonstrate esthetic, functional, and psychological concerns. The present case report is about a 4-year-old female patient with multiple missing (both primary and permanent) teeth with esthetic and social problems. On extraoral examination, the patient demonstrated upper lip relapse due to missing anterior teeth. On physical examination, no other abnormality was detected in relation to the hair, appendages, or presence of a cleft. On intraoral and radiographic examination, 21 teeth were missing, which included both the primary and the permanent tooth buds. To encourage a positive behavioral change, it was decided to carry out prosthetic intervention using a modified fixed Nance appliance and acrylic teeth. After the replacement of the missing teeth, a marked improvement in the profile and esthetics was seen.

1. Introduction

The tooth is one of the most useful tissues in the body. Dentinogenesis is a dynamic process resulting from many instructive and permissive cellular and molecular interactions; any disturbance across these interactions will affect tooth development either partly or entirely [1, 2].

Congenital absence of one or more teeth either in primary or permanent dentition is known as tooth agenesis, which could be partial (hypodontia or oligodontia) or complete (anodontia), excluding the third molar [3, 4]. Oligodontia is a rare condition that can occur either in association with genetic syndromes, as a nonsyndromic isolated familial trait or sporadic finding [5]. It mainly occurs in the permanent dentition but can affect primary dentition also [6]. In the primary dentition, it is seen in the incisal region and is often associated with missing succedaneous teeth [7].

In young patients, the absence of teeth can cause esthetic, functional, and psychological problems, especially when the anterior teeth are involved. This paper presents a unique case of a young child with nonfamilial nonsyndromic oligodontia, present in both primary and permanent dentition, where esthetic, form, and functions of dentition were established through prosthetic intervention.

2. Case Report

A 4-year-old female patient reported to the Department of Pediatric Dentistry at King Fahad Hospital with her father. Her father stated that she demonstrated negative behavioral changes due to multiple missing teeth and avoided social activities. The patient was apprehensive and depicting a negative attitude during a routine dental examination. No significant familial history regarding the absence of teeth was reported. The dental history given by the parents suggested that there was a congenital absence of most of the primary teeth.

Intraoral examination during the first visit revealed that the dentition was spaced, there is absence of 8 primary teeth (tooth numbers 51, 52, 53, 61, 62, 63, 72, and 82), and both right and left lower canines were conical in shape (Figure 1). The alveolus of the upper anterior was very thin, and the teeth present were of standard size, shape, and color. The occlusal view of both maxillary and mandibular (Figure 2) arches revealed the absence of 13 tooth buds (tooth numbers 11, 12, 13, 15, 21, 22, 23, 25, 32, 33, 35, 42, and 45). Provisionally, it was diagnosed as nonfamilial and nonsyndromic oligodontia.

To rule out the syndromic and genetic involvement, the patient was referred to a pediatrician and a genetic consultant, both of whom confirmed that it was a case of nonfamilial and nonsyndromic oligodontia.

3. Treatment Plan

A modified fixed Nance appliance with artificial anterior teeth (Figure 3) was planned for esthetic rehabilitation along with careful behavior management. Since the patient's chief concern was esthetics, it was decided only to rehabilitate the maxillary arch that would help improve her nasolabial profile. This modified appliance was cemented on tooth numbers 55 and 65. With improvement in esthetics, the patient immediately reported a positive change in attitude (Figure 4). After one week, during the follow-up visit, the patient's parents reported a marked improvement in her social interactions and positive behavior.

4. Discussion

The biological basis of tooth agenesis is a sequential and reciprocal series of signaling in a precisely organized manner that leads to the lingual and distal proliferation of the tooth germ from the dental lamina. Any disturbance during this process will affect tooth development either partly or entirely [8, 9].

Various etiological factors have been proposed for tooth agenesis which varies from environmental factors such as radiotherapy, tumors, trauma to the alveolar processes, disturbance in the innervation of the jaw, hormonal influences, rubella, and drugs like thalidomide to hereditary factors such as MSX1 and PAX9, AXIN2, EDA, and EDAR genes [8, 10–15]. The genes responsible for nonsyndromic oligodontia are transforming growth factor-beta (TGF-β), PAX9, and MSX1 [8, 16–18].

Oligodontia (severe partial anodontia) is a developmental dental anomaly that refers to a congenital absence of more than six teeth, excluding third molars [19]. It has been previously reported in both primary and permanent teeth. It can be either associated with syndromes, a nonsyndromic isolated familial trait, or sporadic finding [5]. Gorlin et al. [20] reported that nonsyndromic oligodontia could be sporadic or familial.

Although reports on congenitally missing teeth are not new as these have been reported since ancient times (early reported from the Iron Age) [21], in the history of Saudi Arabia, significantly less data is available (Table 1) [22–29]. The prevalence of nonsyndromic congenitally missing primary teeth (0.24%) in Saudi Arabia has been reported by Yassin [25], which is lower compared to most countries (Table 2) [30–38]. Shilpa et al. [30] suggested that the possible causes for this variation are the difference in age groups included in these studies and geographical locations.

The reported case is unique for several reasons. Firstly, there are very few nonsyndromic nonfamilial cases reported with congenitally missing primary and permanent teeth. Secondly, this is the first nonfamilial and nonsyndromic oligodontia case reported in Saudi Arabia. Gholman et al. [39] reported a case of syndromic oligodontia, and Maganur et al. [40] reported oligodontia in permanent dentition. Thirdly, there are 21 missing teeth in the present case, which makes it an even rarer finding; previously, Venkataraghavan and Anantharaj [41] reported 18 missing teeth.

The diagnosis of oligodontia is usually based on routine clinical examination and radiographic evaluation while detecting missing teeth. Panoramic radiographs are preferred diagnostic aids as these register both the maxillary and mandibular arches and the developmental status of the permanent tooth buds with minimum radiation exposure [42]. For the present case, a diagnostic panoramic radiograph was avoided as the patient was extremely uncooperative, and only intraoral occlusal records were taken to reduce the radiation exposure (Figure 2).

Patients with oligodontia may experience significant psychological, esthetic, and functional issues. Therefore, it is essential to diagnose and treat these patients as soon as possible. The goal of the treatment includes saving the remaining teeth, recovering the masticatory and esthetic functions, improving speech, and restoring emotional and psychological well-being [42, 43]. Dental treatment is based on the severity of the disease and typically involves a multidisciplinary approach. The treatment choice depends on various factors like age of the patient, number and position of present teeth, patient's cooperation and treatment options, orthodontic therapy, implants, adhesive prosthesis, removable prosthesis, fixed prosthesis, and overdentures [42–44]. A treatment option is chosen based on functional and esthetic solutions. It allows the child as normal a lifestyle as possible without damaging or affecting the child's self-esteem, growth, and behavior [45]. In the present case, the treatment goal included behavior management, maintaining optimal oral health, educating about issues that may arise because of the long-term effects of both appliance therapy and spaced dentition, and monitoring of developing occlusion and

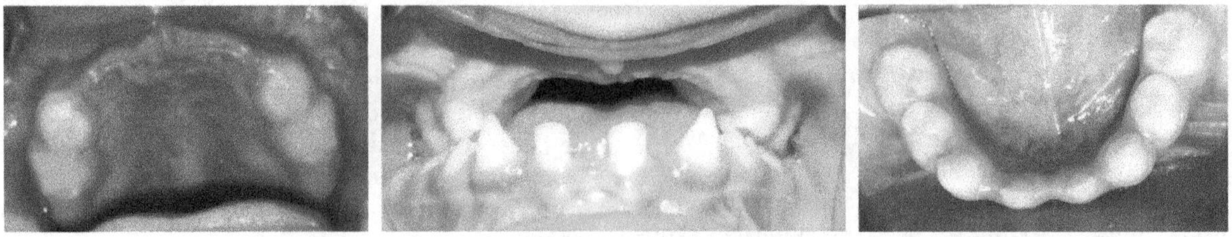

Figure 1: Intraoral pictures demonstrating multiple missing teeth.

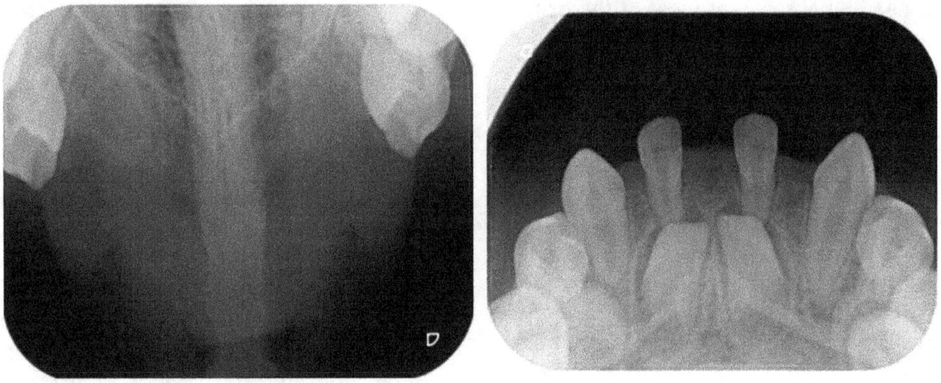

Figure 2: Occlusal view of both the maxillary and the mandibular arches.

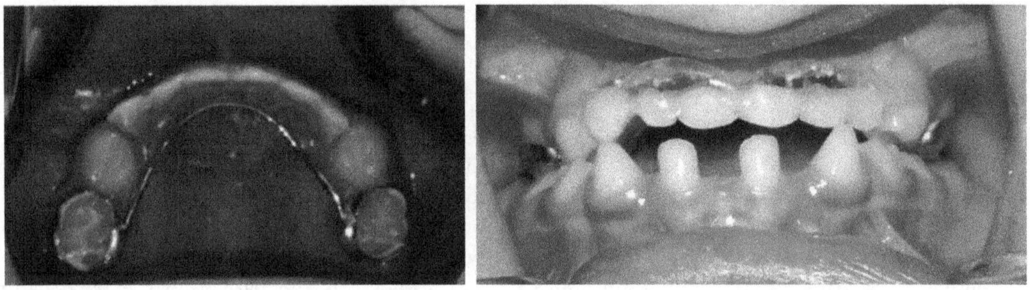

Figure 3: Modified fixed Nance appliance with artificial anterior teeth.

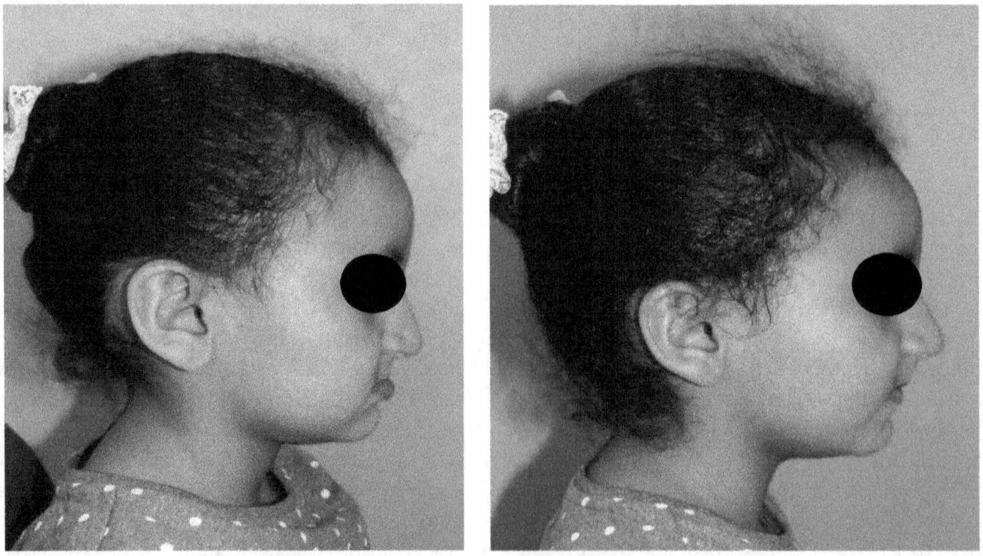

Figure 4: Pretreatment and postplacement of the appliance showing definite improvement in the patient's profile.

Table 1: The prevalence of congenitally missing teeth in the different regions of Saudi Arabia.

S No.	Author name & year	Prevalence	Region
1	Tariq Alswayyed et al. (2018) [22]	33.7%	Riyadh
2	Tareq et al. (2017) [23]	7.42%	Aseer
3	Sajjad et al. (2016) [24]	6.1%	Al-Jouf
4	Yassin et al. (2016) [25]	9.7%	Abha
5	Vani et al. (2015) [26]	5.2%	Jazan
6	Al-Jabaa and Aldrees (2013) [27]	20%	—
7	Ghaznawi et al. (1999) [28]	9.41%	—
8	Salama and Abdel Megid (1994) [29]	2.6%	—

Table 2: The prevalence of nonsyndromic congenitally missing primary teeth worldwide.

S No.	Author name & year	Prevalence	Country
1	Shilpa et al. (2017) [30]	0.88%	South India
2	Mukhopadhyay and Mitra (2014) [31]	0.5%	East India
3	Kapdan et al. (2012) [32]	0.2%	Turkey
4	King et al. (2008) [33]	0.4-4.6%	Southern China
5	Kramer et al. (2008) [34]	0.6%	Brazil
6	Daugaard et al. (1997) [35]	54.9%	Denmark
7	Yonezu et al. (1997) [36]	2.38%	Japan
8	Whittington and Durward (1996) [37]	1.37%	New Zealand
9	Brook (1974) [38]	0.1-1.9%	Britain

eruption of permanent teeth. The treatment option chosen for the patient was a modified fixed Nance appliance with artificial upper anterior teeth.

Very few studies have measured oral health-related quality of life (OHRQoL) that have been carried out to provide some evidence that congenitally missing teeth may have an adverse impact on the quality of life [46]. Hobkirk et al. [47], Locker et al. [48], and Souza et al. [49] have, respectively, suggested that delayed treatment of such patients is likely to impact social and educational development negatively. In the present case, lack of socialization was reported due to missing teeth which was improved within a week after replacing missing teeth. Orthodontic therapy can be life-altering, and esthetically challenging cases such as this can help bring remarkable changes in a patient's esthetic profile [50, 51].

5. Conclusion

Oligodontia may be associated with a systemic condition and a syndrome or occur as an isolated event. Nonsyndromic oligodontia is a rare entity and usually remains undiagnosed till it affects esthetic or masticatory functions. The best way to detect both primary and permanent dentition congenital dental anomalies is through clinical and radiographical examination. A patient with missing teeth suffers not only from masticatory and esthetic problems but also from psychological stress, and it can lower the self-esteem of the individual. This case report illustrates the rare occurrence of oligodontia in both primary and permanent dentitions. An alternative treatment option treated the present case for a 4-year-old patient with agenesis of eight primary teeth. In addition to the effects of dental agenesis, in this situation, the child's mental and psychological health was a significant consideration for early intervention.

References

[1] J. Arechaga, "The tooth as a model in organogenesis," *The International Journal of Developmental Biology*, vol. 39, pp. 13–13, 1995.

[2] I. Thesleff, A. Vaahtokari, S. Vainio, and A. Jowett, "Molecular mechanisms of cell and tissue interactions during early tooth development," *The Anatomical Record*, vol. 245, no. 2, pp. 151–161, 1996.

[3] R. E. Stewart, "The dentition and anomalies of tooth size, form, structure, and eruption," in *Pediatric Dentistry: Scientific Foundations of Clinical Procedures*, p. 91, CV Mosby, St. Louis, Mo, 1982.

[4] B. J. Polder, M. A. van't Hof, F. P. G. M. van der Linden, and A. M. Kuijpers-Jagtman, "A meta-analysis of the prevalence of dental agenesis of permanent teeth," *Community Dentistry and Oral Epidemiology*, vol. 32, no. 3, pp. 217–226, 2004.

[5] E. Kotsiomiti, D. Kassa, and D. Kapari, "Oligodontia and associated characteristics: assessment in view of prosthodontic rehabilitation," *The European Journal of Prosthodontics and Restorative Dentistry*, vol. 15, no. 2, pp. 55–60, 2007.

[6] R. E. Mc Donald and D. R. Avery, "Acquired and developmental disturbances of the teeth and associated oral structures," in

Dentistry for the Child and Adolescent, p. 147, CV Mosby, St. Louis, Mo, 1989.

[7] R. Meon, "Hypodontia of the primary and permanent dentition," *The Journal of Clinical Pediatric Dentistry*, vol. 16, p. 121, 1992.

[8] P. Tangade and M. Batra, "Non syndromic oligodontia: case report," *Ethiopian Journal of Health Sciences*, vol. 22, no. 2, 2012.

[9] M. A. Williams and A. Letra, "The changing landscape in the genetic etiology of human tooth agenesis," *Genes*, vol. 9, no. 5, p. 255, 2018.

[10] B. Bergendal, J. Klar, C. Stecksen-Blicks, J. Norderyd, and N. Dahl, "Isolated oligodontia associated with mutations in EDARADD, AXIN2, MSX1, and PAX9 genes," *American Journal of Medical Genetics. Part A*, vol. 155, no. 7, pp. 1616–1622, 2011.

[11] J. S. Gullikson, "Tooth morphology in rubella syndrome children," *ASDC Journal of Dentistry for Children*, vol. 42, no. 6, pp. 479–482, 1975.

[12] A. Maguire, A. W. Craft, R. G. Evans et al., "The long-term effects of treatment on the dental condition of children surviving malignant disease," *Cancer*, vol. 60, no. 10, pp. 2570–2575, 1987.

[13] M. Nasman, C. M. Forsberg, and G. Dahllof, "Long-term dental development in children after treatment for malignant disease," *European Journal of Orthodontics*, vol. 19, no. 2, pp. 151–159, 1997.

[14] I. Kjaer, G. Kocsis, M. Nodal, and L. R. Christensen, "Aetiological aspects of mandibular tooth agenesis-focusing on the role of nerve, oral mucosa, and supporting tissues," *European Journal of Orthodontics*, vol. 16, no. 5, pp. 371–375, 1994.

[15] E. Andersen, L. T. Skovgaard, S. Poulsen, and I. Kjaer, "The influence of jaw innervation on the dental maturation pattern in the mandible," *Orthodontics & Craniofacial Research*, vol. 7, no. 4, pp. 211–215, 2004.

[16] A. R. Vieira, R. Meira, A. Modesto, and J. C. Murray, "MSX1, PAX9, and TGFα contribute to tooth agenesis in humans," *Journal of Dental Research*, vol. 83, no. 9, pp. 723-727, 2004.

[17] P. J. de Coster, L. A. Marks, L. C. Martens, and A. Huysseune, "Dental agenesis: genetic and clinical perspectives," *Journal of Oral Pathology & Medicine*, vol. 38, no. 1, pp. 1–17, 2009.

[18] G. Galluccio, M. Castellano, and C. la Monaca, "Genetic basis of non-syndromic anomalies of human tooth number," *Archives of Oral Biology*, vol. 57, no. 7, pp. 918–930, 2012.

[19] R. E. Stewart, T. K. Barner, K. C. Troutman, and S. H. Y. Wei, *Pediatric dentistry, scientific foundations and clinical practice*, CV Mosby Co, St Louis, 1st edition, 1982.

[20] R. J. Gorlin, M. M. J. Cohen, and L. S. Levin, Eds., *Syndromes of the Head and Neck*, Oxford University Press, New York, NY, USA, 3rd ed. edition, 1990.

[21] K. Nelsen, N. Tayles, and K. Domett, "Missing lateral incisors in Iron Age South-East Asians as possible indicators of dental agenesis," *Archives of Oral Biology*, vol. 46, no. 10, pp. 963–971, 2001.

[22] T. Alswayyed, A. Q. Manal, A. Al Matrodi et al., "Patterns of dental anomalies in patients attending for orthodontic treatment in King Abdul- Aziz Medical City, Riyadh Saudi Arabia," *International Journal of Oral and Dental Health*, vol. 4, no. 2, pp. 8–13, 2018.

[23] T. Ali, V. S. Nasim, and R. A. Togoo, "Prevalence of congenitally missing permanent teeth in Aseer, KSA," *Journal of Oral & Dental Health*, vol. 1, no. 2, 2017.

[24] A. Sajjad, S. S. Sajjad, N. Husain, and A. M. Al-Enezi, "A retrospective cross-sectional study on the prevalence of hypodontia in a target population of Al-Jouf Province, Saudi Arabia," *Contemporary Clinical Dentistry*, vol. 7, no. 4, pp. 500–505, 2016.

[25] S. M. Yassin, "Prevalence and distribution of selected dental anomalies among Saudi children in Abha, *Saudi Arabia*," *Journal of Clinical and Experimental Dentistry*, vol. 8, no. 5, pp. 485–490, 2016.

[26] N. V. Vani, S. M. Saleh, F. M. Tubaigy, and A. M. Idris, "Prevalence of developmental dental anomalies among adult population of Jazan, Saudi Arabia," *The Saudi Journal for Dental Research*, vol. 7, no. 1, pp. 29–33, 2016.

[27] A. H. Al-Jabaa and A. M. Aldrees, "Prevalence of dental anomalies in Saudi orthodontic patients," *The Journal of Contemporary Dental Practice*, vol. 14, no. 4, pp. 724–730, 2013.

[28] H. I. Ghaznawi, H. Daas, and O. Salakon, "A clinical and radiographic survey of selected dental anomalies and conditions in a Saudi Arabian population," *Saudi Dental Journal*, vol. 11, no. 1, pp. 8–13, 1999.

[29] F. S. Salama and F. Y. Abdel-Megid, "Hypodontia of primary and permanent teeth in a sample of Saudi children," *Egyptian Dental Journal*, vol. 40, no. 1, pp. 625–632, 1994.

[30] G. Shilpa, N. Gokhale, S. K. Mallineni, and S. Nuvvula, "Prevalence of dental anomalies in deciduous dentition and its association with succedaneous dentition: a cross-sectional study of 4180 South Indian children," *Journal of the Indian Society of Pedodontics and Preventive Dentistry*, vol. 35, no. 1, pp. 56–62, 2017.

[31] S. Mukhopadhyay and S. Mitra, "Anomalies in primary dentition: their distribution and correlation with permanent dentition," *Journal of Natural Science, Biology and Medicine*, vol. 5, no. 1, pp. 139–143, 2014.

[32] A. Kapdan, A. Kustarci, B. Buldur, D. Arslan, and A. Kapdan, "Dental anomalies in the primary dentition of Turkish children," *European Journal of Dentistry*, vol. 6, no. 2, pp. 178–183, 2012.

[33] N. M. King, S. Tongkoom, A. Itthagarun, H. M. Wong, and C. K. Lee, "A catalogue of anomalies and traits of the primary dentition of southern Chinese," *The Journal of Clinical Pediatric Dentistry*, vol. 32, no. 2, pp. 139–146, 2008.

[34] P. F. Kramer, C. A. Feldens, S. H. Ferreira, M. H. Spiguel, and E. G. Feldens, "Dental anomalies and associated factors in 2- to 5-year-old Brazilian children," *International Journal of Paediatric Dentistry*, vol. 18, no. 6, pp. 434–440, 2008.

[35] J. Daugaard-Jensen, M. Nodal, and I. Kjaer, "Pattern of agenesis in the primary dentition: a radiographic study of 193 cases," *International Journal of Paediatric Dentistry*, vol. 7, no. 1, pp. 3–7, 1997.

[36] T. Yonezu, Y. Hayashi, J. Sasaki, and Y. Machida, "Prevalence of congenital dental anomalies of the deciduous dentition in Japanese children," *The Bulletin of Tokyo Dental College*, vol. 38, no. 1, pp. 27–32, 1997.

[37] B. R. Whittington and C. S. Durward, "Survey of anomalies in primary teeth and their correlation with the permanent dentition," *The New Zealand Dental Journal*, vol. 92, no. 407, pp. 4–8, 1996.

[38] A. H. Brook, "Dental anomalies of number, form and size: their prevalence in British schoolchildren," *Journal of the International Association of Dentistry for Children*, vol. 5, no. 2, pp. 37–53, 1974.

[39] R. R. Gholman, W. M. Kassar, and O. A. El Meligy, "Dental rehabilitation of a child with ectodermal dysplasia: a case report," *International Journal of Clinical Pediatric Dentistry*, vol. 12, no. 4, pp. 362–365, 2019.

[40] P. C. Maganur, V. Satish, S. Panda, and M. C. Dayanand Saraswathi, "Non-syndromic oligodontia: a rare case report," *Austin Journal of Dentistry*, vol. 4, no. 6, p. 1090, 2017.

[41] K. Venkataraghavan and A. Anantharaj, "Oligodontia in the primary dentition: report of a case," *Journal of Dentistry for Children*, vol. 74, pp. 153–155, 2007.

[42] M. F. Correia, M. N. Nogueira, T. B. Bedran, and D. M. Palomari Spolidorio, "Aesthetic Rehabilitation of Oligodontia in Primary Dentition with Adhesive Partial Denture," *Case Report in Dentistry*, vol. 2013, article 872476, 4 pages, 2013.

[43] N. B. Nagaveni, K. V. Umashankara, N. B. Radhika, and T. S. Satisha, "Non-syndromic oligodontia- report of a clinical case with 14 missing teeth," *Bangladesh Journal of Medical Science*, vol. 10, no. 3, pp. 200–202, 2011.

[44] P. Pannu, V. Galhotra, P. Alhuwalai, and R. S. Gambhir, "Non-syndromic oligodontia in permanent dentition: a case report," *Ghana Medical Journal*, vol. 48, no. 3, pp. 173–176, 2014.

[45] J. Moses, D. Gurunathan, B. N. Rangeeth, and K. S. Kannan, "Non-syndromic oligodontia of primary and permanent dentition: 5 year follow up- a rare case report," *Journal of Clinical and Diagnostic Research*, vol. 7, no. 4, pp. 776–779, 2013.

[46] A. H. Al-Ani, J. S. Antoun, W. M. Thomson, T. R. Merriman, and M. Farella, "Hypodontia: An Update on Its Etiology, Classification, and Clinical Management," *BioMed Research International*, vol. 2017, Article ID 9378325, 9 pages, 2017.

[47] J. A. Hobkirk, J. R. Goodman, and S. P. Jones, "Presenting complaints and findings in a group of patients attending a hypodontia clinic," *British Dental Journal*, vol. 177, no. 9, pp. 337–339, 1994.

[48] D. Locker, A. Jokovic, P. Prakash, and B. Tompson, "Oral health-related quality of life of children with oligodontia," *International Journal of Paediatric Dentistry*, vol. 20, no. 1, pp. 8–14, 2010.

[49] L. D. Souza, N. R. Vaid, E. T. Roy, and G. B. Urs, "Shyness, self-esteem, dental disharmony, and orthodontic treatment," *Indian Journal of Clinical Psychology*, vol. 28, no. 2, pp. 246–251, 2001.

[50] N. Vaid, "Waiting for that big idea!," *APOS Trends in Orthodontics*, vol. 6, no. 2, pp. 55–57, 2016.

[51] A. Venugopal, M. S. Ghoussoub, P. Manzano et al., "Molar protraction on an adult with severe high-angle class III malocclusion and knife-edge residual ridges," *Orthodontic Waves*, pp. 1–9, 2021.

Can Vitamin D Therapy Contribute to the Conservative Resolution of Osteolytic Lesions of the Jaws?

Kamis Gaballah,[1] **Sami Kenz**,[2] **Raeefa Anis**,[3] **and Omar Kujan**[4]

[1]*Department of Oral and Craniofacial Health Sciences, College of Dental Medicine, University of Sharjah, UAE*
[2]*Rashid Centre for Diabetes & Research, Ajman, UAE*
[3]*Ajman University, UAE*
[4]*UWA Dental School, The University of Western Australia, Perth WA6009, Australia*

Correspondence should be addressed to Kamis Gaballah; kamisomfs@yahoo.co.uk

Academic Editor: Kenji Yamagata

Osteolytic lesions of the jaw are not uncommon. Such lesions usually arise from local pathologies, but some have systemic backgrounds. We describe a 12-year-old girl who presented with an asymptomatic left mandibular swelling. The bony swelling was corresponding to a radiolucent lesion in the left premolar/molar region. This lesion could have represented an inflammatory and developmental odontogenic jaw cyst, giant cell lesion, and odontogenic tumor. However, the workup investigations revealed secondary hyperparathyroidism due to vitamin D deficiency. A vitamin D replacement was initiated with a single I.M. injection of 300,000 I.U followed by 10,000 I.U orally, weekly. Six weeks later, her Vitamin D and parathyroid hormone were normalized, and she showed significant clinical and radiological improvement of the jaw lesion. At 18 months, follow-up the panoramic image revealed complete resolution of the radiolucency and stable normal parathyroid hormone and vitamin D levels. In conclusion, Jaw bone lesions can develop secondary to hyperparathyroidism due to vitamin D deficiency, and this should be ruled out before any surgical intervention. Treatment of such lesions lies in the correction of parathyroid excess with a careful and systematic approach. This may prevent unnecessary surgical intervention in such patients.

1. Introduction

Vitamin D deficiency is a health burden that has caused concerns worldwide over the past decades due to implications on bone biology, multiple sclerosis, diabetes, depression, and cardiovascular disease [1]. Despite the sunny climate, a prevalence of 90.9% of hypovitaminosis D was reported in women in the UAE [2, 3]. Likewise, Yammine et al. reported that 57.5% of the UAE general population were vitamin D deficient, and 27.8% had vitamin D levels between 21 and 30 ng/ml, denoting insufficiency below the normal average [4]. Vitamin D deficiency leads to decreased serum calcium levels, resulting in elevated parathyroid hormone (PTH) secretion; therefore, calcium from the bones, kidneys, and intestines will be released. In effect, chronic vitamin D deficiency leads to secondary hyperparathyroidism [5].

Radiolucent lesions of the jaws are not uncommon, often detected in conventional radiography, and could be odontogenic or non-odontogenic [6]. The process of obtaining a definitive diagnosis and formulating a treatment plan is initiated by performing a surgical biopsy of the concerning lesion. However, the exclusion of bone homeostasis abnormalities, such as primary or secondary hyperparathyroidism, should be considered in many cases [6]. Management of the jaw's osteolytic lesions, depending on the diagnosis, ranges from minimal intervention by intralesional corticosteroids, calcitonin therapy, and cryotherapy to surgical intervention followed by jaw reconstruction [7]. We present a rare case of an osteolytic lesion associated with secondary hyperparathyroidism due to vitamin D deficiency, treated with vitamin D supplementation. Our case presentation's findings suggest an altered approach to diagnosing and managing osteolytic lesions before surgical exploration.

2. Case Presentation

A 12-year-old female orthodontist was referred to Dr. Gaballah to assess and treat the radiolucent lesion in the mandibular left premolar-molar area. The lesion was identified during routine workups for orthodontic treatment to address anterior teeth' crowding (Figure 1). Clinically, the patient had an asymptomatic buccal extension of the cortical plate. The lump was roughly 18x22 mm and was not associated with any pocketing of erupted teeth or sinus or cervical lymphadenopathy. There were no neurosensory deficits; the teeth involved were caries-free and not mobile. The case's medical history was unremarkable, although the patient complained of lethargy and general fatigue as defined by the mother.

Panoramic imaging showed a well-defined unilocular ovoid radiolucent lesion with a sclerotic rim extending from the distal aspect of the mandibular second premolar to the distal surface of the distal root of the mandibular first molar (Figure 1 and 2(a)). There was no sign of root resorption. A preliminary differential diagnosis, which included inflammatory and developmental odontogenic jaw cysts, giant cell lesions, and odontogenic tumors, was made because of the clinical and radiological findings. A comprehensive blood test was performed along with the measurement of parathyroid hormone (PTH) and renal function tests (RFT). Laboratory findings were within the range, but PTH was high at 81.3 (15-68) pg/mL and low normal serum calcium at 2.17 mmol/L (2.15-2.6), and low vitamin D 32 (75-200) nmol/L. The primary hyperparathyroidism was excluded with the use of USS thyroid. Thus, the patient was diagnosed with secondary hyperparathyroidism due to vitamin D deficiency and associated with a left mandible lytic lesion.

Vitamin D deficiency was treated as indicated by the endocrinologist before any surgery to correct hyperparathyroidism. As a result, the surgical biopsy was postponed. Treatment was begun correcting the hypovitaminosis with a single injection of Vitamin D3 300,000 I.U complemented by 10,000 I.U orally once a week. Six weeks post-intervention, a repeat vitamin D test showed a vitamin D level of 85 nmol/L with PTH lowered to 38 and serum calcium 2.4 mmol/L suggesting a substantial improvement in parathyroid function and calcium homeostasis. Parents also observed an increase in the patient's physical activity and cognitive performance. The same visit's panoramic follow-up showed some signs of bone formation in the affected region (Figure 2(b)).

The patient was kept on a maintenance dose of 10000 D3 I.U weekly. Based on progress in clinical, laboratory testing, and imaging of the jaw lesions (Figure 2(c)), the parents declined any surgical intervention, including biopsy, and agreed to pursue periodic follow-up. A Radiograph was taken at nine months, followed by further progress with new bone formation (Figure 2(d)). 4Repeat laboratory analysis also showed regular intact PTH 49.3 (15-68) pg./ml, vitamin D (25(OH)D) 73.3 (30-100) ng/ml and calcium 2.5 (2.15-2.60) mmol/L. The patient proceeded with 10,000 D3 I.U weekly and followed up with 18-month post-medical action. The last Panoramic picture showed a full resolution of the lesion (Figure 2(e)), and the laboratory tests confirmed stable values

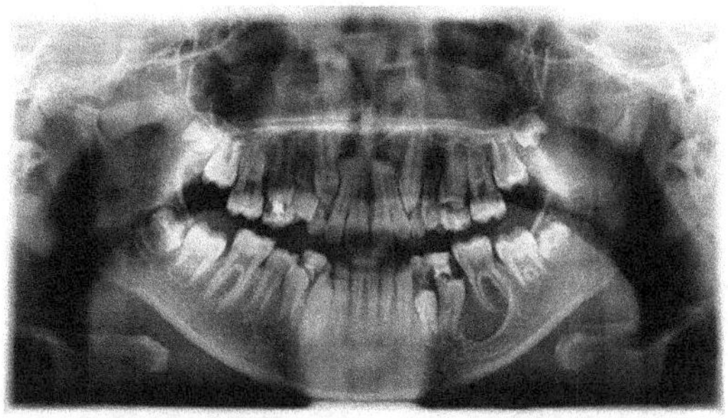

FIGURE 1: Pre-Op Orthopantomograph showing a well-defined radiolucent lesion in the left posterior mandible.

of PTH (31.5 pg/ml), vitamin D (53.53 ng/ml), calcium 2.5 (2.15-2.60) mmol/L. CBC and RFT within the reference scales. Following complete lesion resolution and bone homeostatic parameters correction, the patient was referred back to her orthodontist to resume the treatment. Table 1 summarizes the biochemistry panel of the patient before, after the medical intervention, and eighteen-month follow-up values.

3. Discussion

Despite the favorable latitude and abundance of sunlight in the Gulf region, the UAE population remains vitamin D deficient. Due to excessive heat and humidity in the relatively long summer season, increased sun avoidance, particularly in females, is noticed among the inhabitants [8–10]. Contrary to findings in other regions, increased sun exposure in the UAE occurs during winter when the temperatures are comparatively lower. Females in the UAE and the Middle East may have considerably less sunlight exposure due to their dressing styles covering most or all of the body for cultural or religious reasons [8–10]. Adolescents are at higher risk of vitamin D deficiency due to current trends and preference for indoor activities, computers, mobiles, social media, gaming, and watching television [9]. Vitamin D deficiency results in reduced intestinal calcium absorption and a lower ionized calcium level. This leads to increased secretion of the PTH. The hormone promotes the reabsorption of calcium from renal tubules. It also causes the increased conversion of calcidiol to calcitriol, which leads to increased intestinal calcium absorption and enhanced mobilization of calcium from bone [9]. The secondary hyperparathyroidism that occurs, as a result, maintains serum calcium in the normal range at the expense of mobilization of calcium from the skeleton and an increase in phosphorous wasting in the kidneys [11]. This PTH-mediated rise in osteoclastic activity causes an overall reduction in bone mineral density [11]. In our case, vitamin D deficiency contributed to excessive secretion of PTH, which resulted in an imbalance in osteoclastic-osteoblastic homeostasis, increased mobilization of calcium from bone, and ultimately presented as an osteolytic lesion in the mandible.

Given the clinical and laboratory findings, the biopsy was not performed. We are conscious of the limitation that we were unable to characterize the lesion histopathologically. However, the significant clinical and radiological resolution of the lesion and correction of the secondary hyperparathyroidism bears evidence to the preliminary diagnosis of a

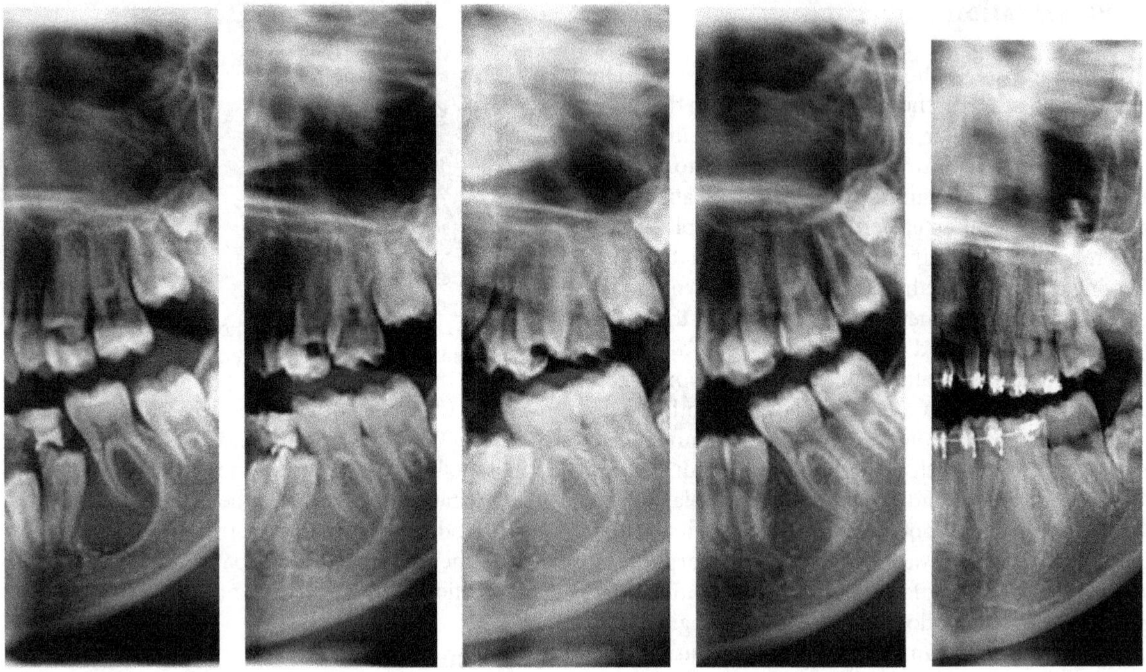

(a) (b) (c) (d) (e)

Figure 2: shows panoramic radiographs taken at initial and subsequent follow-up visits (a). The preoperative imaging referred by the orthodontist. (b) The lesion one-month post-intervention (c) At 3-month follow-up post-intervention. (d) At nine-month follow-up. (e) At 18 months of follow-up post-intervention showing complete resolution.

Table 1: the full biochemistry panel of the patient before, after the medical intervention, and eighteen-month follow-up values.

	Range value	At presentation	Six weeks post-medical intervention	Nine months post-medical intervention	Eighteen months post-medical intervention
PTH	(15-68) pg/mL	81.3	38	49.3	31.5
Serum calcium	(2.15-2.6) mmol/L	2.17	2.4	2.4	2.5
Vitamin D 32	(75-200) nmol/L	32	85	73.3	63.53
Creatinine	49-90 umol/l	50	53	51	54
Urea	2.5-6 mmol/l	4.3	4.3	4.2	4.3
Total CO_2	20-29 mmol/l	23	23	25	23
Sodium	136-145 mmol/l	139	140	140	139
Potassium	3.5-5.1 mmol/l	4.2	4.2	4.1	4.1
Chloride	98-107 mmol/l	101	102	102	101
Calcium	2.15-2.8 mmol/l	2.4	2.4	2.3	2.3
Alkaline phosphatase	28-300 u/l	345	303	191	78

brown tumor of secondary hyperparathyroidism caused by vitamin D deficiency. The biopsy was considered on the initial surgical plan. However, discovering the abnormal bone homeostasis and the improvement noted at the early stage of the Vitamin D replacement make the family deny that option. Keeping in mind, potential complications of surgical biopsy may include damage to surrounding tissue, excessive bleeding, bone fractures, and infection. However, in most cases, biopsy benefit generally overrides the risks in diagnosis and treatment planning. Brown tumor, also known as osteitis fibrosa cystica, is a benign, non-neoplastic, giant cell lesion that arises from excessive PTH levels due to primary or secondary hyperparathyroidism. They are preferentially found in the long bone, ribs, clavicle, pelvic girdle, and mandible. However, They can occur in any skeletal region in the body [12].

In contrast, this manuscript is written a report documented a potential cause of a brown tumor of the left proximal femur in a 16-year-old female treated with calcium vitamin D supplementation [12]. Complete regression of the lesion was noted, and a diagnosis of the brown tumor was considered in the absence of histopathological evaluation due to the treatment's success. Similar to our case report, the authors also advocate biochemical investigations of an osteolytic lesion to rule out brown tumor of hyperparathyroidism before any surgical intervention. This paper sheds light on a potential conservative approach for managing osteolytic lesions associated with hyperparathyroidism reducing morbidity incurred by surgical management, which is commonly practiced.

Abbreviations

PTH: ParaThyroid hormone
RFT: Renal function tests
25(OH)D: 25-hydroxyvitamin D
UAE: United Arab Emirates
CBC: Complete blood count.

References

[1] M. F. Holick, "Vitamin D deficiency," *The New England Journal of Medicine*, vol. 357, no. 3, pp. 266–281, 2007.

[2] S. B. Sridhar, P. G. Rao, S. K. Multani, and M. Jain, "Assessment of prevalence of hypovitaminosis D in multiethnic population of the United Arab Emirates," *Journal of Advanced Pharmaceutical Technology & Research*, vol. 7, no. 2, pp. 48–53, 2016.

[3] H. M. Al Attia and M. A. Ibrahim, "The high prevalence of vitamin D inadequacy and dress style of women in the sunny UAE," *Archives of Osteoporosis*, vol. 7, no. 1-2, pp. 307–310, 2012.

[4] K. Yammine and H. Al Adham, "The status of serum vitamin D in the population of the United Arab Emirates," *Eastern Mediterranean Health Journal*, vol. 22, no. 9, pp. 682–686, 2016.

[5] K. V. Arunkumar, S. Kumar, and D. Deepa, "Brown tumor in mandible as a first sign of vitamin D deficiency: a rare case report and review," *Indian Journal of Endocrinology and Metabolism*, vol. 16, no. 2, pp. 310–315, 2012.

[6] B. L. Dunfee, O. Sakai, R. Pistey, and A. Gohel, "Radiologic and pathologic characteristics of benign and malignant lesions of the mandible," *Radiographics*, vol. 26, no. 6, pp. 1751–1768, 2006.

[7] O. Kujan, A. Z. Al-Shawaf, S. Azzeghaiby, A. AlManadille, K. Aziz, and S. A. Raheel, "Immunohistochemical comparison of p53, Ki-67, CD68, vimentin, α-smooth muscle actin and alpha-1-antichymotry-psin in oral peripheral and central giant cell granuloma," *The Journal of Contemporary Dental Practice*, vol. 16, no. 1, pp. 20–24, 2015.

[8] H. Afrozul and S. Chareles, "Vitamin D deficiency, metabolism and routine measurement of its metabolites [25(O.H.)D2 and 25(O.H.)D3]," *Journal of Chromatography & Separation Techniques*, vol. 6, p. 276, 2015.

[9] A. Haq, S. J. Wimalawansa, P. Pludowski, and F. A. Anouti, "Clinical practice guidelines for vitamin D in the United Arab Emirates," *The Journal of Steroid Biochemistry and Molecular Biology*, vol. 175, pp. 4–11, 2016.

[10] F. Al Anouti, J. Thomas, L. Abdel-Wareth, J. Rajah, W. B. Grant, and A. Haq, "Vitamin D deficiency and sun avoidance among university students at Abu Dhabi, United Arab Emirates," *Dermato-Endocrinology*, vol. 3, no. 4, pp. 235–239, 2011.

[11] M. F. Holick, N. C. Binkley, H. A. Bischoff-Ferrari et al., "Evaluation, treatment, and prevention of vitamin D deficiency: an Endocrine Society clinical practice guideline," *The Journal of Clinical Endocrinology and Metabolism*, vol. 96, no. 7, pp. 1911–1930, 2011.

[12] A. Goyal, H. Boro, and R. Khadgawat, "Brown tumor as an index presentation of severe vitamin D deficiency in a teenage girl," *Cureus*, vol. 10, article e2722, 2018.

27

Conservative Approach of a Dentigerous Cyst

Farah Chouchene,[1] Wassim Ben Ameur,[1] Habib Hamdi,[2] Maissa Bouenba,[1] Fatma Masmoudi,[1] Ahlem Baaziz,[1] Fethi Maatouk,[1] and Hichem Ghedira[1]

[1]*Pediatric and Preventive Dentistry Department, Faculty of Dental Medicine of Monastir, Laboratory of Biological, Clinical and Dento-Facial Approach, University of Monastir, Monastir, Tunisia*
[2]*Dental Surgery Department, Faculty of Dental Medicine of Monastir, Monastir, Tunisia*

Correspondence should be addressed to Farah Chouchene; farah.pedo@gmail.com

Academic Editor: Márta Radnai

Dentigerous cysts (DC) are the most common odontogenic cystic lesions of inflammatory origin occurring in children. These lesions can be treated by enucleation with or without related impacted teeth or marsupialization/decompression. The latter procedures have been used successfully for many years, but decompression is increasingly recommended in children because of its good outcomes and the preservation of the developing tooth. This conservative surgical technic allows simultaneously the normal eruption of the involved permanent teeth and the ossification of the bony defect. The present report describes an 8-year-old female patient with an inflammatory DC associated with an endodontically treated primary molar accidentally discovered on panoramic radiograph. Decompression of the cyst was performed, by means of a removable space maintainer acting as an acrylic obturator after removal of teeth 83 and 84. Ten months after the decompression procedure, a complete resolution and regression of the cystic lesion with full spontaneous eruption of the premolar were observed.

1. Introduction

From the age of 5 to 12 years, children are in mixed dentition. At this age, to ensure proper eruption of the permanent dentition and to prevent arch length deficit and loss of space, it is important to preserve the primary teeth [1].

Several disturbances can cause either infection or necrosis of the pulp tissue of primary teeth, and since pulp therapy is not always easy to perform on these teeth because of their complex anatomy, the preservation of primary teeth can induce undesirable effects on the permanent successor, such as the formation of inflammatory DC [2].

These cysts are caused by the accumulation of fluid between the reduced enamel epithelium and the crown of the tooth [3]. Although the canines and molars are the most affected, cystic formations involving the crown of the premolars and incisors are rare [4, 5].

Enucleation with or without impacted teeth or marsupialization/decompression are the treatments of choice of inflammatory DC. Both procedures, marsupialization and decompression, have been used successfully for many years, but decompression is increasingly recommended because of its successful outcomes and preservation of the developing tooth structure [6].

Since these cysts are more common in children, conservative management by decompression may be recommended, allowing the conservation of the permanent involved tooth [7, 8].

The present report is aimed at describing a complete regression of an inflammatory DC with full spontaneous eruption of the premolar ten months after a decompression procedure in an 8-year-old female patient.

2. Case Presentation

The present clinical case report was reported according to the CARE (CAse REport) Guidelines [9].

An eight-year-old female patient consulted the Department of Pediatric and Preventive Dentistry at the Faculty of Dental Medicine of Monastir for dental malocclusion management.

Written informed consent was obtained from the child's parents for all imaging exams, treatment modalities, and data publications.

The panoramic radiograph performed for the interceptive orthodontic treatment revealed a large unilocular radiolucency repressing the dental germ of the first lower-right premolar (#44) including the lower-right deciduous canine (#83), and associated with a treated root of nonvital lower-right first primary molar (#84) (Figure 1).

The medical history of the patient did not reveal any specific systematic diseases or previous traumatic injuries in the affected area.

The extraoral examination seemed to show no abnormalities while the intraoral examination revealed an imperceptible expansion of the buccal cortical on the alveolar ridge in relation to teeth 83 and 84.

Inspection showed a normal looking mucosa (Figure 2). Palpation was painless with boney consistence. There was no motor or/and sensorial deficit at the orofacial structures.

A retroalveolar radiograph was performed and showed a well-defined surrounded by a slight peripherical radiopaque thickening lesion apical to the lower-right first primary molar (#84) (Figure 3).

To confirm the lesion limits, a cone-beam computed tomography (CBCT) was requested.

The sagittal and coronal views of the CBCT revealed a 12 mm diameter well-demarcated unilocular radiolucency (Figures 4 and 5).

The lesion was identified in the mandibular right region causing expansion of the buccal cortical with no signs of root resorption in the adjacent tooth and surrounding the crown of the unerupted first premolar (tooth 44).

The first lower-right premolar germ was forced against the lingual cortical with a mesial angulation. Based on the above-mentioned clinical and radiological findings, a provisional diagnosis of inflammatory DC was made.

The second primary molar and canine were extracted under local anesthesia, and a conservative approach by decompression to preserve the mandibular first premolar was followed.

The extraction socket was extended to establish a communication between the cyst and the oral cavities without disturbing the erupting premolar (Figure 6).

The cystic fluid was evacuated under irrigation with normal saline solution through the socket.

An iodoform gauze was then packet into the lesion cavity, and sutures were placed.

The patient and her parents were advised to follow post-surgical instructions, rinsing the opening cyst twice a day with saline solution.

For the first 48 hours, postoperative care included the use of a cold pack. For pain management, 200 mg dexibuprofen three times a day was prescribed for the young patient.

Two days postoperatively, an impression was made before gently removing the gauze which helped to prevent the alginate from getting the bone cavity. Then, a removable space maintainer acting as an acrylic obturator was designed (Figure 7).

During the surgical procedure, a tissue sample was taken for biopsy. Microscopically, the cyst was lined with cuboidal nonkeratinized stratified epithelium resembling reduced enamel epithelium, and the underlying connective tissue capsule showed chronic inflammatory cell infiltration. The histopathological examination confirmed the initial diagnosis of the inflammatory DC.

The acrylic obturator remained until the eruption of tooth 44 was visualized using a subsequent radiographic evaluation.

The follow-up appointments were scheduled every three months postsurgery.

The three-month postoperative radiograph showed a reduction in radiolucency associated with a gradual spontaneous eruption of the tooth (Figure 8).

After 10 months follow-up, the radiographic and clinical findings showed that the affected teeth successfully erupted without any intervention.

The tooth was vital with almost a complete root formation (Figures 9 and 10).

3. Discussion

According to the World Health Organization (WHO) classification of odontogenic lesions, odontogenic cysts were divided into developmental and inflammatory cysts. The inflammatory odontogenic cysts included radicular cysts and inflammatory collateral cysts while the developmental odontogenic and nonodontogenic cysts included dentigerous cysts, lateral periodontal cysts, botryoid odontogenic cysts, gingival cysts, glandular odontogenic cysts, orthokeratinized odontogenic cysts, and nasopalatine duct cysts [10].

The DCs constitute the most frequent maxillary cystic lesions (30% of the odontogenic cysts) [11], with sometimes important local consequences that can cause dental shifts and root resorptions and even interrupt dental eruptions in the child. Therefore, early intervention is needed [12].

These cysts are also very common in mixed dentition and are usually associated with the roots of a nonvital or necrotic primary tooth and the crown of an unerupted permanent tooth [3], such described in the present report.

The pathogenesis of DC is still controversial. However, three possible mechanisms were proposed in the literature [4].

The first mechanism suggested that the developmental DC might form a dental follicle and might become inflamed later [4]. The second mechanism suggested that the formation of DC of extrafollicular origin may occur following the formation of a radicular cyst at an apex of a nonvital primary tooth followed by eruption of its permanent successor [4].

The follicle of permanent successor might get secondarily infected from either periapical inflammation of a nonvital primary tooth or other source leading to a DC formation, and this inflammatory process may explain the DC development in the present report [4].

For this reason, especially in mixed dentition, it is very important to establish not only a clinical but also a

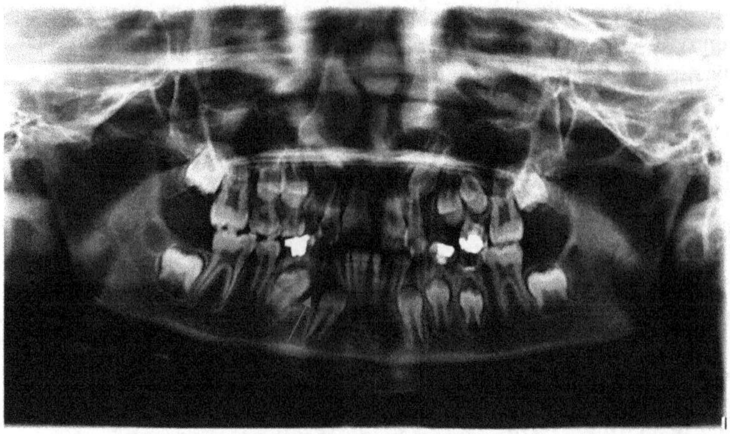

Figure 1: Preoperative panoramic radiograph (red arrow).

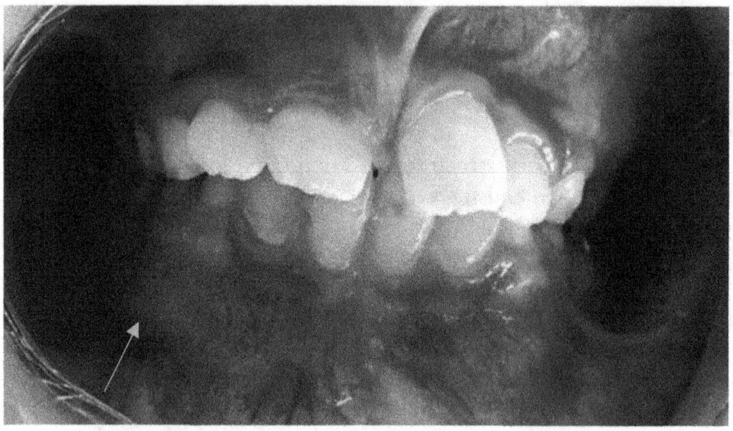

Figure 2: Intraoral view showing buccal hard swelling (blue arrow).

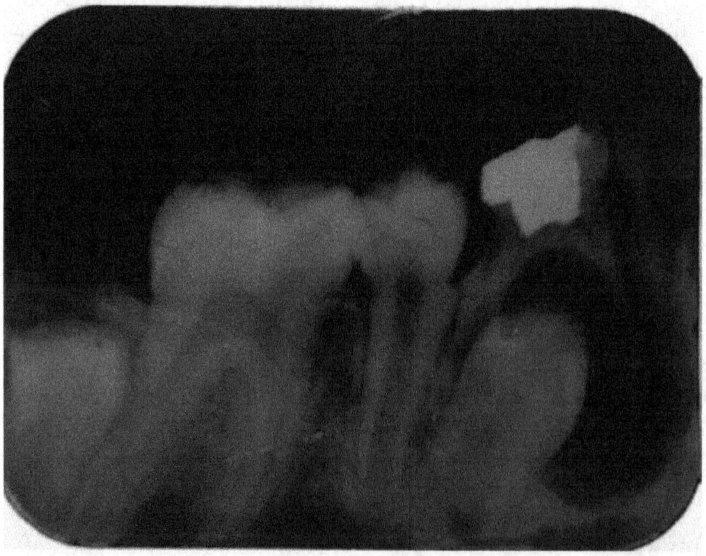

Figure 3: Retroalveolar radiograph showing radiolucency associated with an endodontically treated first right primary molar (tooth 84).

radiological follow-up of the endodontically treated primary molars until the eruption of permanent successors to be able to detect as soon as possible the side effects of pulp therapy and to manage them in prompt time.

Usually, DCs are asymptomatic and are discovered during routine dental radiographies [13].

Radiographically, these developmental cysts are characterized by the presence of a radiolucent, well-defined,

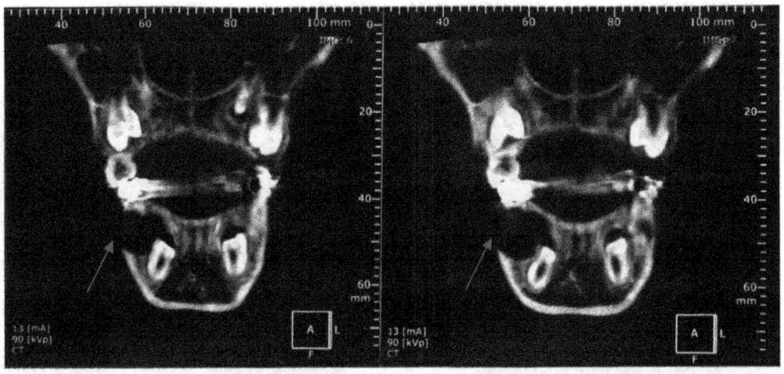

FIGURE 4: Sagittal sections showing a 12 mm diameter well-defined radiolucent lesion surrounding the crown of the unerupted first premolar (# 44) (red arrow).

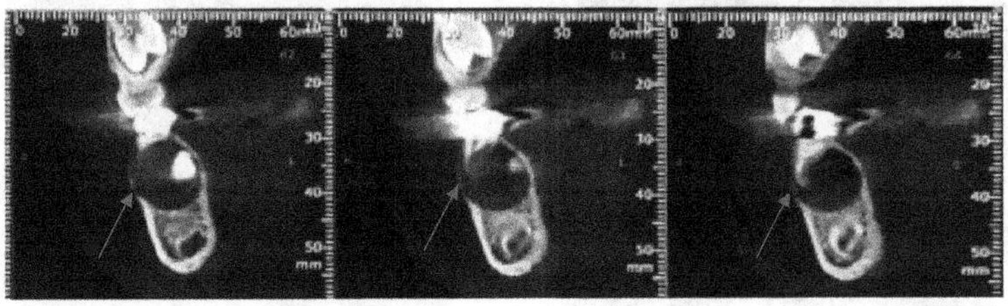

FIGURE 5: Coronal sections showing a well-defined radiolucent lesion surrounding the crown of the unerupted first premolar (# 44) (red arrow).

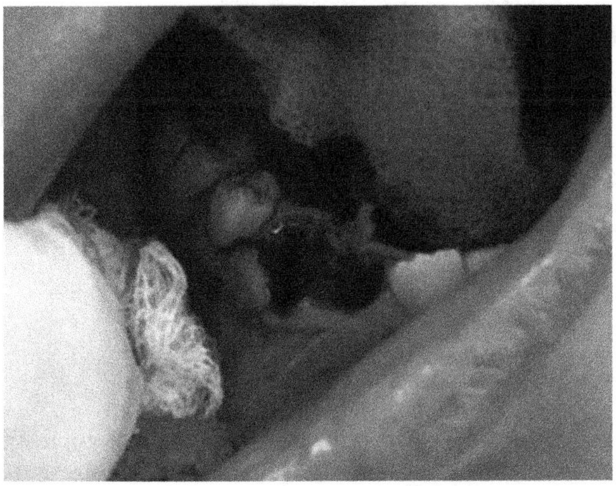

FIGURE 6: Decompression of the cyst and inspection of the right first premolar (tooth 44).

unilocular lesion around the crown of an unerupted permanent tooth. They can be reported in the presence of exformation of the maxillaries, dental structures shifting, or delays in dental eruptions [14]. In the present case, the cyst lesion was discovered accidentally after a routine panoramic radiograph.

According to the literature, the DC management is exclusively surgical, and two treatment techniques have been suggested: the enucleation or the marsupialization/decompression.

In their retrospective study, Iatrou et al. choose the technique of enucleation, reserving the marsupialization to large cysts. An association of both techniques can be suggested for the more aggressive cysts to reduce the volume of the lesion, before surgical removal [15].

Conservative techniques for the treatment of odontogenic cysts have evolved gradually the last decades.

Marsupialization and decompression are minimal surgical intervention but decompression is less invasive because it requires a smaller bony window.

Decompression may envelop marsupialization, and it includes any method that keeps an opening into the exterior by using a conduit to decrease intracystic pressure [16].

The benefits of decompression are maintenance of pulp vitality, prevention of maxillary fractures, preservation of the inferior alveolar nerve or maxillary sinus, and low risk of recurrence [16].

In the present reported case, since the patient and her parents were cooperative, the decompression was recommended.

After decompression, the cystic cavity must remain open; numerous means have been described such as stents, stents fixed by mini-screws, packs of iodoform gauze, tubes for decompression, and retainers [17].

Ghandour et al. recommended the placement of a gauze during the first two days after the surgery to keep the surgical site open [18]. Preserving the fenestration open may allow to reduce the size of the cystic lesion postoperatively; to reduce the infection, iodoform can be used [19].

In mixed dentition, a loss of space may occur during the first three weeks following the extraction of the primary teeth; for this reason, maintaining the space is necessary to avoid the decrease in the arch length [20]. In the reported case, a removable partial denture was indicated both to keep the cyst cavity opening and intracystic pressure at a reduced level and to keep the space of the first premolar while guiding its eruption.

A clinical and radiographic follow-up will be necessary, every three months initially, then every six months, until

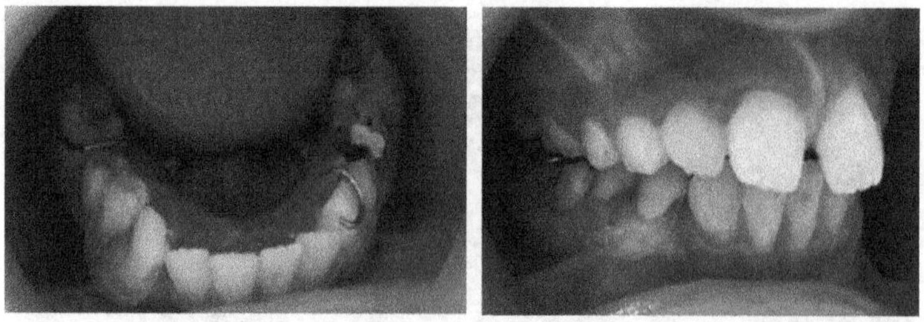

FIGURE 7: Removable space maintainer acting as an acrylic obturator used to guide the eruption of the premolar.

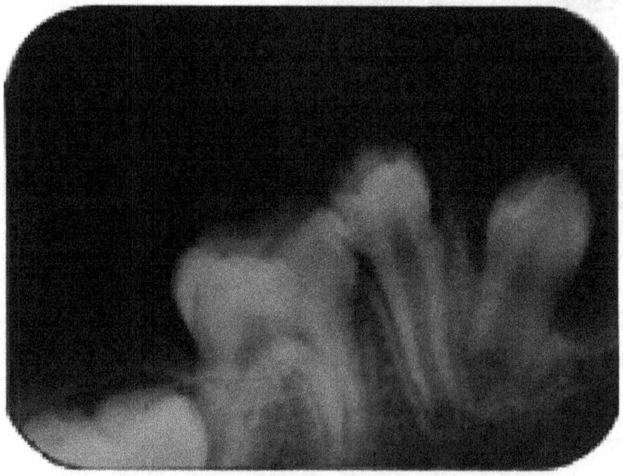

FIGURE 8: Three-month postoperative radiograph.

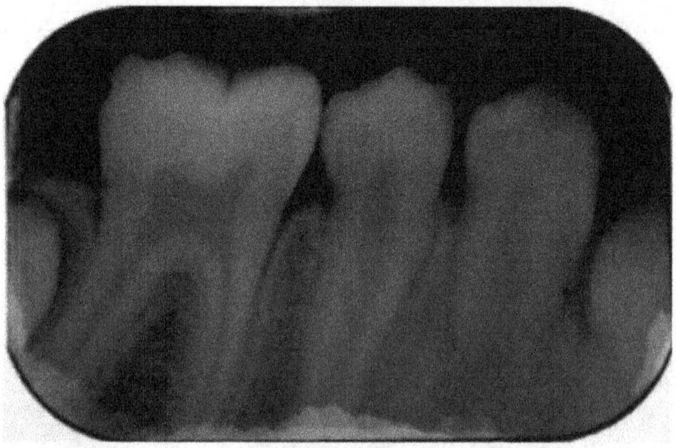

FIGURE 9: Twelve-month postoperative radiograph showing spontaneous eruption of the tooth 44.

the end of the eruption of the tooth and the healing of the bone [15].

Both radiological and clinical findings after 10 months showed in the present report that the first premolar had successfully erupted without any orthodontic intervention.

Although the predictive criteria for this eruption remain unknown, the size of the cystic lesion does not constitute a risk factor for the eruption.

In fact, the most favorable predictive factors are essentially the age of the patient (less than ten years old), the depth of the inclusion (less is better), and the angulation of the germ (inferior to 25°) [21].

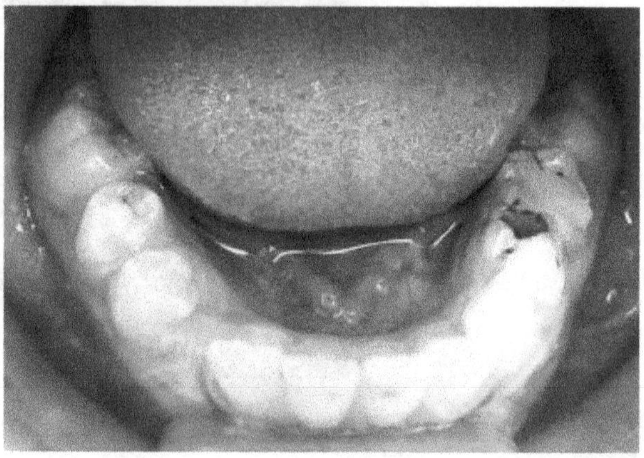

FIGURE 10: Intraoral view showing complete eruption of tooth 44 after 12 months follow-up.

After minimal surgical intervention, the spontaneous eruption may occur in approximately 70% to 90 of cases. The length of the eruption is very variable, ranging from seven months to five years, and orthodontic traction can be associated [15, 21].

4. Conclusion

Extraction of the primary infected tooth and decompression is the treatment of choice for infected dentigerous cyst in mixed dentition.

The surgical procedure can be followed by wearing of an acrylic resin obturator, incorporating features of space maintainer especially when primary molars are involved, both to maintain the surgical opening during healing and to prevent the arch length deficiency.

This report highlights the interest of performing a systematic radiological examination during the child's first visit.

Consent

Written informed consent was obtained from the legal guardian of the patient (the father of the child) for publication of this case report and any accompanying images.

References

[1] R. R. Bijoor and K. Kohli, "Contemporary space maintenance for the pediatric patient," *The New York State Dental Journal*, vol. 71, no. 2, pp. 32–35, 2005.

[2] G. d. A. C. Lautenschläger, M. C. Gallina, O. Ferreira Júnior, and V. S. Lara, "Primary failure of tooth eruption associated with secondarily inflamed dental follicle: inflammatory follicular cyst?," *Brazilian Dental Journal*, vol. 18, no. 2, pp. 144–147, 2007.

[3] D. Sardana, A. Goyal, and K. Gauba, "Management of an inflamed dentigerous cyst in a patient with an anterior crossbite, using a modified obturator," *South African Dental Journal*, vol. 71, no. 6, pp. 266–269, 2016.

[4] R. M Shetty and U. Dixit, "Dentigerous cyst of inflammatory origin," *International Journal of Clinical Pediatric Dentistry*, vol. 3, no. 3, pp. 195–198, 2010.

[5] R. Kumar, R. K. Singh, R. K. Pandey, S. Mohammad, and H. Ram, "Inflammatory dentigerous cyst in a ten-year-old child," *National Journal of Maxillofacial Surgery*, vol. 3, no. 1, pp. 80–83, 2012.

[6] F. Ugurlu, S. Akyuz, and A. Mentes, "Outcome of mandibular dentigerous cysts 1 to 10 years after decompression using a custom-made appliance," *Journal of Oral and Maxillofacial Surgery*, vol. 79, no. 1, pp. 152–163, 2021.

[7] R. dos Santos Pinheiro, G. F. Castro, M. Roter et al., "An unusual dentigerous cyst in a young child," *General Dentistry*, vol. 61, no. 2, pp. 62–64, 2013.

[8] M. Picciotti, L. Divece, S. Parrini, M. Pettini, and G. Lorenzini, "Replantation of tooth involved in dentigerous cyst: a case report," *European Journal of Paediatric Dentistry*, vol. 13, no. 4, pp. 349–351, 2012.

[9] CARE Case Report Guidelines, "CARE Case Report Guidelines," 2021, https://www.care-statement.org.

[10] B. Sivapathasundharam, P. G. Biswas, and S. Preethi, "The World Health Organization classification of odontogenic and maxillofacial bone tumors: an appraisal," *Journal of Oral and Maxillofacial Pathology*, vol. 23, no. 2, pp. 178–186, 2019.

[11] N. Martin-Duverneuil and M. Auriol, *Les tumeurs maxillofaciales: imagerie, anatomopathologie*, Sauramps Médical, 2004.

[12] V. Koželj and B. Sotošek, "Inflammatory dentigerous cysts of children treated by tooth extraction and decompression—report of four cases," *British Dental Journal*, vol. 187, no. 11, pp. 587-590, 1999.

[13] M. Al-assaf, A. Al-awad, A. Al-Mandily, M. Al-Khen, and A. Farhoud, "Huge inflammatory dentigerous cyst: case report," *International Journal of Dentistry and Oral Science*, vol. 7, no. 2, pp. 723–726, 2014.

[14] Y. Anavi, G. Gal, H. Miron, S. Calderon, and D. M. Allon, "Decompression of odontogenic cystic lesions: clinical long-term study of 73 cases," *Oral Surgery, Oral Medicine, Oral Pathology, Oral Radiology, and Endodontics*, vol. 112, no. 2, pp. 164-169, 2011.

[15] I. Iatrou, N. Theologie-Lygidakis, and M. Leventis, "Intraosseous cystic lesions of the jaws in children: a retrospective analysis of 47 consecutive cases," *Oral Surgery, Oral Medicine, Oral Pathology, Oral Radiology, and Endodontology*, vol. 107, no. 4, pp. 485-492, 2009.

[16] J. Castro-Núñez, "An innovative decompression device to treat odontogenic cysts," *Journal of Craniofacial Surgery*, vol. 27, no. 5, p. 1316, 2016.

[17] U. Ertas and M. S. Yavuz, "Interesting eruption of 4 teeth associated with a large dentigerous cyst in mandible by only marsupialization," *Journal of Oral and Maxillofacial Surgery*, vol. 61, no. 6, pp. 728–730, 2003.

[18] L. Ghandour, H. F. Bahmad, and S. Bou-Assi, "Conservative treatment of dentigerous cyst by marsupialization in a young female patient: a case report and review of the literature," *Case Reports in Dentistry*, vol. 2018, Article ID 7621363, 6 pages, 2018.

[19] N. Marwah, K. A. Bishen, V. Prabha, and P. Goenka, "A conservative approach in the management of inflammatory dentigerous cyst in transitional dentition: a case report," *Journal of the Massachusetts Dental Society*, vol. 61, no. 1, pp. 18–21, 2012.

[20] K. Park, D.-W. Jung, and J.-Y. Kim, "Three-dimensional space changes after premature loss of a maxillary primary first molar," *International Journal of Paediatric Dentistry*, vol. 19, no. 6, pp. 383–389, 2009.

[21] Y. Yahara, Y. Kubota, T. Yamashiro, and K. Shirasuna, "Eruption prediction of mandibular premolars associated with dentigerous cysts," *Oral Surgery, Oral Medicine, Oral Pathology, Oral Radiology, and Endodontics*, vol. 108, no. 1, pp. 28–31, 2009.

28

Restoration of Primary Anterior Teeth with Glass Fiber-Reinforced Post and Core: 3-Year Follow-Up Case Report

Salah Afraa,[1] Hashim Raghad,[1] Khalid Ayam,[2] and Hamid Aeshah[1]

[1]*Growth and Development Department, Ajman University, UAE*
[2]*Basic Science Department, Ajman University, UAE*

Correspondence should be addressed to Salah Afraa; a.salah@ajman.ac.ae

Academic Editor: Gianrico Spagnuolo

Background. Esthetic appearance of primary anterior teeth is one of the major demands in the dental field. Destructed anterior primary teeth due to caries is considered a major issue due to the difficulty in regaining the esthetic crowns and attaching them until the normal exfoliation time. There have been many attempts and tools used to attach the composite crowns to the treated canals of primary anterior teeth. The study evaluates endodontic treatment for destructed primary maxillary incisors with a glass fiber-reinforced post as a retentive tool to hold the esthetic composite crowns until the normal exfoliation time of primary incisors. *Case Presentation.* A four-year-old child attending a dental clinic complained of pain of maxillary incisors. Dental examination showed irreversible pulpitis of four maxillary incisors indicated for root canal treatment and crown placement. Endodontic treatment was carried out, and a glass fiber-reinforced post was used to get successful retention for the composite crowns. Follow-up was carried out for 3 years. The 3 crowns were retained successfully until replaced by permanent incisors. One crown fell during the treatment course. *Conclusion.* Retention of primary teeth is one of the challenges in pediatric dentistry. Restoration of primary decayed incisors is important for child medical, physical, and psychological conditions. A glass fiber-reinforced post and core is a strong retentive tool for composite crown retention for primary incisors. This procedure opens the door for a strong tool to retain composite crowns for a long time. The glass fiber-reinforced post and core is a strong retentive tool for composite crown retention for primary incisors.

1. Background

The restoration of primary anterior teeth represented a great challenge in dentistry [1]. Many factors affect the treatment outcome of the restoration of primary teeth incisors and laterals: teeth, small size, child behavior cooperation, child's age, and cost of the treatment. Dental caries is the main causative factor in tooth structure destruction. The thin enamel and dentin layer enhance caries extension and tooth destruction with or without pulp involvement. Child behavior affects the selection of the treatment options and the treatment setting: either in a local environment or in treatment under general anesthesia [2]. The age factor will put the shadow of selecting the treatment with longevity rather than the option for the short term. With all the previously mentioned factors, the treatment cost will guide the parents to the treatment option, especially with the absence of dental insurance.

The maxillary primary incisors are the anterior primary teeth most affected by dental caries [1, 3, 4]. The caries pattern may affect all surfaces in a short time, leaving the tooth with the complete destruction of the tooth structure with or without pulp involvement. Esthetic satisfaction and the longevity of the restoration of anterior primary teeth were the main concerns for the parents and the dentist [5]. According to the American Academy of Pediatric Dentistry (AAPD), restoration techniques for the anterior primary teeth include the following: open-faced stainless steel crowns, full-coverage composite, strip crowns, and full white ceramic crowns [6].

The most conservative treatment (in primary and permanent dentition) is a direct restoration performed with resin-based composites. This treatment has always been preferred due to it being esthetically pleasing [7], reparable [8, 9], conservative [4], and economically affordable. Direct restorations can also be performed in an endotreated tooth with

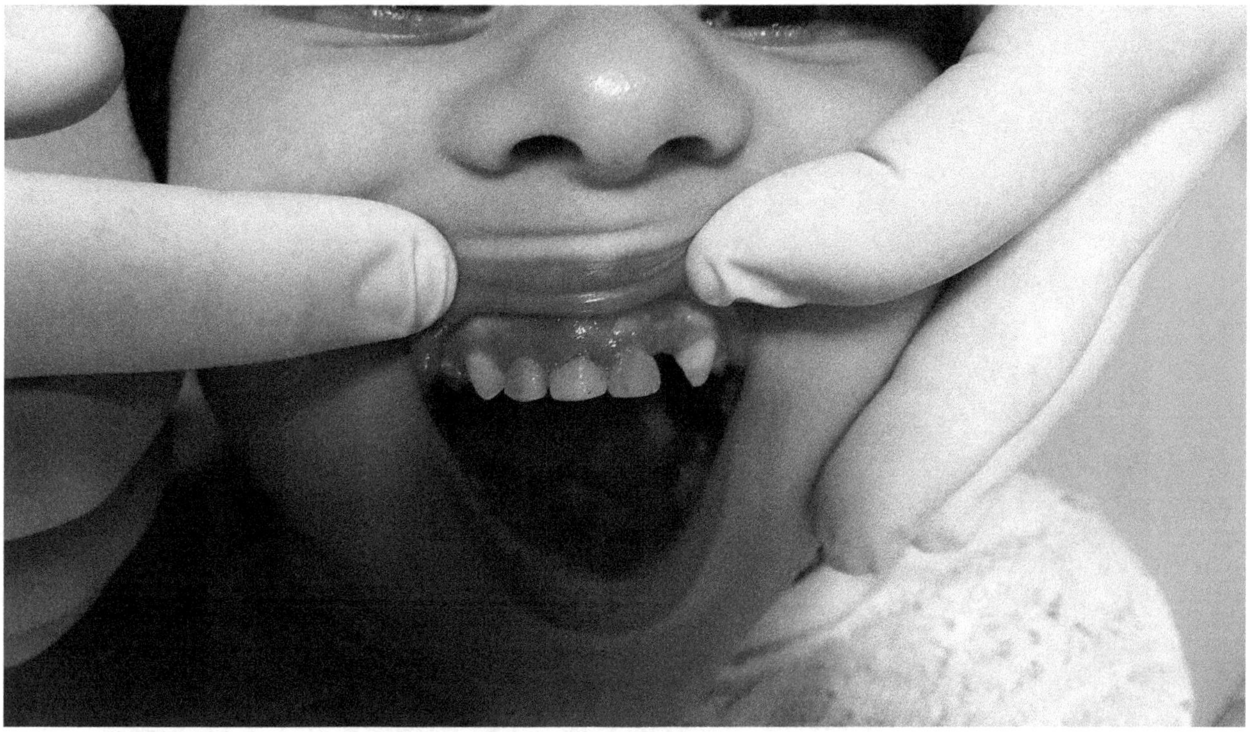

FIGURE 1: Final coronal restoration.

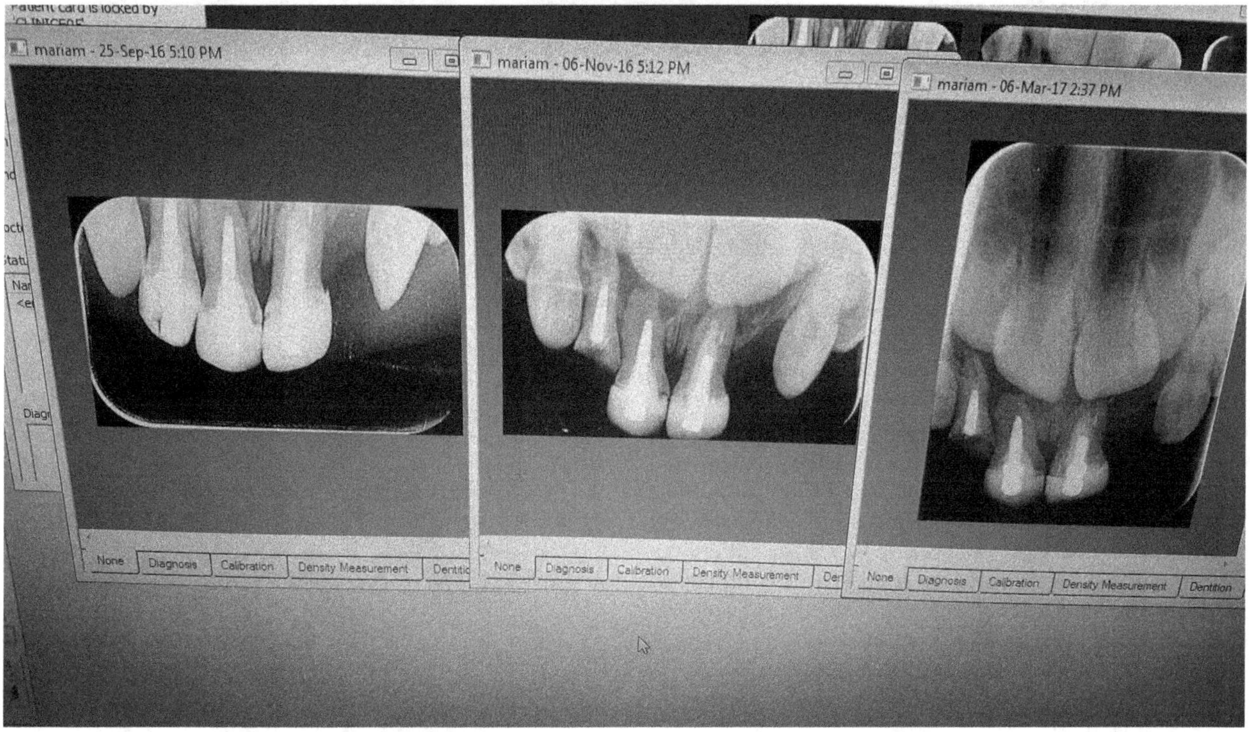

FIGURE 2: Radiographic follow-up of treated teeth.

success following basic principles [4]. In addition to the revised challenges, restorations could be very difficult when the crown structure is destroyed completely with pulp involvement as well as for younger ages. For conditions that represent poor retention and poor oral hygiene, there will be no benefit to proceeding with this challenge. The best treatment will be extraction and replacement with kiddie partial [2, 7]. However, some parents' wish to keep the

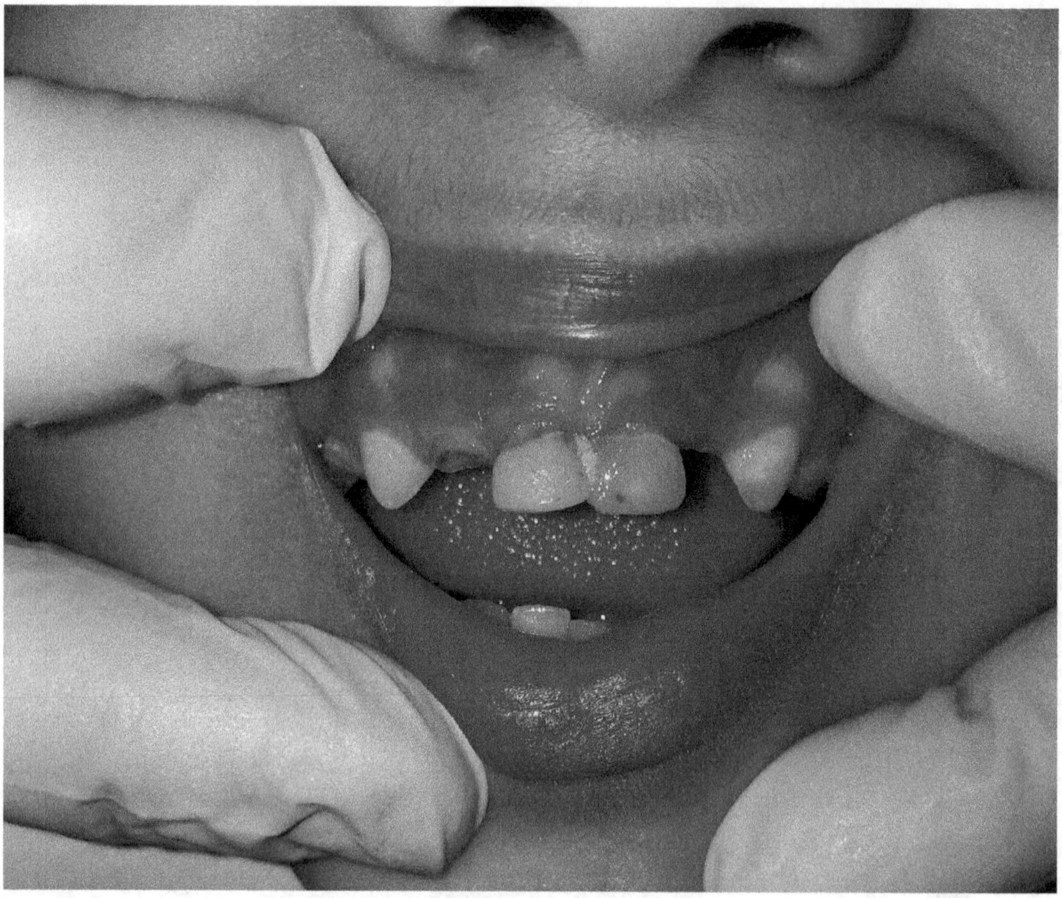

Figure 3: Clinical crowns of central incisors.

affected teeth may play a big role in going through this challenge. The main concern of anterior primary teeth restorations with root canal filling is the retention of the coronal restoration to the remaining tooth structure and the root canal filling [4]. This concern is the same for permanent dentition, and several classifications have been proposed for restoration according to the residual structure [10], and fiber posts appear to be the best build-up retention procedure [11].

The absence of primary anterior teeth for children in their young ages will affect their eating, smiling, pronunciation, and psychological interaction with others. Oral health neglect could be pronounced, but in many conditions, most of the parents prefer to keep the primary teeth instead of removing them and ask for alternative treatment rather than extraction of the anterior primary teeth. The present condition represents a special challenge where the dentist prepares four root canals with special retentive mean and coronal restoration for the maxillary incisors and laterals with a follow-up for 3 years until the eruption of the permanent incisor teeth [1, 4, 7].

2. Case Presentation

A 4-year-old female patient attended a pediatric dental clinic at the Dental College of Ajman University on September 2016. The patient was complaining of dental pain in the anterior maxillary teeth. The parents asked for a treatment to

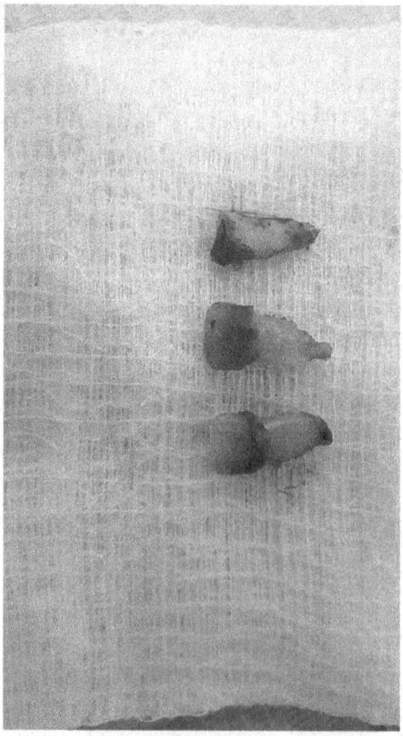

Figure 4: Extracted anterior primary teeth.

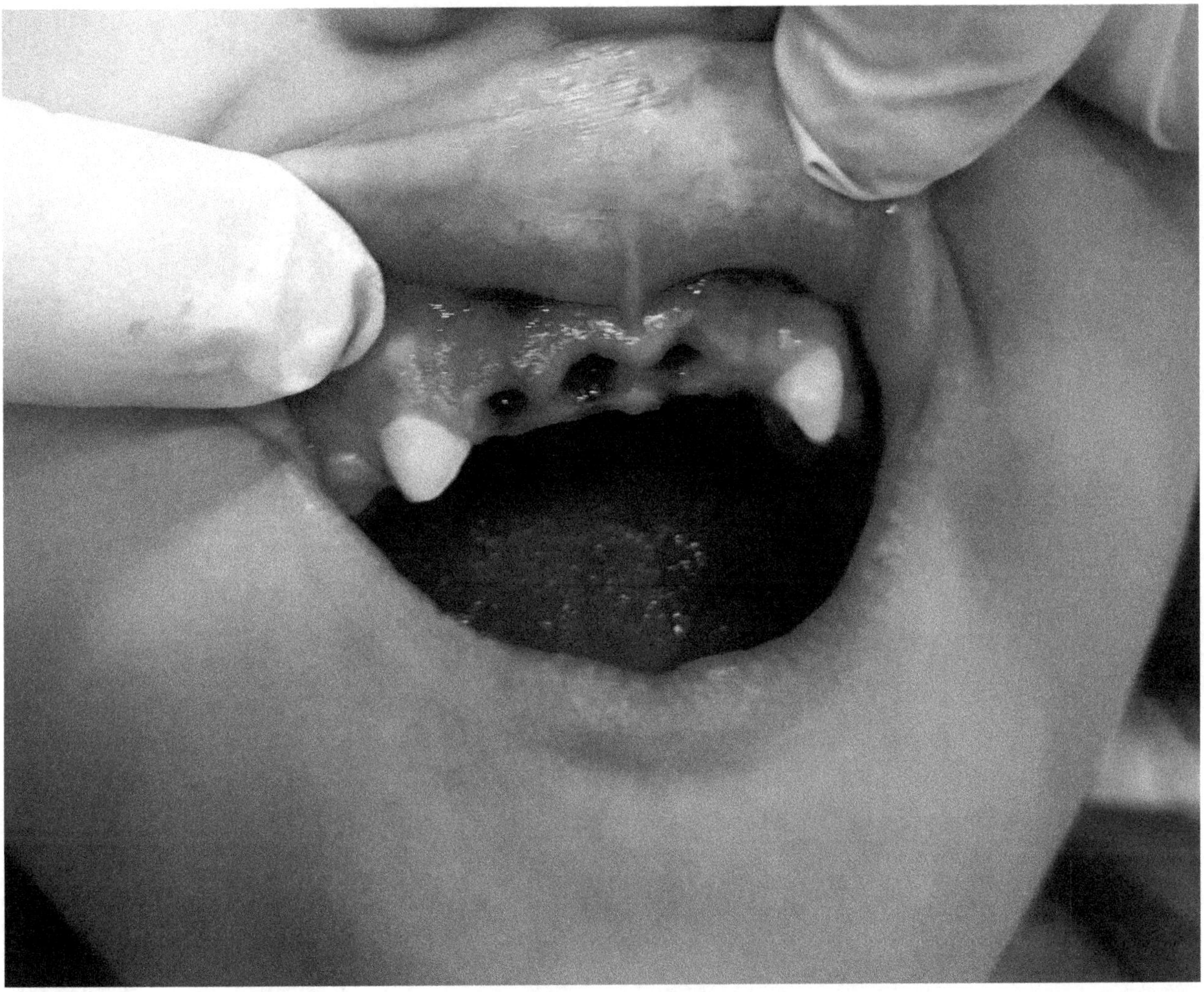

FIGURE 5: Extraction of primary anterior teeth.

relieve the dental pain and restore the esthetic appearance for the patient. A dental examination showed destructed anterior maxillary teeth and bad oral hygiene of the remaining teeth. The dental history explained the bad oral hygiene and destructed anterior teeth due to bottle-feeding for 3 years and parental neglect in addition to the expensive dental treatment, which the parents could not afford. The dental examination showed retained roots of 51, 52, 61, and 62. The 62nd root showed great mobility and a bad prognosis for any future restoration. The intraoral radiograph revealed pulp involvement of 51, 52, 61, and 62 and showed root resorption.

3. Treatment Plan

The dentist decided to do a root canal filling for 51, 52, and 61 with fiber post and strip composite crown and extraction of 62. Labial and palatal infiltration was carried out for 51, 52, and 61, and gross carious lesions were removed. The pulp chamber was opened, pulp tissue was extirpated, and working length determination was carried out by IAPA film. The preparation of the canal was carried out for 51, 52, and 61, and proper irrigation with 2.5% of NaOCl and normal saline was performed for all the canals. The canals were dried using paper points, and the thick endo paste of Vitapex was used to fill the canals as much as possible and condensed by a Lentulo spiral into the canal; the opened canals were closed with a temporary filling. After 1 week, the patient came back for the dental appointment and the preparation of the fiber post space.

The fiber post preparation required the removal of 4-5 mm of the endo paste from the canal and cleaning with saline and dried with air. The spaces made for the post were acid etched, rinsed, and dried; a light-cured bonding agent was brushed on the etched surfaces and dispersed by an air blast. Before the placement of the fiber post, flowable composites were inserted in the post spaces, and then, the post was introduced to the space with the composite inside. Then, both were light-cured for 60 seconds.

The coronal area was etched, washed, and bonded using a light cure. Strip crowns were prepared according to the final post placement and filled with composite. Next, they were

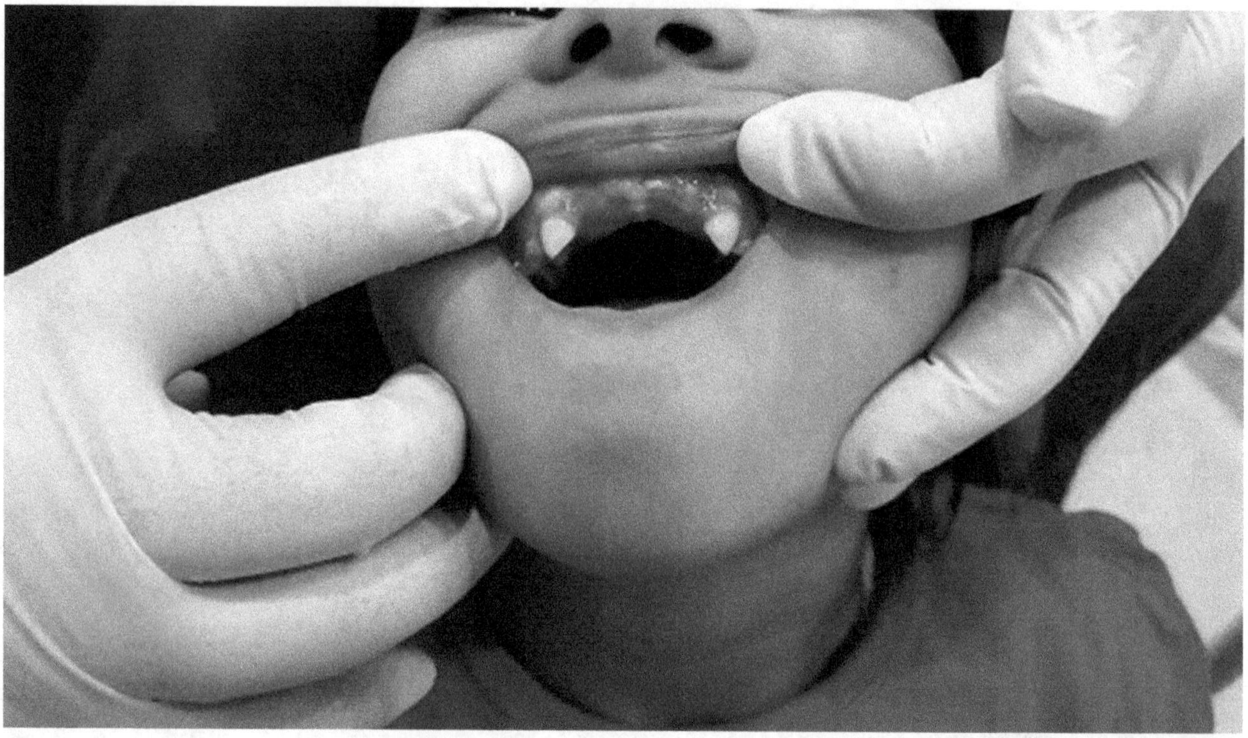

Figure 6: Clinical healing of anterior maxillary area.

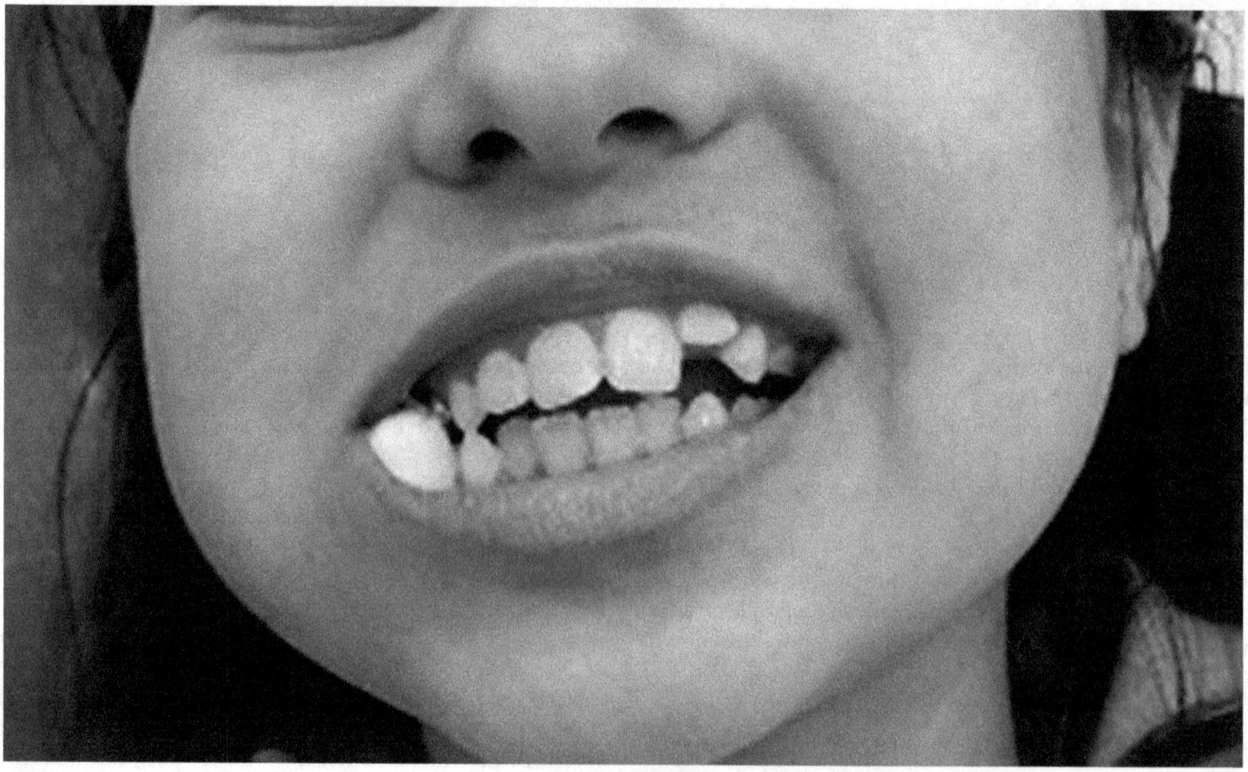

Figure 7: Eruption of anterior permanent incisors.

placed on 51, 52, and 61. Then, the final coronal restoration was cured with a light cure, 62 was extracted, and an IOAR was taken to keep the follow-up record (Figures 1 and 2).

The patient returned after 2 months for IOAR and a checkup, and the parents were satisfied with the result with no pain or discomfort. However, the crown of 52 fell and was lost. The canal obturated, and the efforts for repeating the crown failed (Figure 3).

On March 2017, the patient returned for another visit, and the dentist took IOAR. The radiograph showed evidence of normal physiological root resorption with no complaint or mobility. On June 2018, the patient complained of the mobility of the three teeth, which required the extraction of these teeth since it caused problems for her during eating (Figures 4 and 5).

On July 2018, the patient came with complete healing of the anterior maxillary area (Figure 6).

The next visit was on November 2018. Her centrals erupted. The patient's last visit was on May 2019 when the four anterior teeth, both maxillary centrals and laterals, fully erupted in the oral cavity (Figure 7).

4. Discussion

Esthetic restorations of primary anterior teeth represent a great challenge for most pediatric dentists. Small crown size, caries pattern, and the behavior of the patient plays a big role in successful treatment for restoring the esthetic appearance for young patients. Destructed anterior primary teeth with root canal treatment need a retentive post to hold the coronal crown on the treated canal [1, 2, 12, 13]. However, post selection is not an easy or successful procedure. Omega-shaped orthodontic wires and nickel-chromium cast posts did not meet the esthetic requirements as well as the adaptation to the canal shape [1]. A resin composite post building up directly did not achieve the required retention for the long term.

A glass fiber post is one of the posts used in some cases of primary anterior teeth [2, 13]. With root canal treatment and coronal placements, it can be used as an alternative to other post types for root canals. It has great advantages over the other posts, with greater flexural strength, easy application and handling, applications in high stress-bearing areas, esthetically acceptable, and the ability to bond to any composite [14]. According to the present study, it shows great retention within the canal for a long time. Due to these reasons, this method is considered superior to other types of posts for primary anterior teeth [15–18]. By the end of the treatment, parents were so happy with the results and on how we could keep the teeth until the permanent teeth erupted without affecting the child's appearance.

Restoration of child esthetics became one of the main concerns for parents as well as for children. Improving root canal post selections for a root canal-treated tooth will make the restoration of the coronal crown a successful one. The treatment of this case and the follow-up at 3 years until the primary is removed on time. The case has interesting, promising results for future treatments for traumatic or carious anterior primary teeth.

References

[1] L. Verma and S. Passi, "Glass fibre-reinforced composite post and core used in decayed primary anterior teeth: a case report," *Case Reports in Dentistry*, vol. 2011, Article ID 864254, 4 pages, 2011.

[2] P. Agarwal, R. Nayak, and G. Elangovan, "A predictable aesthetic rehabilitation of deciduous anterior teeth in early childhood caries," *Case Reports in Dentistry*, vol. 2018, Article ID 1742529, 5 pages, 2018.

[3] A.-H. Muhamad, W. Nezar, A. Azzaldeen, and A.-S. Hanali, "Anterior dental esthetics in primary teeth," *International Journal of Public Health Research*, vol. 3, no. 1, pp. 25–36, 2015.

[4] N. Gugnani, I. K. Pandit, M. Gupta, and J. Nagpal, "Esthetic rehabilitation of primary anterior teeth using temporization material: a novel approach," *International journal of clinical pediatric dentistry*, vol. 10, no. 1, pp. 111–114, 2017.

[5] M. Burykina, O. Admakin, E. Skatova, T. Medvedeva, and N. Kozlova, "Indirect restoration of primary teeth with individual crowns," *International Journal of Paediatric Dentistry*, vol. 23, pp. 53-54, 2013.

[6] V. Dhar, K. L. Hsu, J. A. Coll et al., "Evidence-based update of pediatric dental restorative procedures: dental materials," *Journal of Clinical Pediatric Dentistry*, vol. 39, no. 4, pp. 303–310, 2015.

[7] G. Orsini, V. Tosco, R. Monterubbianesi, G. Orilisi, and A. Putignano, "A new era in restorative dentistry," *The First Outstanding 50 Years of "Università Politecnica delle Marche": Research Achievements in Life Sciences*, pp. 319–334, 2020.

[8] N. Mohamed, M. Rasdi, N. Atiqah, C. Lah, and N. F. Izzati, "A survey of knowledge and clinical consideration on fiber post for restoration of endodontically treated tooth among undergraduate dentistry students," *Int J Dentistry Oral Sci.*, vol. 8, no. 3, pp. 2094–2098, 2021.

[9] E. Conserva, U. Consolo, A. Gimenez Sancho et al., "Stress distribution in carbon-post applied with different composite core materials: a three-dimensional finite element analysis," *Journal of Adhesion Science and Technology*, vol. 31, no. 22, pp. 2435–2444, 2017.

[10] M. Paryab, H. Afshar, B. Seraj, S. Shakibapoor, and M. J. Kharazifard, "Fracture strength of severely damaged primary anterior teeth after restoration with composite resin and resin-modified glass ionomer cement," *Journal of Islamic Dental Association of Iran*, vol. 28, no. 2, pp. 57–63, 2016.

[11] A.-H. Muhamad and A. Azzaldeen, "Strip crowns technique for restoration of primary anterior teeth: case report," *Journal of Dental and Medical Sciences*, vol. 14, no. 12, pp. 48–53, 2015.

[12] M. C. S. Marquezin, B. R. Zancopé, L. F. Pacheco, M. B. D. Gavião, and F. M. Pascon, "Aesthetic and functional rehabilitation of the primary dentition affected by amelogenesis imperfecta," *Case reports in dentistry*, vol. 2015, Article ID 790890, 6 pages, 2015.

[13] S. M. Sholapurmath and S. Anand, "Use of polyethylene fiber in pediatric esthetics clinical reports of two cases," *Journal of International Oral Health*, vol. 2, no. 2, 2010.

[14] P. Babaji, *Crowns in pediatric dentistry*, Jaypee Brothers Medical Publishers, New Delhi, 2015.

[15] D. Ram and A. B. Fuks, "Clinical performance of resin-bonded composite strip crowns in primary incisors: a retrospective study," *International journal of paediatric dentistry*, vol. 16, no. 1, pp. 49–54, 2006.

[16] G. Paolone, "Direct composites in anteriors: a matter of substrate," *International journal of esthetic dentistry*, vol. 4, 2017.

[17] G. Paolone, E. Moratti, C. Goracci, E. Gherlone, and A. Vichi, "Effect of finishing systems on surface roughness and gloss of full-body bulk-fill resin composites," *Materials*, vol. 13, no. 24, p. 5657, 2020.

[18] A. Talekar, "Clinical efficacy of zirconia crown (Nusmile Zr) and glass fiber reinforced composite crown (Figaro) in primary molar teeth," *International Journal of Paediatric Dentistry*, vol. 29, Supplement 1, pp. 39–43, 2019.

29

Orthodontic, Maxillofacial Surgery, and Prosthodontic Rehabilitation Supported by Miniscrew in a Patient with Cleft Lip and Palate

Alberto De Stefani, Giovanni Bruno, Martina Barone, and Antonio Gracco

Department of Neuroscience, School of Dentistry, University of Padua, 35100 Padua, Italy

Correspondence should be addressed to Alberto De Stefani; alberto.de.stefani@hotmail.it

Academic Editor: Asja Celebic

Aim. This paper is aimed at reporting the clinical case of a patient with cleft lip and palate treated with a multidisciplinary approach. *Case Report.* An 11-year-old patient presented cleft lip and palate, with persistent oronasal communication, tooth displacement, and upper and lower crowding with a deep curve of Spee. He was treated with metal bracket orthodontic therapy, graft surgery, and prosthetic rehabilitation supported by miniscrews. *Conclusions.* Cleft lip and/or palate patients require adequate management of the case to resolve the anomalies connected to their condition and to improve their quality of life.

1. Introduction

Cleft lip and/or cleft palate is one of the most common congenital deformities of the face, with an incidence of approximately 1 : 1000 live births [1–3] and usually caused by failure of the facial process fusion during embryogenesis, with altered embryological development of the orofacial structures [3]. The exact etiology of this defect is unknown, but genetic, nutritional, and environmental factors seem to be implicated [3, 4]. While a severe cleft could be diagnosed during the prenatal period, with the prenatal ultrasound inspection, a small cleft is generally diagnosed at birth [5]. Cleft lip and/or palate have a great impact on the quality of life of patients, because they influenced facial growth, dental development, function, aesthetics, and psychological status [1, 2]. Moreover, patients affected by cleft lip and palate often present deviations in facial morphology, speech problems, and a higher prevalence of dental anomalies than the general population, such as tooth agenesis [3, 6–10], which can affect their oral health-related quality of life, i.e., the impact that oral conditions can have on the individual's daily functioning, health, and quality of life [11]. This category of patients has reported lower oral health-related quality of life than the general population [9]. Patients with cleft lip and/or palate require careful management starting from their birth. The treatment is electively surgical, but the approach has necessary to be multidisciplinary, involving figures as a maxillofacial surgeon, ENT, plastic surgeon, orthodontist, pedodontist, oral surgeon, prosthodontist, and implantologist. The protocol applied for the treatment of this category of patients is structured in different phases, based on the patient's age [12]. At the patient's birth, a passive palate plate made of soft resin can be placed to help the child's feeding. Then, at 3 months of age, a surgeon can perform soft palate surgery and lip and nostril surgery to obtain the definitive lip repair. This surgery can be followed by a rhinoplasty at 6 months of age. Speech therapy is important for this cleft lip and/or palate patient: it is recommendable to start it at 8-12 months of age and to continue it even after hard palate surgery, which can be performed at 18-20 months of age. At 5 years of age, orthopedic therapy can start, by placing a rapid palate expander and a maxillary traction device (as a Delaire mask), to resolve the transverse contraction of the maxilla resulting from its underdevelopment and induce its growth forward. At the end of the period of palate expander activation, which depends on the

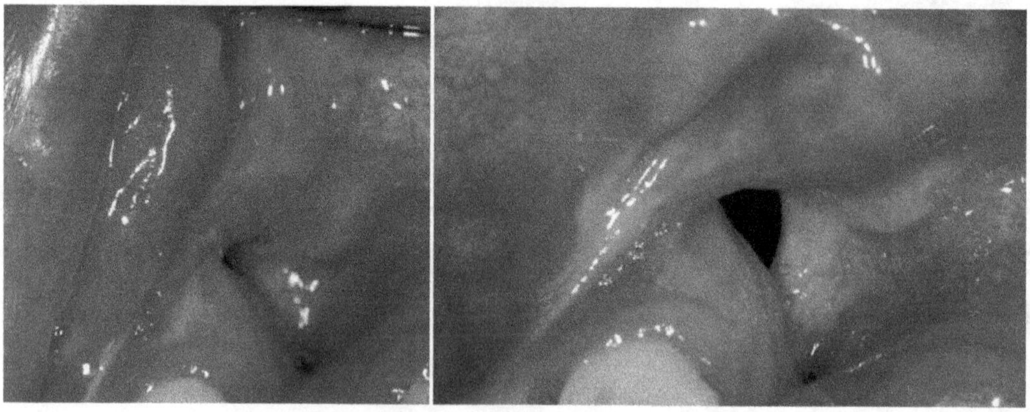

Figure 1: Persistent oronasal communication.

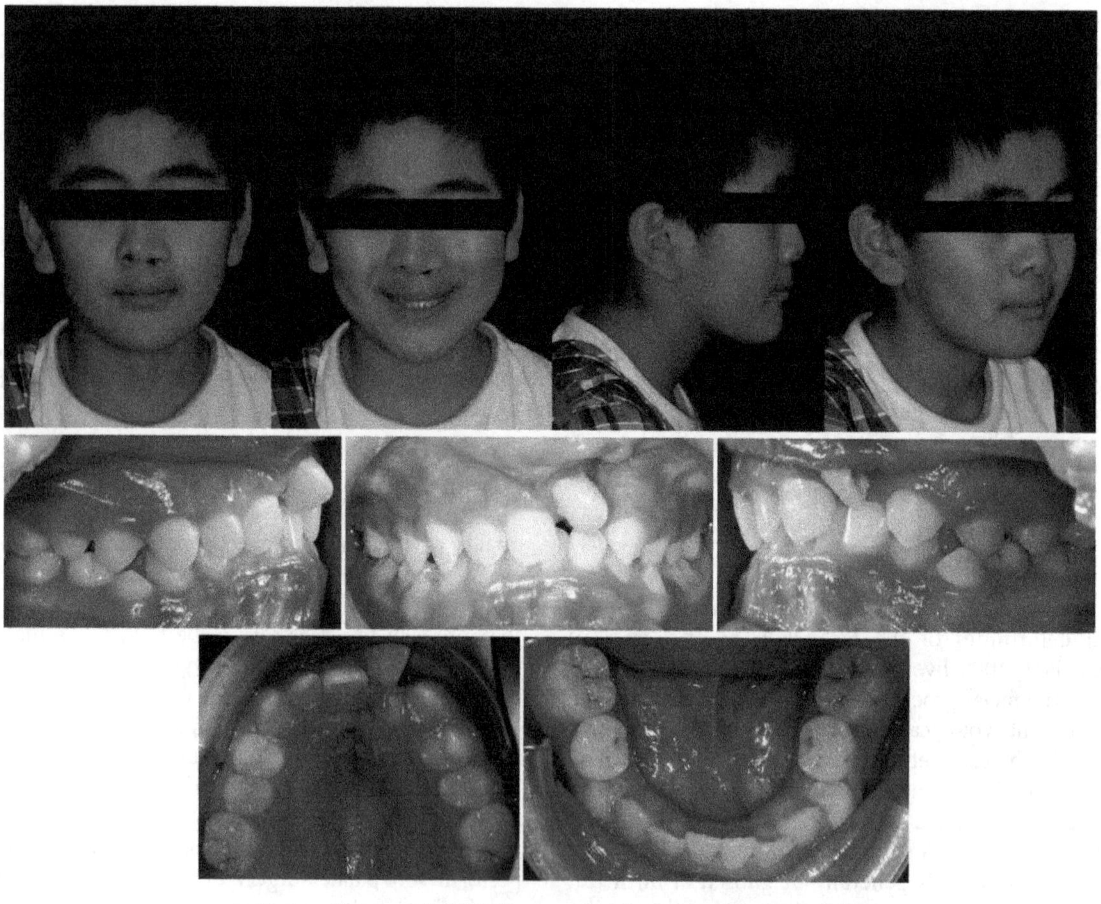

Figure 2: Initial photographic documentation.

degree of maxillary constriction, it has to be passively maintained in the mouth for about 1 year. During this period, speech therapy has to continue. At 9-11 years of age, ideally, when canine root development was between one-fourth and two-thirds of its final root length, graft surgery can be performed: an alveolar graft is placed in the cleft side. The bone graft can be sampled from the iliac crest. If the patient presents malocclusion and dental misalignment, an orthodontic fixed therapy can start at 9-15 years of age, with the objective to obtain alignment, leveling, malocclusion correction, and eventual tooth repositioning in the arch. If necessary, when the patient reaches 18 years of age, other procedures can be performed, as maxillofacial surgery (in the presence of a skeletal malocclusion), plastic surgery, or dental implants (to replace missing teeth). Patients with cleft lip and/or palate often present severe maxillary retrusion, transversal contraction of the maxilla, and skeletal class III malocclusion [10], because of the maxillary underdevelopment due to the cleft. If the skeletal malocclusion cannot be adequately corrected only with orthodontic therapy, in

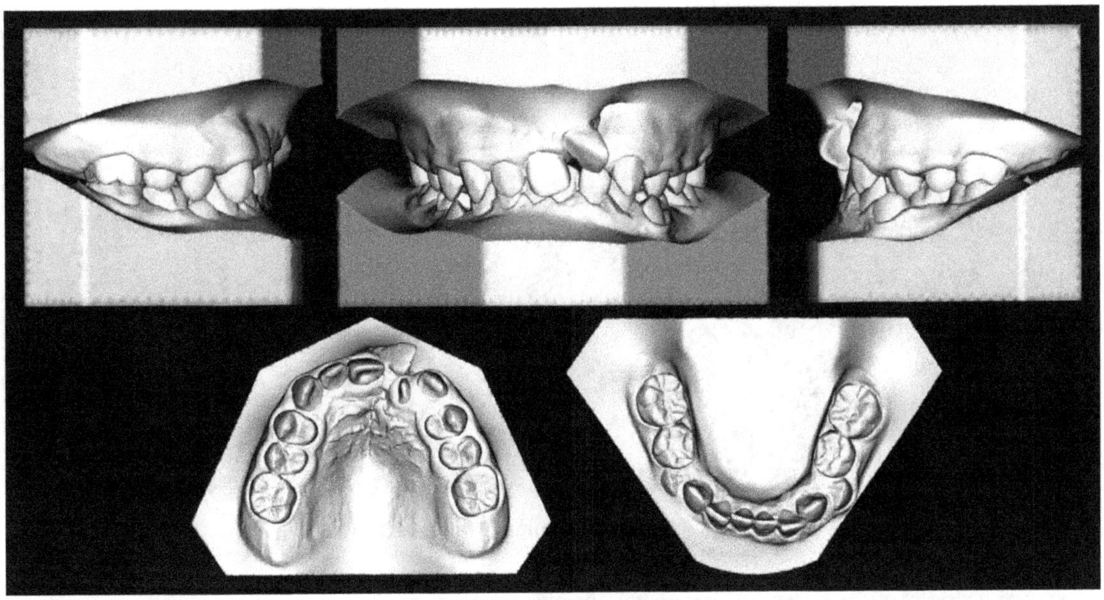

FIGURE 3: Initial dental casts.

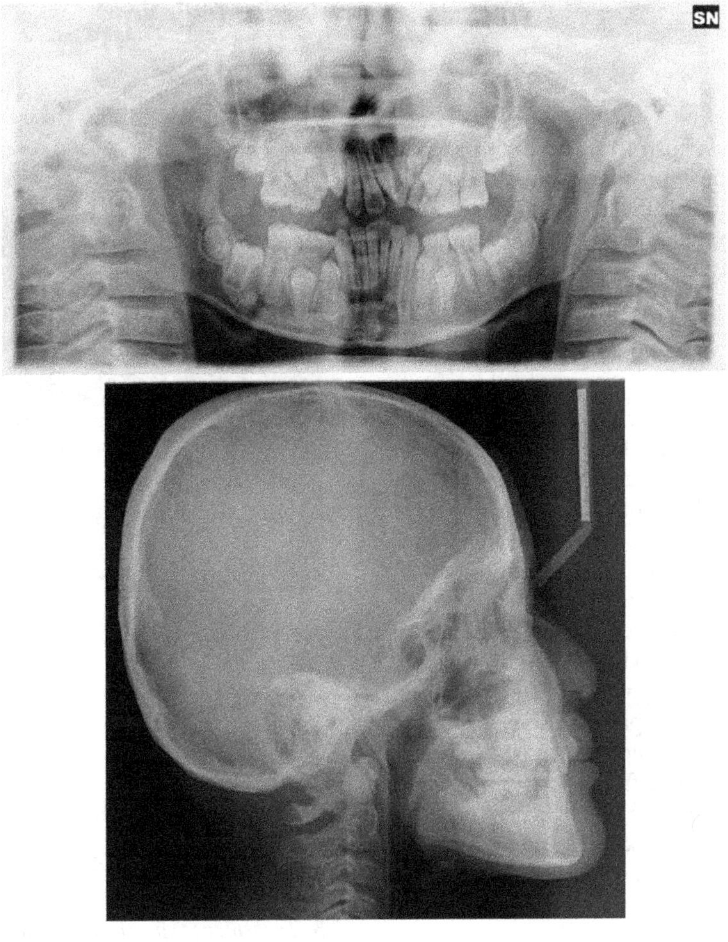

FIGURE 4: Initial panoramic radiograph and lateral cephalogram of the skull.

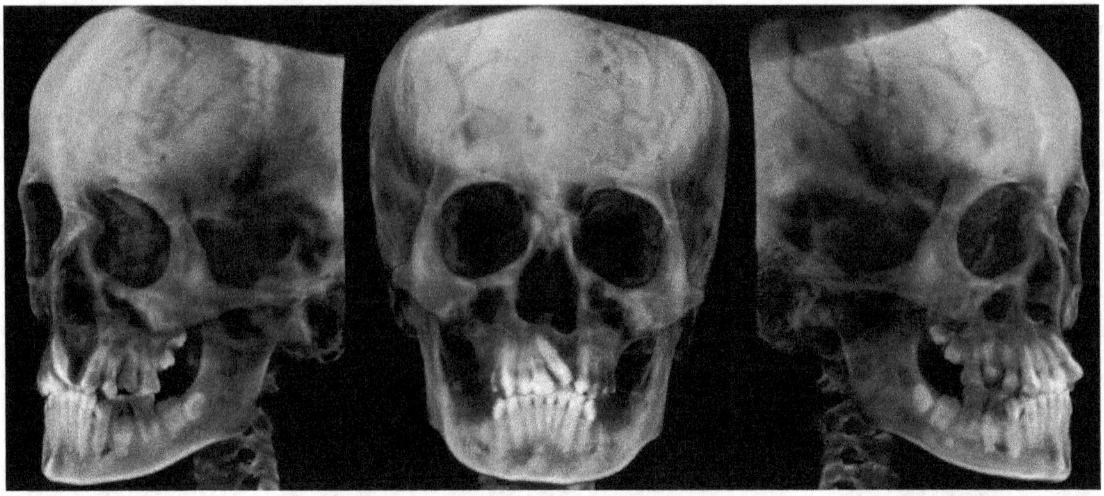

FIGURE 5: Cone-beam computed tomography.

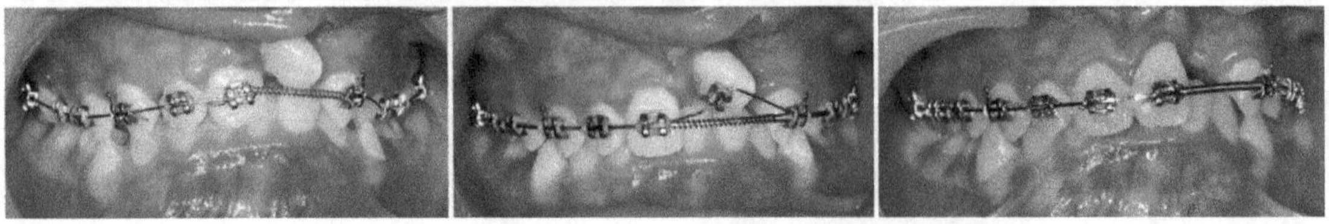

FIGURE 6: Tooth 21 recovery in the dental arch.

adulthood the orthodontic-surgical treatment, with orthognathic surgery, represents the approach of choice [13].

This paper is aimed at describing the clinical case of a patient with cleft lip and palate treated at the orthodontic department of the Dental Clinic of Padua University Hospital in Italy.

2. Material and Methods

2.1. Diagnosis and Etiology. The case presented is that of an 11-year-old patient that arrived at the orthodontic department of the Dental Clinic of Padua University Hospital. He was born in China and adopted by an Italian family, so his family anamnesis was unknown. The patient presented with a cleft lip and palate, a condition for which he underwent the first surgery in China, but with persistent oronasal communication (Figure 1). Moreover, during this surgery, he was unfortunately infected with B hepatitis. At the clinical and radiological (panoramic radiograph and lateral cephalogram of the skull) examination, the patient also presented an ectopic tooth 21, an ectopic and conoid tooth 22 positioned at the level of the left unilateral cleft, and upper and lower crowding with a very deep curve of Spee (Figures 2–4). As the presence of strong bone dehiscence, the orthodontic team decided to require a cone-beam computed tomography (CBCT) to a better definition of the bone condition (Figure 5).

2.2. Treatment Objectives. The treatment plan provided:

(i) Tooth 21 orthodontic recovery in the dental arch

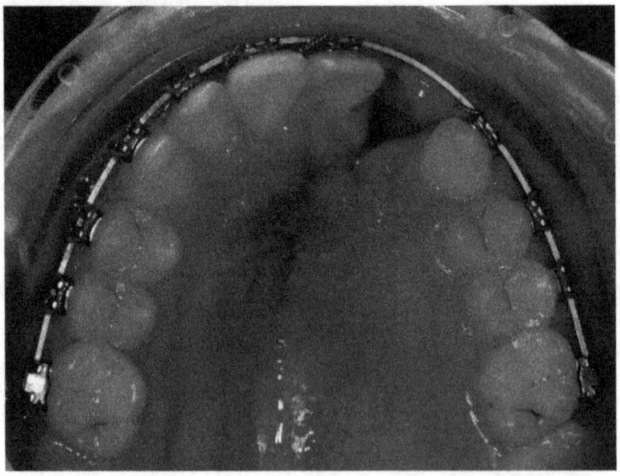

FIGURE 7: Tooth 22 extraction.

(ii) Graft surgery in the cleft area

(iii) Tooth 22 extraction, to limit possible dehiscence after the graft surgery planned in the cleft area

(iv) Malocclusion resolution

(v) Prosthetic rehabilitation of tooth 22

2.3. Treatment Alternatives. Metal bracket orthodontic therapy was considered the most adequate therapeutic option to obtain the recovery of tooth 21 in the dental arch, dental alignment, and malocclusion resolution. To achieve satisfactory aesthetics, by replacing tooth 22 avulsed, the therapeutic

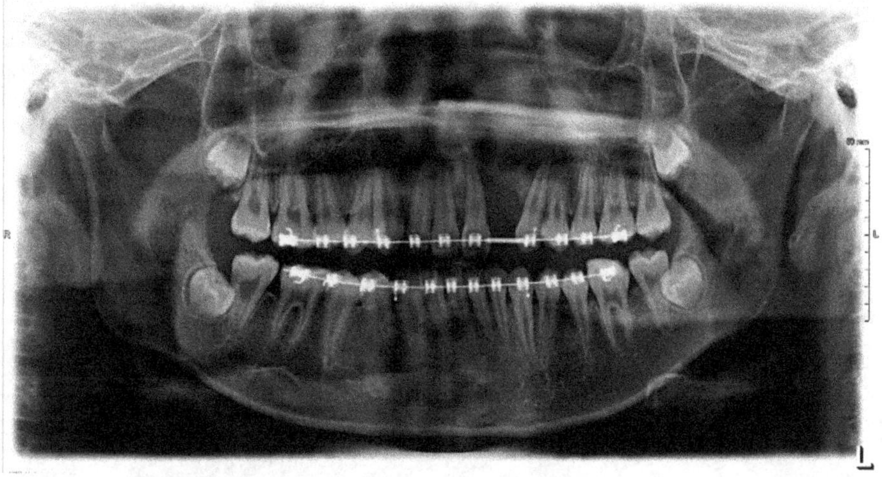

FIGURE 8: Panoramic radiograph after graft surgery.

alternative evaluated were implant-prosthetic rehabilitation, Maryland single-wing bridge supported by tooth 21, and a temporary prosthetic tooth supported by orthodontic palatal miniscrews.

2.4. Treatment Progress. The treatment started with upper dental arch bonding using Victory Low Profile 3M brackets (slot 0.22 × 0.28 MBT prescription) and a 0.16 NiTi archwire. An open spring in compression between teeth 11 and 23 was applied. After 3 months of treatment, the archwire is replaced with a 0.19 × 0.25 NiTi archwire, a bracket is applied on tooth 21, and an accessory 0.16 NiTi archwire was applied for extruding and distorting the tooth (Figure 6). After another 3 months of treatment, a 0.14 NiTi archwire and a slightly active spaced chain to bring tooth 21 to tooth 11 were applied. After 4 months, a carious lesion of tooth 21 was treated with conservative reconstruction; moreover, a 0.19 × 0.25 steel archwire is applied. The maxillofacial surgeon then proceeded with tooth 22 extraction (Figure 7) and bone graft surgery (Figure 8). After the surgery, the lower dental arch bonding was performed by using the same bracket typology of the upper dental arch and by application of the following archwire sequence: 0.16 NiTi, 0.19 × 0.25 NiTi, and 0.19 × 0.25 steel. With the sequential application of chains, open spring, and intraoral elastics, the treatment continued to optimize the occlusal class and to center the midlines.

Once the achievement of these objectives, the team decided to prosthetically rehabilitate the avulsed tooth 22 with the application of a temporary prosthetic tooth supported by orthodontic miniscrews applied on the patient palate using the Easy Driver system (Figure 9). This method consisted of the application of the miniscrews and the structure for the support of the prosthetic tooth during the same session, by using a surgical template produced by the dental laboratory. Then, the debonding was performed.

2.5. Treatment Results. At the end of the therapy, all the treatment objectives were achieved: the patient presented a first molar and canine class, an adequate overjet and overbite, a correct dental alignment in the upper and lower dental arch, good aesthetics, midline centering, and a flattened curve of Spee. Figures 10–12 showed the therapeutic result obtained.

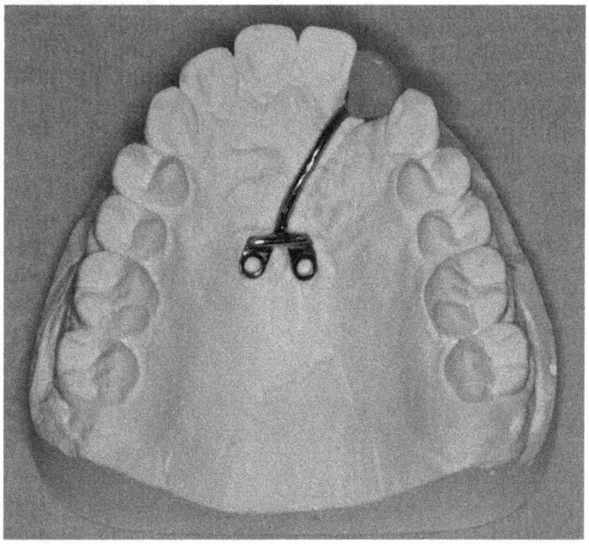

FIGURE 9: Temporary prosthetic tooth supported by orthodontic palatal miniscrews.

3. Discussion

This paper reports the clinical case of a young patient with a cleft lip and palate who sought surgical-orthodontic treatment. The patient needed a treatment that, according to his age and stage of growth, led him to an occlusal, functional, and aesthetic improvement. This case report shows how the team was able to obtain satisfactory rehabilitation for the patient treated.

The complexity of the case was due to various motivations, firstly the ectopic position of tooth 21, which needed to be recovered in the dental arch, then the persistence of the residual oronasal communication, which was connected

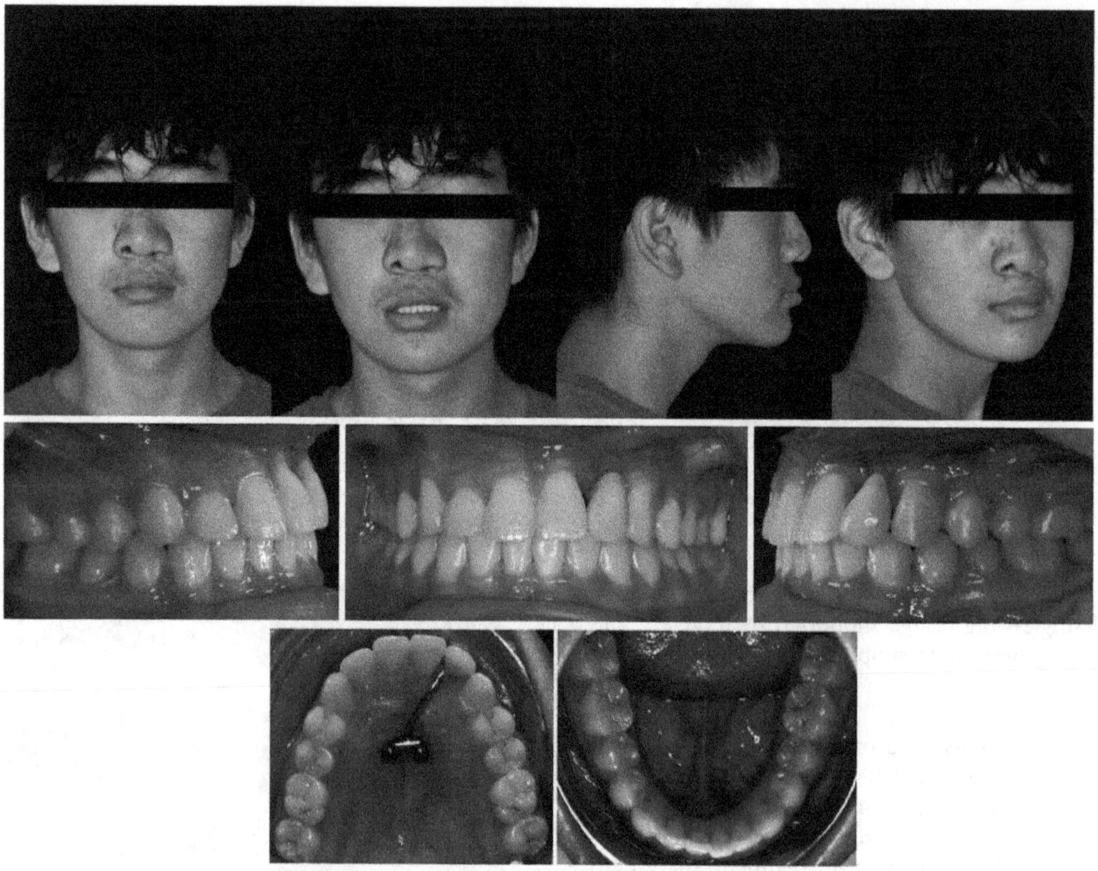

FIGURE 10: Final photographic documentation.

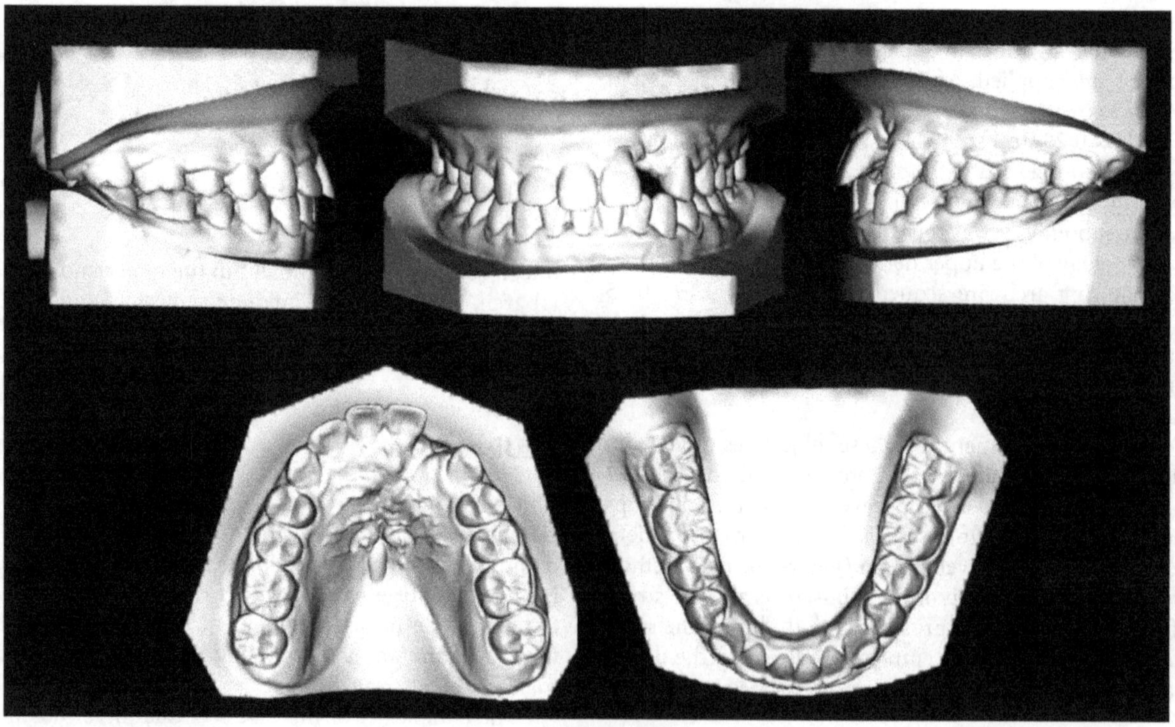

FIGURE 11: Final stone models.

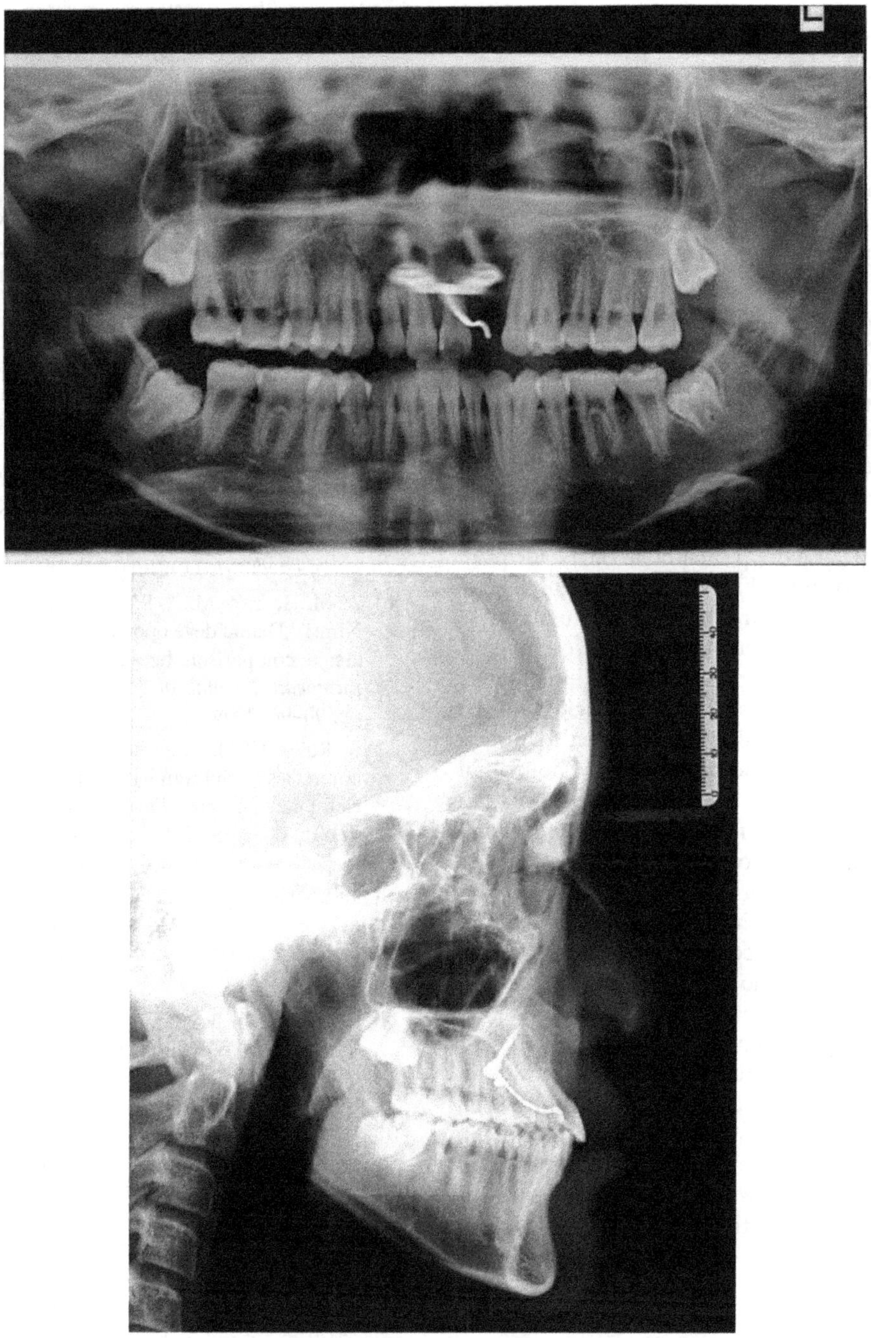

FIGURE 12: Final panoramic radiograph and lateral cephalogram of the skull.

to the evaluation of the tooth 22 prognosis. The possible dehiscence that could have been verified after the graft surgery planned in the cleft area led to the tooth 22 extraction decision. Moreover, the patient presented a malocclusion with a deep curve of Spee, which had to be resolved.

As the persistence of the oronasal communication after the first surgery performed in China, the patient needed a graft surgery to resolve the condition. The positioning of the alveolar bone graft permits restoring the function and continuity of the maxillary arch at the cleft site. The presurgical orthodontics has an important role in the correction of the central incisors' position or repositioning of displaced maxillary alveolar segments, allowing better access for the maxillofacial surgeon for the placement of the graft and the closure of the soft tissue [1]. Alveolar bone grafting seems to show a higher rate of success when performed before the canine eruption, as well as when presurgical orthodontics is performed [1, 12]. Ma et al. reported long-term success rates of 72-95% for bone grafts performed before the canine eruption and of 67-91% for bone grafts performed after the canine eruption. Nevertheless, for this patient, there was no choice: the eruption of 23 already occurred when the patient arrived at the attention of the orthodontic department. Anyway, graft surgery had a satisfactory result.

Taken the clinical decision to extract tooth 22, an important strategy of treatment that the team had to evaluate was how to prosthetically rehabilitate the extracted tooth 22. Since the patient was very young, the implant-prosthetic rehabilitation was discarded; in fact, the maxillary bone growth has to be completed to perform the implant insertion. Therefore, this therapeutic option could be considered in adulthood. Another considered option, as provisional prosthetic proposals, was the application of a Maryland single-wing bridge supported by tooth 21; the team decided to discard this option too, because of the little residual overjet presented by the patient at the end of orthodontic treatment. Finally, the rehabilitation choice was the application of a temporary prosthetic tooth supported by orthodontic miniscrews inserted on the patient's palate. This therapeutic option was chosen because the palatal bone offers adequate anchorage for the structure that supports the prosthetic dental tooth. It is compliance-free, as it is a nonremovable device. It offers a satisfactory aesthetic result and can be useful to allow gingival conditioning and the formation of interdental papillae between the prosthetic dental tooth and the adjacent teeth; this can be useful especially given the future implant insertion. The maintenance of adequate home oral hygiene can be considered easy for the patient, as this can be obtained by using the common device for home oral hygiene, i.e., brushing with toothpaste, using dental floss and/or brush, and mouth rinses with chlorhexidine (particularly in the event of soft tissue inflammation). The removal of the device for eventual necessary modification to the prosthetic dental tooth by the dental laboratory can be performed rapidly, as well as if the patient in adulthood should decide to undergo implant-prosthetic for the definitive replacement of the missing tooth. This option represents a temporary modality of missing tooth replacement, which needs a periodic follow-up during the growth of the patient. Possible side effects can be represented by inflammation of the gingiva surrounding the prosthetic dental tooth, mucositis in the area of insertion of the miniscrews, mobility or detachment of the miniscrews, and detachment of the prosthetic tooth.

4. Conclusions

Cleft lip and/or palate patients require multidisciplinary treatment to resolve all the anomalies connected to their condition. And adequate management of the case can substantially improve the quality of life of the patients.

References

[1] L. Ma, Y. Hou, G. Liu, and T. Zhang, "Effectiveness of presurgical orthodontics in cleft lip and palate patients with alveolar bone grafting: a systematic review," *Journal of Stomatology, Oral and Maxillofacial Surgery*, vol. S2468-7855, no. 20, pp. 30173–30177, 2020.

[2] F. Topolski, R. B. de Souza, A. Franco, O. A. Cuoghi, L. R. da Silva Assunção, and A. Fernandes, "Dental development of children and adolescents with cleft lip and palate," *Brazilian Journal of Oral Sciences*, vol. 13, pp. 319–324, 2014.

[3] A. De Stefani, G. Bruno, P. Balasso, S. Mazzoleni, U. Baciliero, and A. Gracco, "Prevalence of hypodontia in unilateral and bilateral cleft lip and palate patients inside and outside cleft area: a case-control study," *The Journal of Clinical Pediatric Dentistry*, vol. 43, no. 2, pp. 126–130, 2019.

[4] P. Defabianis, "Pre-surgical orthopedics in newborns affected by clefts of the lip, alveolus and palate. Report of two cases," *European Journal of Paediatric Dentistry*, vol. 18, no. 3, pp. 237–242, 2017.

[5] V. Lehtonen, V. Anttonen, L. P. Ylikontiola, S. Koskinen, P. Pesonen, and G. K. Sándor, "Dental anomalies associated with cleft lip and palate in Northern Finland," *European Journal of Paediatric Dentistry*, vol. 16, no. 4, pp. 327–332, 2015.

[6] A. M. Hazza'a, M. A. Rawashdeh, G. Al-Jamal, and K. S. Al-Nimri, "Dental development in children with cleft lip and palate: a comparison between unilateral and bilateral clefts," *European Journal of Paediatric Dentistry*, vol. 10, no. 2, pp. 90–94, 2009.

[7] R. Rullo, V. M. Festa, R. Rullo et al., "Prevalence of dental anomalies in children with cleft lip and unilateral and bilateral cleft lip and palate," *European Journal of Paediatric Dentistry*, vol. 16, no. 3, pp. 229–232, 2015.

[8] A. De Stefani, G. Bruno, P. Balasso, S. Mazzoleni, U. Baciliero, and A. Gracco, "Teeth agenesis evaluation in an Italian sample of complete unilateral and bilateral cleft lip and palate patients," *Minerva Stomatologica*, vol. 67, no. 4, pp. 156–164, 2018.

[9] M. Corcoran, S. Karki, V. Harila et al., "Oral health-related quality of life among young adults with cleft in northern Finland," *Clinical and Experimental Dental Research*, vol. 6, no. 3, pp. 305–310, 2020.

[10] V. Montanari, G. Bruno, F. Cavallin, U. Baciliero, A. De Stefani, and A. Gracco, "Cephalometric evaluation of patients with unilateral and bilateral complete cleft lip and palate," *Minerva Pediatrica*, 2020.

[11] A. De Stefani, G. Bruno, G. Irlandese, M. Barone, G. Costa, and A. Gracco, "Oral health-related quality of life in children using the child perception questionnaire CPQ11-14: a review," *European Archives of Paediatric Dentistry*, vol. 20, no. 5, pp. 425–430, 2019.

[12] D. Toscano, U. Baciliero, A. Gracco, and G. Siciliani, "Long-term stability of alveolar bone grafts in cleft palate patients," *American Journal of Orthodontics and Dentofacial Orthopedics*, vol. 142, no. 3, pp. 289–299, 2012.

[13] M. Barone, A. De Stefani, U. Baciliero, G. Bruno, and A. Gracco, "The accuracy of jaws repositioning in bimaxillary orthognathic surgery with traditional surgical planning compared to digital surgical planning in skeletal class III patients: a retrospective observational study," *Journal of Clinical Medicine*, vol. 9, no. 6, p. 1840, 2020.

30

Management and Follow-Up of Complicated Crown Fractures with Intrusive Luxation of Maxillary Incisors in an 8-Year-Old Boy

Niusha Abazarian,[1] Shabnam Milani,[2] Moahammad Hassan Hamrah,[3] and Marzieh Salehi Shahrabi[2]

[1]Department of Pediatric Dentistry, Dental School, AJA University of Medical Sciences, Tehran, Iran
[2]Department of Pediatric Dentistry, Tehran University of Medical Sciences, Tehran, Iran
[3]Department of Pediatric Dentistry, School of Dentistry, Tehran University of Medical Sciences Tehran, Iran

Correspondence should be addressed to Marzieh Salehi Shahrabi; salehipegah7@gmail.com

Academic Editor: Andrea Scribante

Intrusive luxation is a severe form of dental injury which causes damage to the pulp and supporting structures of a tooth because of its dislocation into the alveolar process. This paper shows the case of the reeruption of maxillary incisors accompanied by complicated crown fractures after 3 months. An 8-year-old boy patient was referred to the Department of Pedodontic Dentistry of Tehran University of Medical Science, Tehran, Iran, 18 hours after a fall at school. Clinical and radiographic examinations revealed intrusive luxation of both incisors with complicated crown fractures. Cervical pulpotomy is the treatment of choice for traumatized immature intruded teeth with pulp exposure. Two months later, the right central incisor teeth reerupted to a normal position and the final aesthetic restorations were done. The left central incisor was spontaneously repositioned with external root resorption, and the team decided to use interim medication (calcium hydroxide) in the root canal for stopping the process of resorption, and by the 9-month follow-up, the process of resorption had been stopped. An MTA plug was placed into the canal, and the final esthetic restorations were done.

1. Introduction

The most frequent traumatic dental injuries involving permanent teeth are complicated and uncomplicated crown fractures, and the most affected teeth are maxillary central incisors (93.3%) especially in children [1]. The most severe form of traumatic dental injury is intrusive luxation that accounts for 15–61% of traumas in permanent teeth and is defined as apical displacement of the tooth in its socket. The etiological factors include falling, bicycle injury, sports accidents, and fights [2, 3].

Intrusive luxation of permanent teeth is a rare dental injury when compared with other types of luxation injuries. It comprises of 3% of all traumatic injuries in the permanent teeth [1]. The displacement results in the damage to the alveolar bone, the periodontal ligament, the cementum, and the pulp. Healing subsequent to trauma is complex. Complications include pulp necrosis, inflammatory root resorption, dentoalveolar ankylosis, loss of marginal bone support, calcification of pulp tissue, paralysis or disturbance of root development, and gingival retraction [1, 4]. Intrusive luxations are associated with a high risk of complications during healing, including pulpal necrosis and calcification, external inflammatory resorption, replacement resorption, gingival retraction, and marginal bone loss [4]. The incidence of pulp necrosis for intruded teeth with open apex is significantly lower compared to closed apex, and it occurs between 63% and 68% in open apex and 100% for teeth with closed apex [1]. Depending on the severity of intrusion, the frequency of replacement resorption in intruded incisors ranges from 5% to 31% [2, 3] and appears to be more in mature than in immature teeth [5]. Although 97% of all inflammatory

Table 1: Patient characteristics.

Age	Sex	Chief complaint	Clinical examination (extraoral examination)	Clinical examination (intraoral examination)	Radiographic examination
8 years old	Male	Trauma of the central incisors following a fall at school 18 hours ago	Abrasion on the skin of the chin inflammation and bleeding of the labial gingival of the central incisors	Complicated crown fracture of the central incisors with no mobility and percussive metallic sound	An intact periodontal ligament space, incomplete root formation, no root fracture

resorption are arrested after long-term calcium hydroxide therapy, there is no effective treatment for replacement resorption [1].

There are numerous ways to manage complicated crown fractures, such as direct pulp capping, partial pulpotomy, cervical pulpotomy, or pulpectomy. Furthermore, the treatment option for intruded teeth up to 7 mm for open apex is spontaneous repositioning [5].

Cervical pulpotomy is the treatment of choice for traumatized immature intruded teeth with pulp exposure. It allows the development of the roots to continue, with apical closing and strengthening of the root structure [6].

The present case report describes the management and follow-ups of traumatized immature intruded teeth with complicated crown fractures.

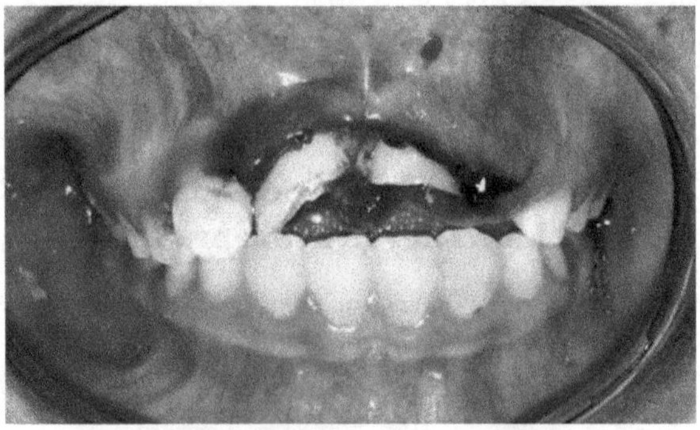

Figure 1: Intraoral examinations.

2. Case Presentation

An 8-year-old boy patient was referred to the Department of Pedodontic Dentistry of Tehran University of Medical Science, Tehran, Iran, with the chief complaint being trauma of the central incisors following a fall at school 18 hours ago. The general medical, dental, and traumatic incident histories were recorded. There was no systemic disease history. Extraoral examination revealed abrasion on the skin of the chin and inflammation and bleeding of the labial gingival of the central incisors (Table 1). Intraoral examination revealed complicated crown fracture of the central incisors with no mobility and percussive metallic sound, indicating intrusion [1] (Figure 1).

Periapical radiographic examination showed an intact periodontal ligament space, incomplete root formation of both central incisors, and no root fracture (Figure 2).

The periapical radiographies were taken using Xgenus (de Gotzen S.r.l device, distributed by Satelec-Acteon Group, Italy).

Cervical pulpotomy using white mineral trioxide aggregate (BioMTA, Seoul, Republic of Korea) was done for both incisors after under local anesthesia and rubber dam isolation; all coronal pulp tissues were gently removed by using a high-speed sterile round diamond bur (Dentsply Maillefer, Tulsa, OK, USA) under water cooling. Hemorrhage was controlled with sterile cotton pellets and sterile saline solution to avoid clot formation. When pulpal bleeding stopped within 3 min, MTA powder was mixed with distilled water according to the recommended consistency and placed without any pressure to cover the exposed pulps. A moist cotton pellet was placed on the MTA, and the cavity was sealed temporarily with RMGI (Fuji IX, GC Corporation, Tokyo, Japan) (Table 2 and Figure 3).

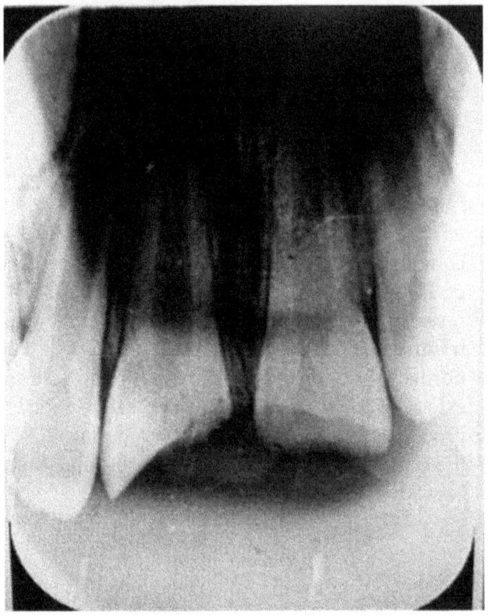

Figure 2: Radiographic examinations.

Follow-up after 4 weeks showed left central incisor percussion with spontaneous eruption, and the right central incisor percussion was metallic sound with no signs and symptoms. Radiographic evaluations have demonstrated a PDL widening in the middle third of the root in both central incisors (follow-up after 1 month) (Figure 4).

After 2 months of follow-up, the left center incisor was spontaneously repositioned with external root resorption and had a sensitive percussion. And the right central incisor with no signs and symptoms showed normal percussion and mobility with a normal radiography, and so, it was decided to do a composite buildup (Figure 5).

Treatment used to stop the external resorption of the left central incisor was irrigation with sodium hypochlorite

Table 2: Clinical passages.

Phase number	Treatment steps
1	Under local anesthesia and rubber dam isolation, all coronal pulp tissues were gently removed by using a high-speed sterile round diamond bur (Dentsply Maillefer, Tulsa, OK, USA) under water cooling.
2	Hemorrhage was controlled with sterile cotton pellets and sterile saline solution to avoid clot formation.
3	When pulpal bleeding stopped within 3 min, MTA powder was mixed with distilled water according to the recommended consistency and placed without any pressure to cover the exposed pulps.
4	A moist cotton pellet was placed on the MTA, and the cavity was sealed temporarily with RMGI (Fuji IX, GC Corporation, Tokyo, Japan).

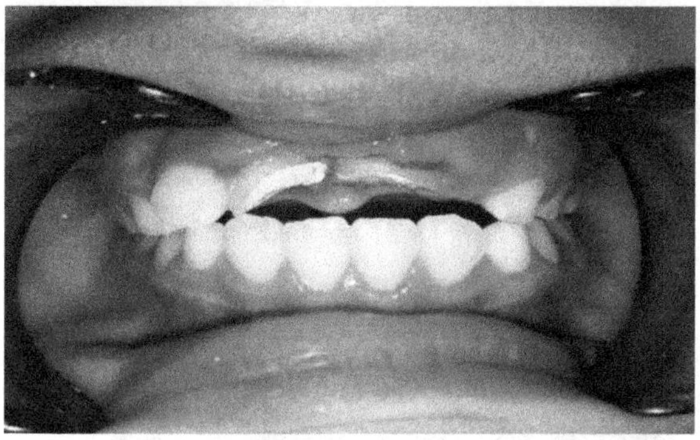

Figure 3: Cervical pulpotomy white MTA for both incisors.

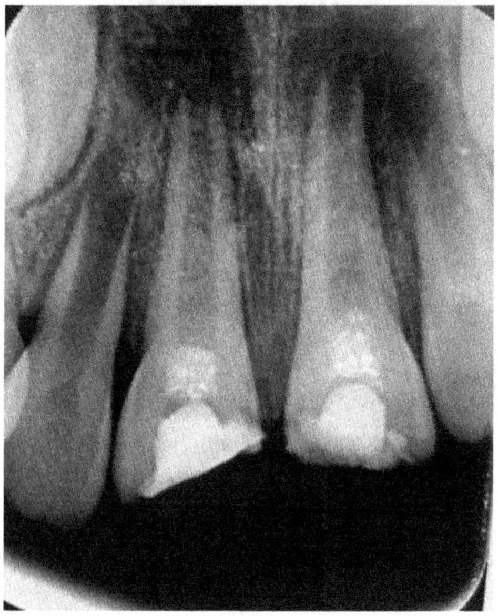

Figure 4: Follow-up after 4 weeks.

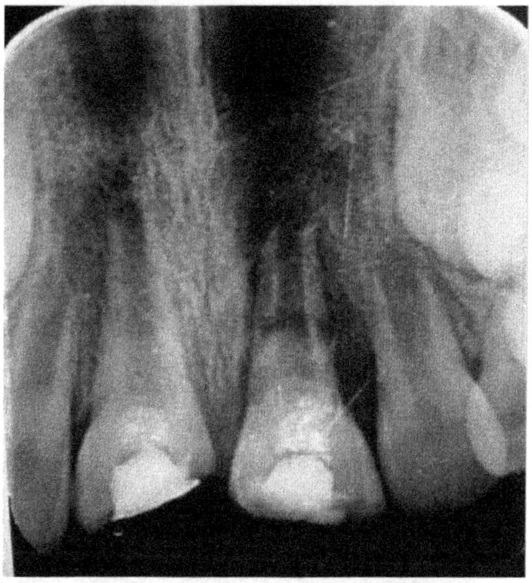

Figure 5: Follow-up after 8 weeks.

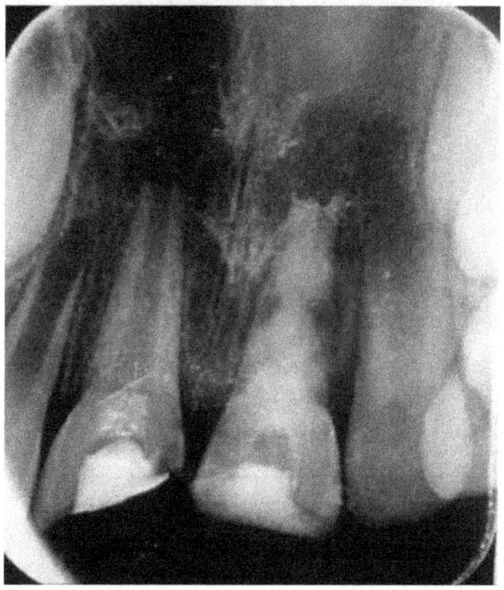

Figure 6: Calcium hydroxide was applied as intracanal medicament to stop the external resorption.

(Beyond Technology Corp., Beijing, China) and saline. The CaOH (Prevest Denpro, Golchai, Iran) was positioned within the canal and dressed with RMGI (Fuji II LC, GC, Tokyo, Japan) (Figure 6).

After 3 months, CaOH (Prevest Denpro, Golchai, Iran) was replaced. At the 9-month follow-up, the resorption process had stopped, and an MTA (BioMTA, Seoul, Republic of Korea) plug was placed in the canal and dressed with RMGI (Fuji II LC, GC, Tokyo, Japan). After one week, obturation, done with gutta-percha (reoko, Langenau, Germany) and composite (Filtek Z350 XT, 3 M ESPE, St. Paul, MN, USA) buildup, was performed (Figures 7(a) and 7(b)).

At the 22-month recall, the teeth were asymptomatic and showed no signs of resorption, clinically and radiographically (Figures 8(a) and 8(b)).

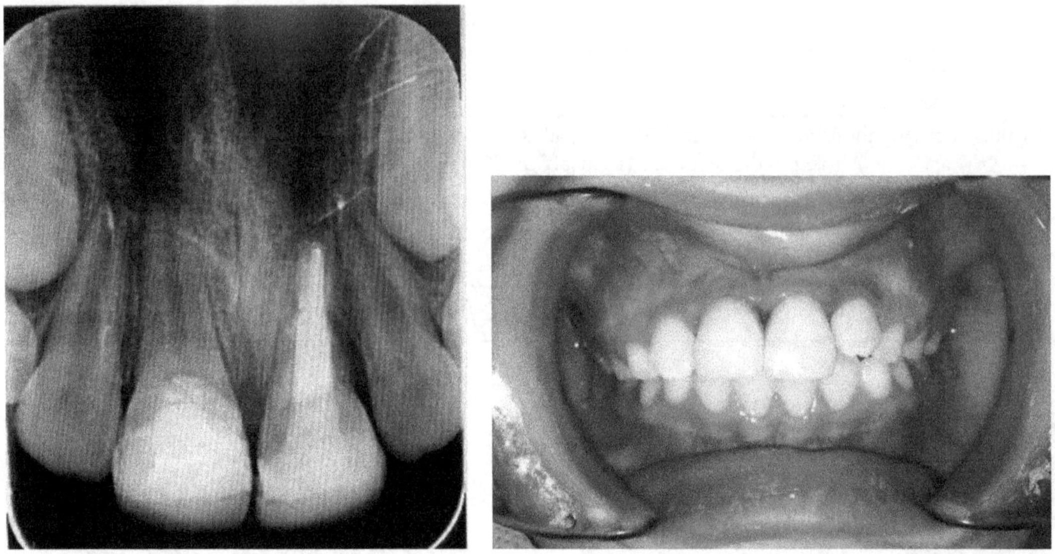

(a) (b)

Figure 7: (a) MTA apical plug of 4-5 mm thickness and final obturation. (b) Final restoration of the tooth.

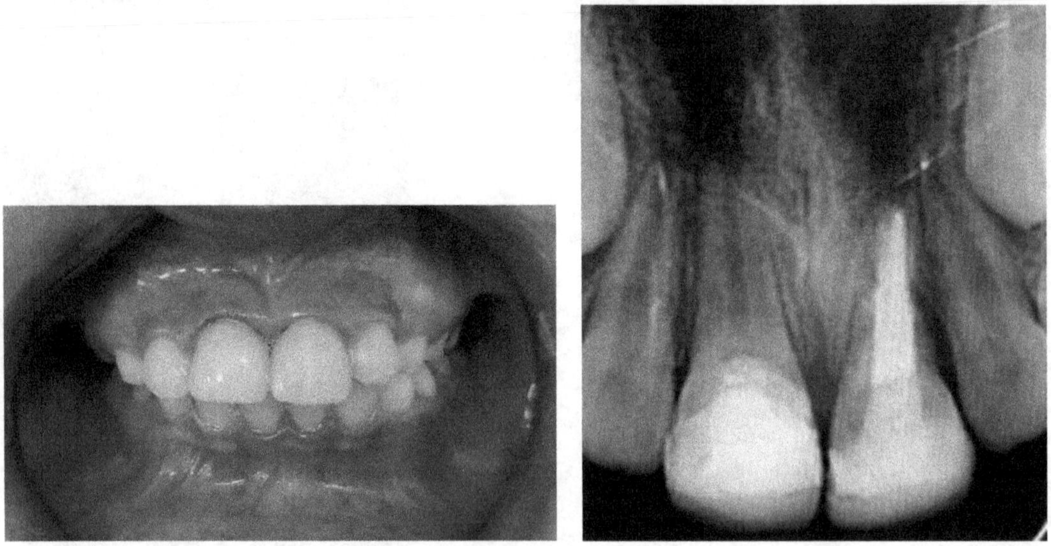

(a) (b)

Figure 8: (a) Follow-up after 22 months. (b) Radiography after 22-month follow-up.

Table 3: Clinical procedures.

Phase number	Treatment steps
First session	Cervical pulpotomy white MTA for both incisors
Follow-up after 4 weeks	(i) Left central incisor percussion with spontaneous eruption (ii) Right central incisor percussion was metallic sound with no signs and symptoms (iii) Radiographic evaluations have demonstrated a PDL widening in the middle third of the root in both central incisors
Follow-up after 8 weeks	(i) The left center incisor was spontaneously repositioned with external root resorption and had a sensitive percussion, and calcium hydroxide was applied as intracanal medicament (ii) The right central incisor with no signs and symptoms showed normal percussion and mobility with a normal radiography
Follow-up after 36 weeks	The resorption process had stopped, and an MTA plug was placed in the canal and dressed with RMGI.
Follow-up after 37 weeks	Obturation, done with gutta-percha and composite buildup, was performed
Follow-up after 22 months	The teeth were asymptomatic and showed no signs of resorption, clinically and radiographically.

The patient has been followed for the last 22 months showing the success of the treatment (Table 3).

3. Discussion

Complicated crown fractures are defined as fractures involving enamel and dentin with pulp exposure. These injuries produce changes in the exposed pulp tissues, and a biological and functional restoration represents an important clinical challenge [1].

Dental traumas may include numerous injuries, including intrusion (33.5%), an associated crown fracture intrusion (60.5%), or a combination of intrusion and coronal or root fractures (6%) [2]. In most cases, it affects only one tooth (46.3%), followed by two teeth (32.4%) and three or more teeth (21.3%) [7]. Most of the intruded teeth are displaced from 1 to 8 mm into the alveolar bone by a traumatic force [8].

Intrusive luxation is a type of severe trauma that results in injury to the tooth structure, cells and fibers of periodontal ligament, pulp tissue, and alveolar bone [9].

Intrusive luxation is associated with a high risk of complications during healing and considered as one of the most difficult types of injury to treat as there are differing opinions on what constitutes as treatment. It was previously believed that the stage of development of the root was the determining factor for prognosis of intruded teeth [10]. Current dental literature suggests different treatment approaches for the management of intrusive luxation injuries including passive repositioning, allowing the tooth to reerupt, and active repositioning, either surgically or by use of orthodontic appliances [2]. Miniscrews are effective orthodontic devices for various orthodontic movements of the intruded teeth; it is recommended for dental extrusion without involving other teeth, implant side effects, or gingival margin cosmetic disability [11]. In case of intrusive luxation, the miniscrew-assisted orthodontic repositioning has been proposed [11]. In fact, orthodontic miniscrews demonstrated excellent mechanical properties and also with small diameters so they can be used also in hard to reach areas [12].

Root resorption after an intrusion is a commonly occurring scar complication. Inflammatory root resorption and replacement root resorption are classified as invasive or progressive root resorption [11, 12]. External root resorption has been reported and cited to be between 28% and 66% [1, 13, 14]. Andreasen et al. reported a total incidence of 86% of external resorption (38% inflammatory, 24% surface, and 24% replacement resorption). They also found a higher incidence of resorption in teeth with closed apices (70%) than in those with open apices (58%) [1].

It has been shown that calcium hydroxide stops the inflammatory resorption with a high degree of success [15]. Calcium hydroxide paste should be maintained in the root canal for 1 to 6 months before obturation with gutta-percha points. In this case, we applied calcium hydroxide (Prevest Denpro, Golchai, Iran) paste when the external root resorption has been started. After 9 months of follow-up, the resorption process had been stopped. In support of this, dressing to allow the healing should be kept for 6–9 months [16].

The long-term use of calcium hydroxide has some drawbacks. The treatment requires multiple appointments and takes anywhere from 3 to 18 months [17, 18]. It demands high cooperation and motivation from the patient. In addition, the long-term presence of calcium hydroxide in root canal space can increase the brittleness of the root dentin and the risk of future cervical root fractures especially in open apex teeth [11]. In spite of these disadvantages, it is still the preferred treatment protocol due to its high success rate [1, 11].

This case report shows that within the limitations of this study is a successful outcome. However, there were weaknesses on follow-up of the patient due to the COVID-19 pandemic lockdown and delay in attending patient to hospital after injury.

4. Conclusion

The findings in this case report suggest that calcium hydroxide stops the inflammatory resorption with a high degree of success.

References

[1] J. O. Andreasen, L. K. Bakland, R. C. Matras, and F. M. Andreasen, "Traumatic intrusion of permanent teeth. Part 1. An epidemiological study of 216 intruded permanent teeth," *Dental Traumatology*, vol. 22, no. 2, pp. 83–89, 2006.

[2] J. O. Andreasen, F. M. Andreasen, and L. Andersson, *Textbook and color atlas of traumatic injuries to the teeth*, John Wiley & Sons, 2018.

[3] V. Chacko and M. Pradhan, "Management of traumatically intruded young permanent tooth with 40-month follow-up," *Australian Dental Journal*, vol. 59, no. 2, pp. 240–244, 2014.

[4] J. M. Humphrey, D. J. Kenny, and E. J. Barret, "Clinical outcomes for permanent incisor luxations in a pediatric population. I. Intrusions," *Dental traumatology*, vol. 19, no. 5, pp. 266–273, 2003.

[5] A. W. Raut, V. Mantri, V. I. Shambharkar, and M. Mishra, "Management of complicated crown fracture by reattachment using fiber post: minimal intervention approach," *Journal of natural science, biology, and medicine*, vol. 9, no. 1, pp. 93–96, 2018.

[6] A. Nosrat and S. Asgary, "Apexogenesis treatment with a new endodontic cement: a case report," *Journal of Endodontics*, vol. 36, no. 5, pp. 912–914, 2010.

[7] V. Faus-Matoses, M. Martínez-Viñarta, T. Alegre-Domingo, I. Faus-Matoses, and V. J. Faus-Llácer, "Treatment of multiple traumatized anterior teeth associated with an alveolar bone fracture in a 20-year-old patient: a 3-year follow up," *Journal of clinical and experimental dentistry*, vol. 6, no. 4, 2014.

[8] R. F. Cunha, "Early treatment of an intruded primary tooth: a case report," *The Journal of Clinical Pediatric Dentistry*, vol. 25, no. 3, pp. 199–202, 2001.

[9] C. Y. Yu and P. V. Abbott, "Responses of the pulp, periradicular and soft tissues following trauma to the permanent teeth," *Australian dental journal.*, vol. 61, pp. 39–58, 2016.

[10] A. L. C. S. D. Omena, I. A. Ferreira, C. L. Ramagem, K. M. S. Moreira, I. Floriano, and J. C. Imparato, "Severe trauma in young permanent tooth: a case report," *RGO-Revista Gaúcha de Odontologia*, vol. 68, 2020.

[11] R. F. Horliana, A. C. Horliana, A. D. Wuo, F. E. Perez, and J. Abrão, "Dental extrusion with orthodontic miniscrew anchorage: a case report describing a modified method," *Case reports in dentistry*, vol. 2015, Article ID 909314, 6 pages, 2015.

[12] M. F. Sfondrini, P. Gandini, R. Alcozer, P. K. Vallittu, and A. Scribante, "Failure load and stress analysis of orthodontic miniscrews with different transmucosal collar diameter," *Journal of the mechanical behavior of biomedical materials*, vol. 87, pp. 132–137, 2018.

[13] A. Rovira-Wilde, N. Longridge, and S. McKernon, "Management of severe traumatic intrusion in the permanent dentition," *BMJ Case Reports CP*, vol. 14, no. 3, p. e235676, 2021.

[14] C. J. Pearce, "Recent developments in equine dentistry," *New Zealand veterinary journal*, vol. 68, no. 3, pp. 178–186, 2020.

[15] H. Al-Saffar and S. V. Stefanescu, "Management of non-vital open apex in a lateral incisor using calcium hydroxide and reverse GP cone cold lateral compaction in a general practice setting," *Journal of Dental Research*, vol. 2, no. 1, pp. 1–12, 2021.

[16] R. M. Darley, C. Fernandes e Silva, F. D. Costa, C. B. Xavier, and F. F. Demarco, "Complications and sequelae of concussion and subluxation in permanent teeth: a systematic review and meta-analysis," *Dental traumatology*, vol. 36, no. 6, pp. 557–567, 2020.

[17] D. D. Müller, R. Bissinger, M. Reymus, K. Bücher, R. Hickel, and J. Kühnisch, "Survival and complication analyses of avulsed and replanted permanent teeth," *Scientific Reports*, vol. 10, no. 1, pp. 1–9, 2020.

[18] C. Bourguignon, N. Cohenca, E. Lauridsen et al., "International Association of Dental Traumatology guidelines for the management of traumatic dental injuries: 1. Fractures and luxations," *Dental Traumatology*, vol. 36, no. 4, pp. 314–330, 2020.

31

Orthodontic Treatment for a Patient with Root Resorption of All Four Maxillary Incisors due to Bilaterally Impacted Canines

Makoto Yanoshita, Naoto Hirose, Azusa Onishi, Sayuri Nishiyama, Naoki Kubo, Daiki Kita, and Kotaro Tanimoto

Department of Orthodontics and Craniofacial Developmental Biology, Hiroshima University Graduate School of Biomedical and Health Sciences, Kasumi 1-2-3 Minami-ku, Hiroshima-shi, Hiroshima Prefecture, Japan

Correspondence should be addressed to Naoto Hirose; hirose@hiroshima-u.ac.jp

Academic Editor: Sivakumar Nuvvula

Maxillary canines require the longest period from the generation of the tooth germ to the completion of eruption, and they have more difficulties in eruption than other teeth. The incisor roots are often resorbed due to malpositioned canines. An 11-year-old girl presented with an extremely rare case of root resorption of four maxillary incisors due to bilaterally impacted maxillary canines, which were located excessively mesially. The case was managed through oral surgery and orthodontic treatment over five years. After extracting the maxillary deciduous canines, the maxillary bilateral canines were surgically exposed. The bimaxillary lateral incisors were extracted, and the canines were orthodontically tracted over 8 months. All teeth were then aligned using edgewise brackets. No further root resorption of the central incisors was observed for 5 years after canine traction. This case demonstrates the importance of early detection of abnormally positioned canines.

1. Introduction

Maxillary canines are important in terms of function and esthetics. Canines have the greatest frequency of impaction, second only to third molars [1, 2]. There is a 1–3% chance that canines fail to erupt and become impacted [3]. The period between the formation of the tooth germ and completion of tooth eruption is the longest for maxillary canines; they also experience more difficulty in eruption compared with other teeth [3]. The causes of impaction of maxillary canines include crowding, trauma, root curvature, odontoma, cysts, and supernumerary teeth [4–8].

Impacted canines can cause root resorption in permanent incisors. This root resorption is assumed to be caused by physical contact between the incisor roots and canine crown [9]. Root resorption associated with ectopic eruption of maxillary canines occurs in 48 of patients with impacted canines aged 9 to 15 years [10].

Deciduous root resorption is a normal physiological process that precedes permanent tooth eruption. Root resorption of permanent teeth is considered the result of complex biological processes; however, the exact mechanism remains unclear. In case of root resorption of the permanent maxillary incisors due to an impacted maxillary canine, prompt decisions must be made regarding the need for surgical exposure of the canine, traction of the canine, and extraction of the resorbed incisors should be extracted, followed by orthodontic alignment.

This report describes the surgical and orthodontic management of a case of root resorption of the bilateral maxillary central and lateral incisors due to maxillary canines erupting in an abnormal direction.

2. Case Report

An 11-year-old girl with impacted bilateral maxillary canines with an aberrant direction of eruption was referred to our department for orthodontic consultation. Root resorption of the four maxillary incisors had been detected on panoramic radiography at the previous dental clinic.

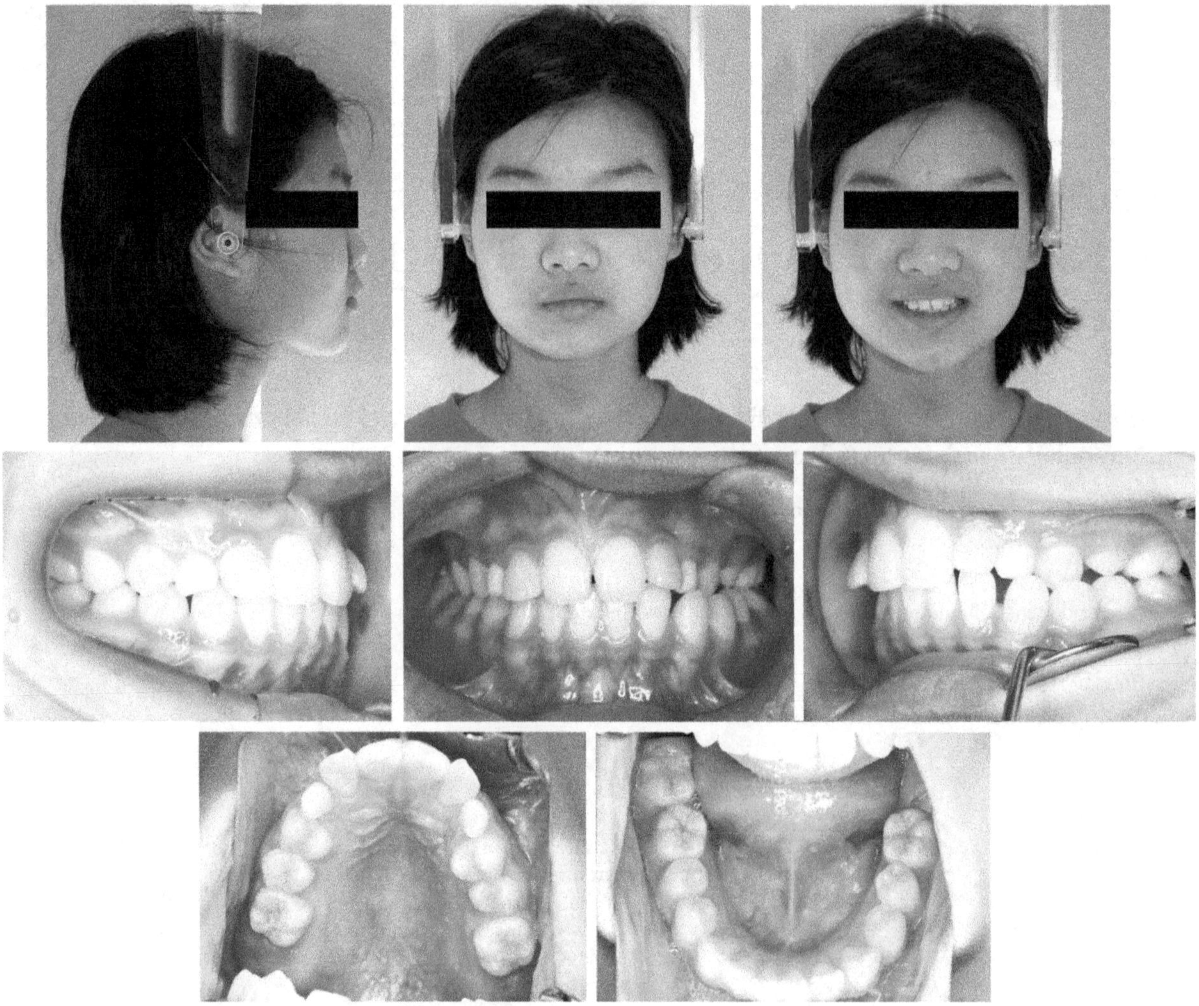

FIGURE 1: Pretreatment facial and intraoral photographs.

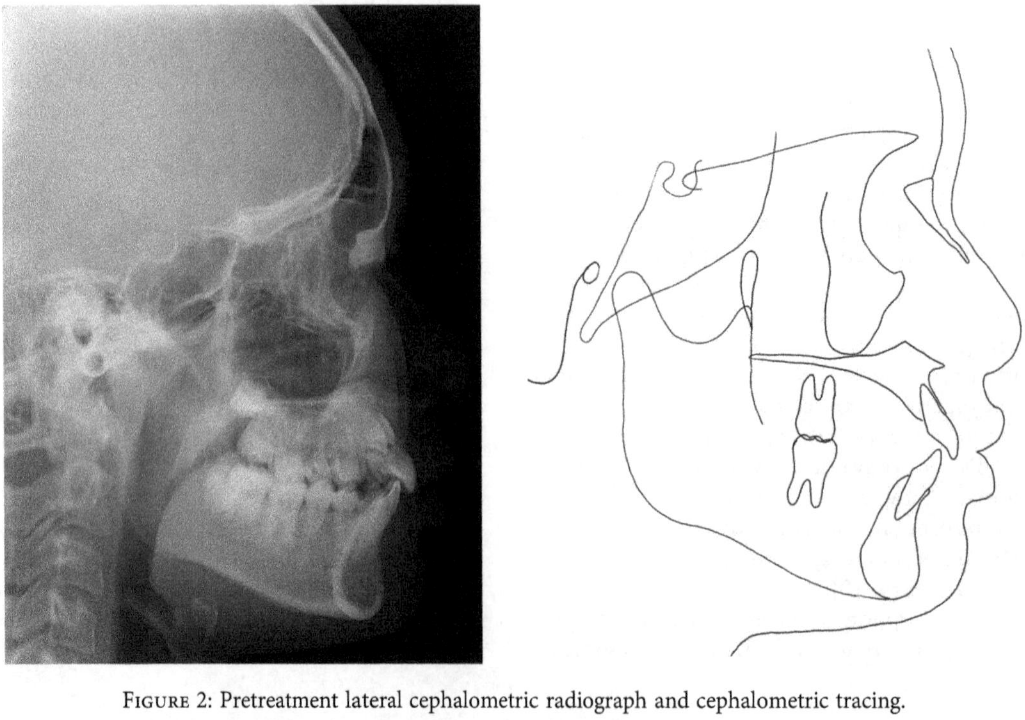

FIGURE 2: Pretreatment lateral cephalometric radiograph and cephalometric tracing.

Table 1: Superimposition of pre- and post-cephalograms.

Location	Measurement	Pretreatment	Posttreatment	Norm
Skeletal				
Maxilla to cranial base	SNA (°)	88.8	88.8	79.9 ± 2.4
Mandible to cranial base	SNB (°)	85.6	85.8	77.7 ± 2.7
Maxillomandibular	ANB (°)	3.2	3.0	2.9 ± 1.8
	FMA (°)	18.3	18.5	28.8 ± 5.6
Dental				
Maxillary dentition	U1 to SN (°)	114.9	118.7	104.5 ± 7.0
Mandibular dentition	IMPA (°)	102.1	93.4	91.3 ± 5.4
	FMIA (°)	59.7	68.1	59.9 ± 10.6
Intermaxillary dental relationship	Interincisal angle (°)	123.8	127.3	124.5 ± 11.6

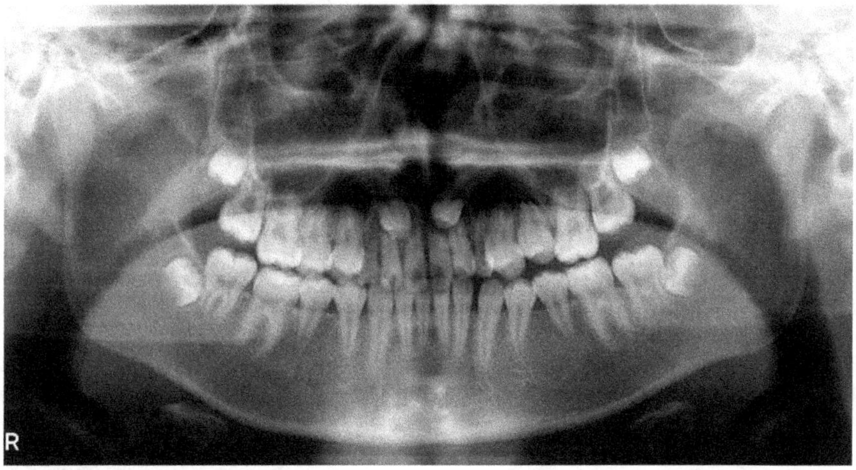

(a)

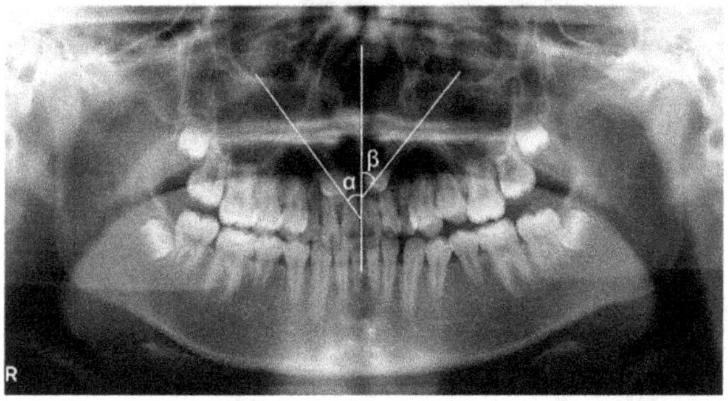

(b)

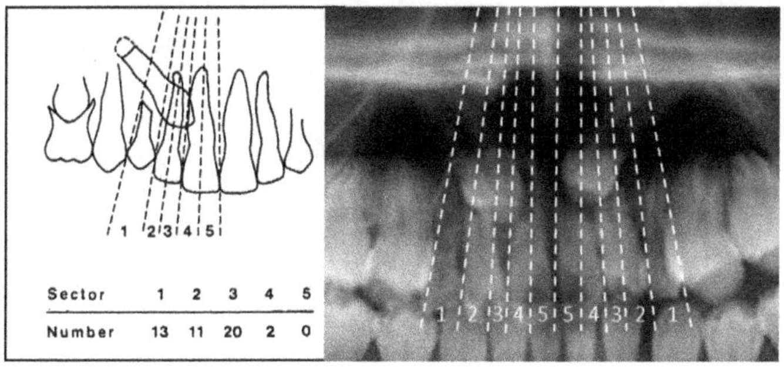

(c)

Figure 3: Continued.

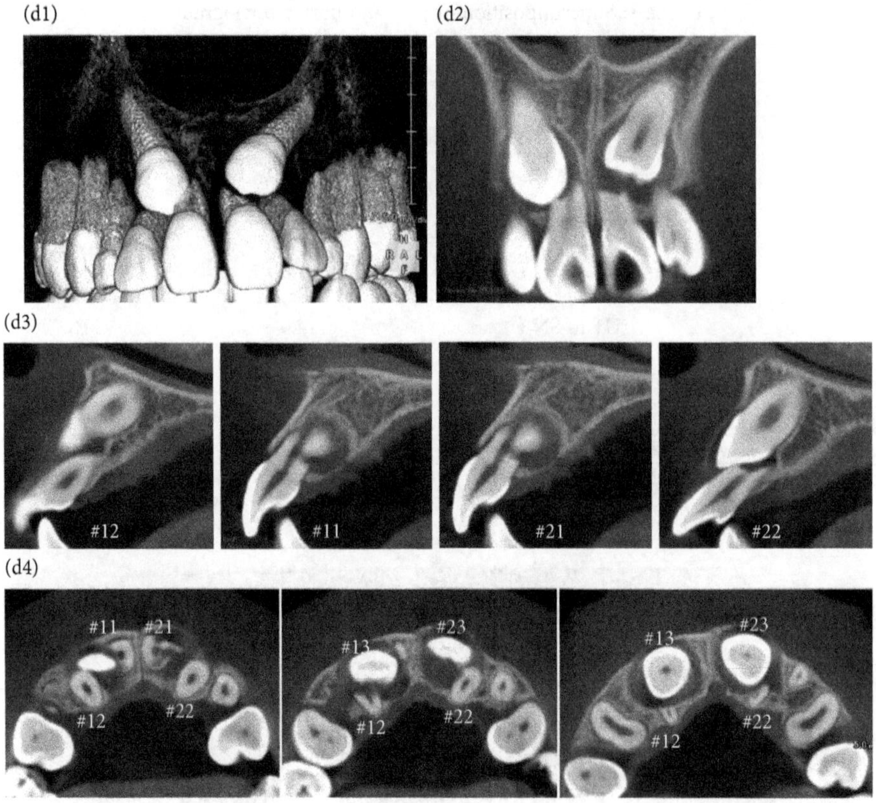

(d)

Figure 3: Pretreatment panoramic radiograph and cone-beam computed tomography (CBCT) images. (a) The impacted bilateral canines were mesially inclined. (b) The angle of inclination to the maxillary dental midline was 33° on the right side (α) and 43° on the left side (β). (c) According to Ericson and Kurol's classification, tooth 13 had grade 4 impaction and tooth 23 had grade 5 impaction. (d) Both canines were located on the buccal side and the roots of the four incisors were resorbed (D1; three dimensional CBCT image, D-2; coronal view, D-3; sagittal view, D-4; axial view).

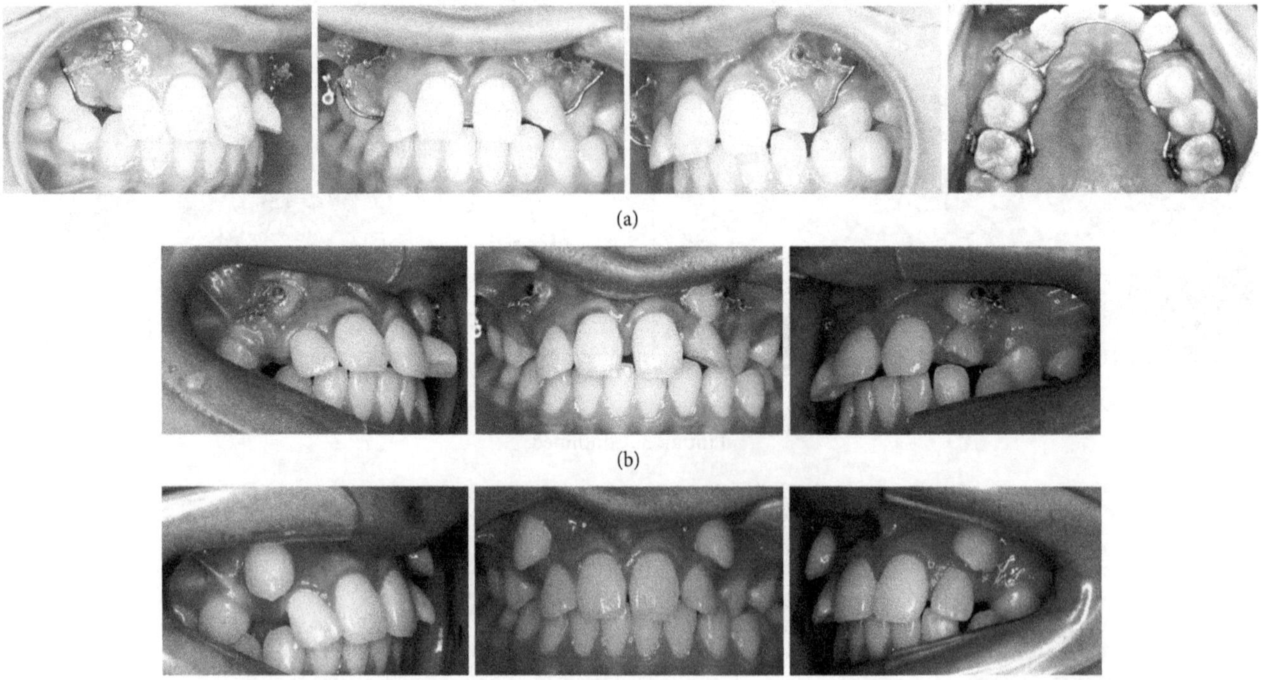

(c)

Figure 4: Treatment progress: (a) at the beginning of canine traction, (b) six months after canine traction, and (c) on completion of canine traction.

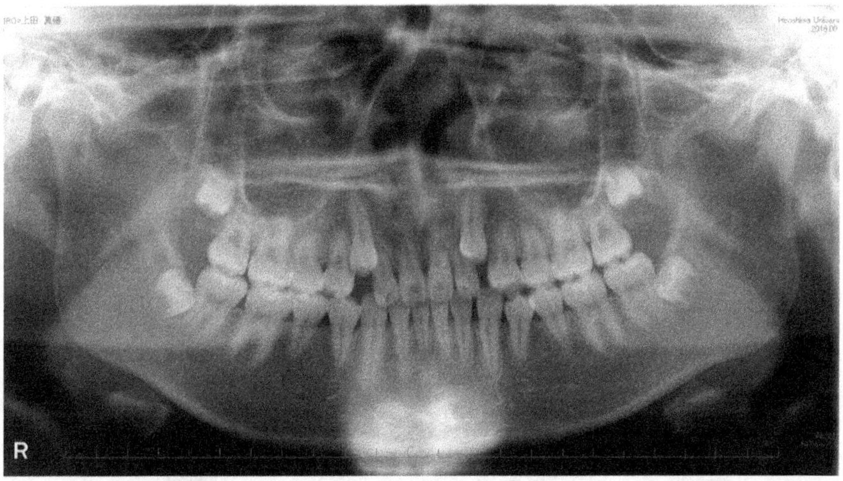

(a)

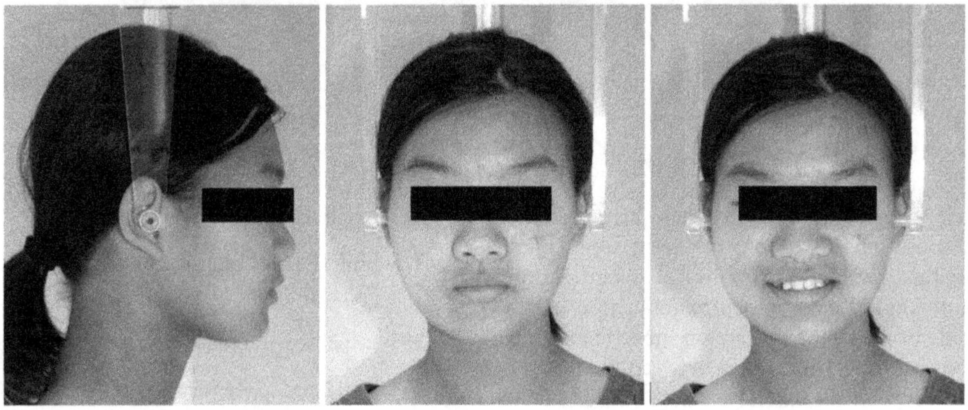

(b)

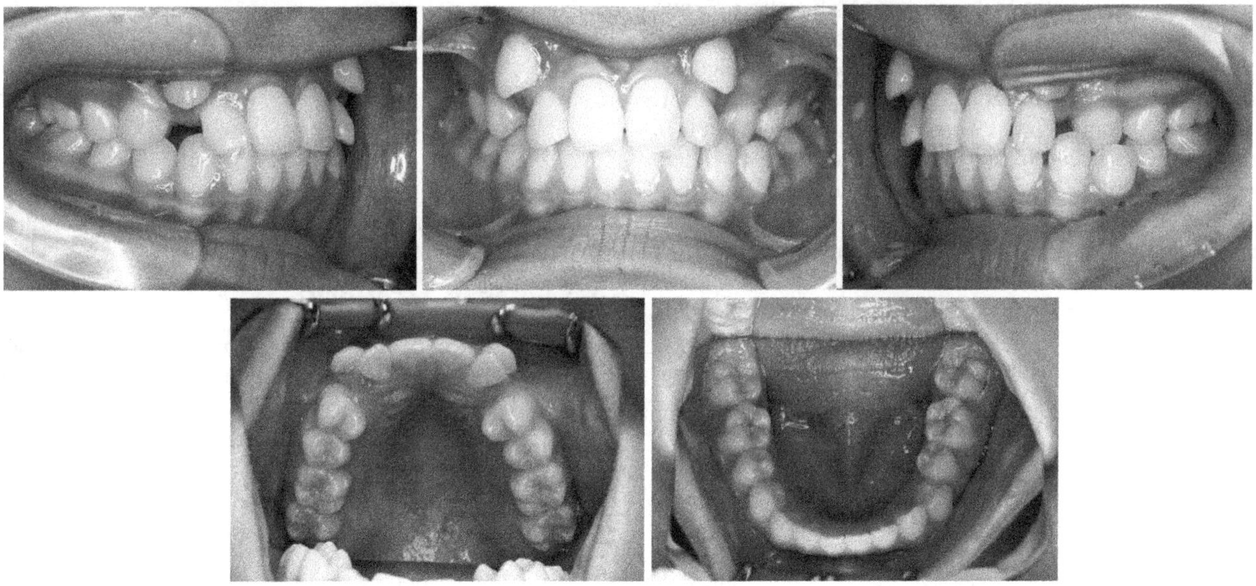

(c)

Figure 5: Continued.

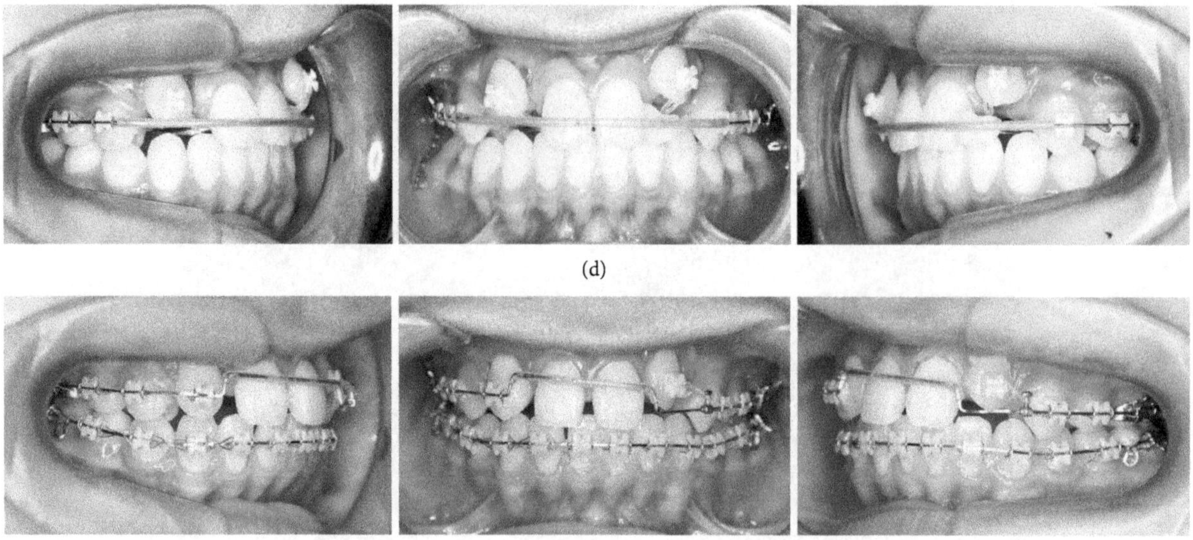

(d)

(e)

FIGURE 5: (a–c) Following completion of canine reposition. Facial and intraoral photographs and panoramic radiograph, (d and e) treatment progress.

She had no relevant medical and family history. The patient's general condition was good with regard to nutrition and psychosomatic development. Clinical examination revealed a bilateral Angle Class II molar relationship, overjet of 4.5 mm, overbite of 3.6 mm, crossbite on the left side, and bilateral deciduous canines. The contact between the permanent canines and roots of the lateral incisors caused labial inclination of the incisors (Figure 1). Cephalometric analysis revealed a skeletal Class I relationship (ANB angle 3.2°) and normal inclination of the angle of the upper and lower central incisors (U1 to SN angle 114.9°/FMIA 59.7°) (Figure 2 and Table 1). Panoramic radiography revealed that the bilateral maxillary canines were mesially inclined (Figure 3(a)), and the angle between the tooth axis and the maxillary dental midline was 33° on the right side and 43° on the left side (Figure 3(b)). According to Ericson and Kurol's classification 3, the medial displacement of the crown of the canine in relation to the long axis of the incisors reflected grade 4 impaction of tooth 13 (Federation Dentaire Internationale tooth numbering system) and grade 5 impaction of tooth 23 (Figure 3(c)). Cone-beam computed tomography showed that the canine crowns with cystic changes were located on the buccal aspect, between the maxillary bilateral central incisors, and that the lateral incisor roots were resorbed (Figure 3(d)).

Written informed consent was obtained from the patient and her parents. The statement of ethics approval by the ethics committee is not required as it is a single case report.

3. Diagnostic Summary

Diagnosis: Crowding with bilaterally impacted maxillary canines causing root resorption of the four maxillary incisors.

(1) Angle Class II molar relationship.

(2) Buccal cross bite on the left side of numbers 63, 24, 33, and 34.

(3) Impacted maxillary bilateral permanent canines.

(4) Deficient space for the maxillary canines in the maxillary arch.

4. Treatment Objectives

(1) Surgical exposure and alignment of the bilateral maxillary canines.

(2) Lateral crossbite correction.

(3) Achievement of balanced and functional occlusion.

5. Course of Treatment

After extraction of the deciduous maxillary canines, both maxillary canines were surgically exposed. Full-thickness mucoperiosteal flaps were raised to gain access, and the soft tissue and bone around the crown were removed to facilitate orthodontic traction. The buttons attached to the ligature wire to tract the canines were bonded to the labial surface of the tooth. Initially the canines were tracted buccally to prevent further damage using elastics from the arm of the lingual arch. After confirming that part of the crown was exposed, the canines were tracted distally (Figures 4(a) and 4(b)). It took eight months to tract the maxillary canines to the correct vertical position, and the labial inclination of the lateral incisors improved spontaneously (Figure 4(c)). All incisors had Miller classification grade 2 mobility after the completion of canine traction. Panoramic radiography showed that the roots

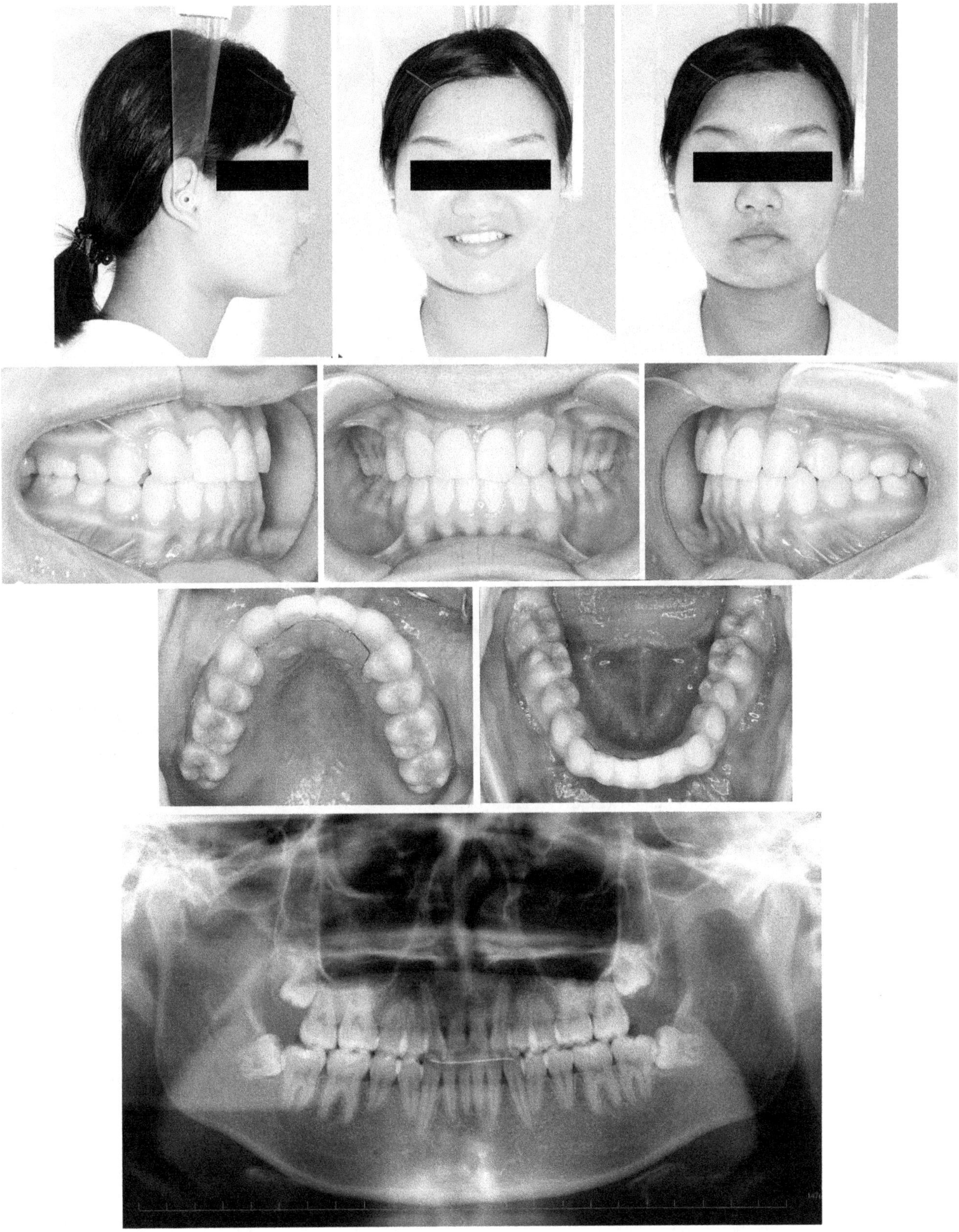

Figure 6: Posttreatment facial and intraoral photographs and panoramic radiograph.

of the central and lateral incisors were equally resorbed (Figure 5(a)). After observing the mandibular growth for 6 months, multi-bracket treatment was initiated (Figures 5(b) and 5(c)). Extracting the lateral incisors was necessary to gain space for maxillary canine alignment. In addition, excessive force on the incisors must be avoided to

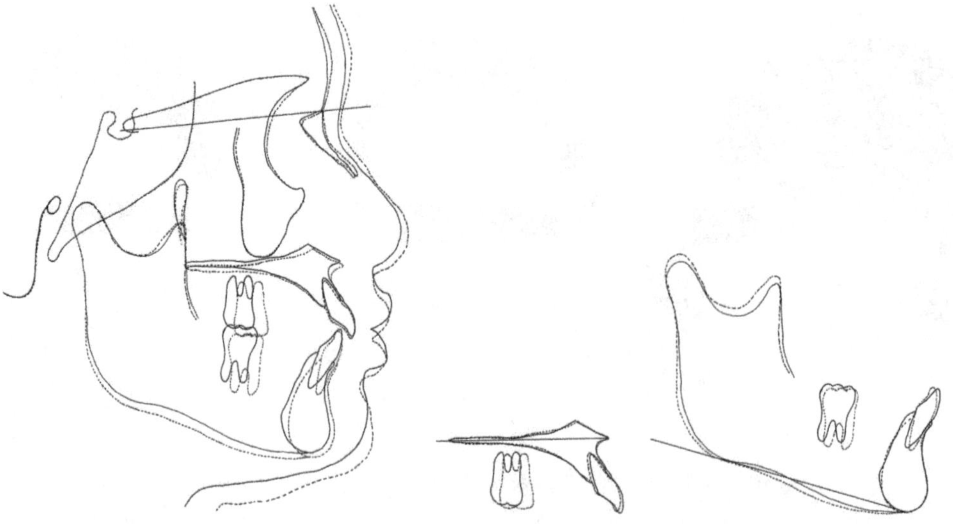

FIGURE 7: Superimposed tracing of the pretreatment and posttreatment lateral cephalometric radiographs: (a) overall, (b) maxilla, and (c) mandible.

prevent further root resorption. The canines, which were positioned superiorly, were pulled toward the occlusal plane with the hook of the lingual arch and arch-wire with elastic chains (Figure 5(d) and 5(e)). The crossbite on the left side was corrected, and all teeth were aligned with $0.018 \times 0.25''$ edgewise brackets. The treatment duration was 30 months. After achieving a well-balanced and functional occlusion (Figure 6), a wrap-around retainer was placed on the upper dentition, and the Hawley retainer was placed on the lower dentition. Superimposing the pre- and post-treatment cephalograms revealed that the treatment goals were mostly accomplished (Figure 7 and Table 1). Root resorption of the maxillary central incisors has not progressed for five years since the initial condition (Figure 8).

6. Discussion

For this report, a case of bilateral maxillary incisor root resorption caused by ectopic maxillary canines was presented. The maxillary canines deviate from their natural path of eruption more often than other teeth [11]. The maxillary canine tooth germ is located in a relatively crowded site in the maxilla, and the period between the generation of the tooth germ and completion of eruption is prolonged. Some studies have indicated that impacted canines and their ectopic formation might cause dental crowding, bony obstructions, tumors or cysts, and delayed replacement of deciduous canines [12, 13]. In this case, the patient had no relevant previous history, systemic factors, or local factors, such as trauma, inflammation, bad habits, or lesions in the maxilla. It is unclear why the canines had deviated from their natural path of eruption. It was speculated that the mesial malpositioning of the canines was a result of a lack of guidance.

In most cases, malpositioned canines avoid the incisor roots during eruption. Root resorption has been reported in approximately 12% of incisors adjacent to ectopic maxillary canines. Maxillary root resorption of permanent incisors was reported to occur in 48% of 9- to 15-year-old children with ectopic maxillary canine eruption [14]. The average angle of inclination of the maxillary canines on the panoramic radiograph was 18.6° in the group with root resorption and 29.5° in the group without [15]. There are few reports according to which central incisors, and not only the bilateral lateral incisors, can be affected. As stated in a previous report, in three out of 40 assessed patients, bilateral lateral incisors were affected by root resorption, however, none of the evaluated patients reported root resorption of all four incisors [16].

It was important to confirm the location and direction of erupted canines by radiography at the age of 10 years because no cases of root resorption have been observed before that age. However, in some cases, root resorption of the lateral incisors can extend to the pulp after the age of 10 years [17]. Early intervention to prevent malpositioning of maxillary canines could prevent severe root resorption of the maxillary incisor roots [18].

It was also reported that the extraction of deciduous canines in patients with displaced canines was an effective interceptive approach to correct ectopically erupting maxillary canines and prevent incisor root resorption [15]. In this case, if ectopic maxillary canines had been confirmed by panoramic radiography earlier and the deciduous canines had been extracted at the age of 10 years, the maxillary incisor root resorption may have been prevented.

Some studies have reported that when an ectopic maxillary canine is severely malpositioned in the horizontal and mesial direction, their extraction is considered because orthodontic traction may be a significant risk factor for incisor root resorption [18]. In this case, because the horizontal

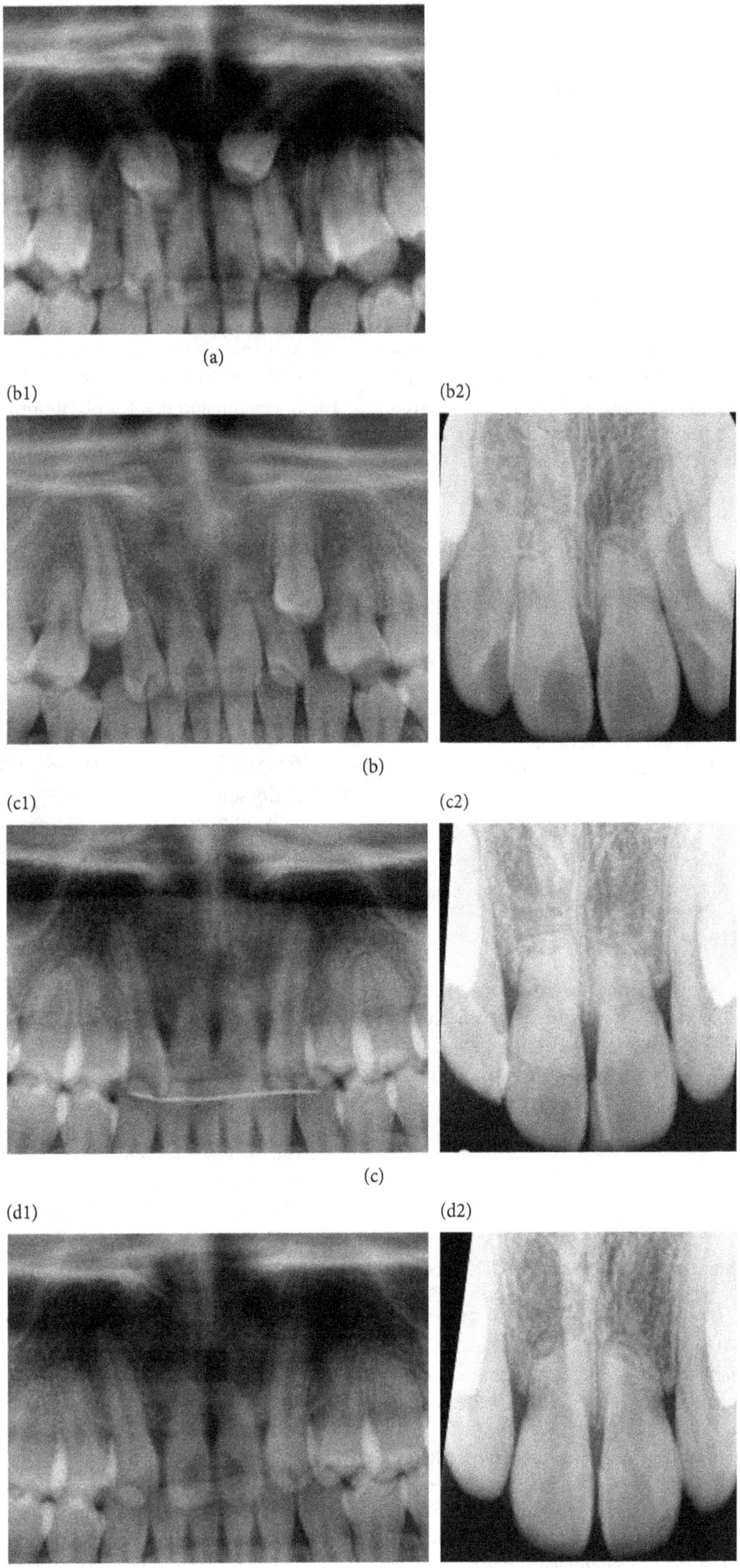

(a) (b1) (b2) (b) (c1) (c2) (c) (d1) (d2) (d)

FIGURE 8: Panoramic radiograph revealing root resorption of maxillary incisors: (a) pretreatment, (b) post-canine traction, (c) posttreatment, and (d) two years posttreatment.

angle of the canines was not severe, traction and alignment of the bilateral canines after surgical exposure and extraction of the bilateral incisors with root resorption.

Many case reports indicate that orthodontically-induced resorption ceases when the force is removed; similarly, when an ectopic canine is maintained at an adequate distance from incisor roots, root resorption ceases [17, 19]. Furthermore, an apparent increase in maxillary incisor root resorption in cases of ectopic canines was not observed 10 years after orthodontic treatment [20]. For this case, the patient was advised to monitor the resorbed incisor as a precautionary measure. However, after consulting with a specialist, root canal treatment was deemed to be inappropriate as a means of reducing further resorption [21]. Therefore, it is necessary to evaluate the long-term status of teeth that have undergone root resorption during active orthodontic treatment.

7. Conclusions

This report described the case of an 11-year-old Japanese girl with root resorption of the bilateral central and lateral incisors, which was caused by impacted bilateral maxillary canines and maxillary crowding. Orthodontic treatment helped achieve the functional and esthetic goals through extraction of the bilateral lateral incisors with root resorption. Early detection and diagnosis through radiographic examinations could efficiently help prevent root resorption.

Authors' Contributions

Makoto Yanoshita and Naoto Hirose involved in writing and editing. Azusa Onishi, Sayuri Nishiyama, Naoki Kubo, and Daiki Kita involved in patient management and revision of the final text. Kotaro Tanimoto involved in patient management, scientific revision, editing, and supervision.

References

[1] I. G. Gisakis, F. D. Palamidakis, E.-T. R. Farmakis, G. Kamberos, and S. Kamberos, "Prevalence of impacted teeth in a Greek population," *Journal of Investigative and Clinical Dentistry*, vol. 2, no. 2, pp. 102–109, 2011.

[2] K. Aitasalo, R. Lehtinen, and E. Oksala, "An orthopantomography study of prevalence of impacted teeth," *International Journal of Oral Surgery*, vol. 1, no. 3, pp. 117–120, 1972.

[3] H. Jacoby, "The etiology of maxillary canine impactions," *American Journal of Orthodontics*, vol. 84, no. 2, pp. 125–132, 1983.

[4] B. Thilander and S. O. Jakobsson, "Local factors in impaction of maxillary canines," *Acta Odontologica Scandinavica*, vol. 26, no. 1-2, pp. 145–168, 1968.

[5] A. Becker, P. Smith, and R. Behar, "The incidence of anomalous maxillary lateral incisors in relation to palatally-displaced cuspids," *The Angle Orthodontist*, vol. 51, no. 1, pp. 24–29, 1981.

[6] A. Becker, I. Gillis, and N. Shpack, "The etiology of palatal displacement of maxillary canines," *Clinical Orthodontics and Research*, vol. 2, no. 2, pp. 62–66, 1999.

[7] S. Leifert and I. E. Jonas, "Dental anomalies as a microsymptom of palatal canine displacement," *Journal of Orofacial Orthopedics*, vol. 64, no. 2, pp. 108–120, 2003.

[8] A. Becker and S. Chaushu, "Dental age in maxillary canine ectopia," *American Journal of Orthodontics and Dentofacial Orthopedics*, vol. 117, no. 6, pp. 657–662, 2000.

[9] A. Becker, N. Casap, and S. Chaushu, "Conventional wisdom and the surgical exposure of impacted teeth," *Orthodontics and Craniofacial Research*, vol. 12, no. 2, pp. 82–93, 2009.

[10] S. Ericson and P. J. Kurol, "Resorption of incisors after ectopic eruption of maxillary canines: a CT study," *The Angle Orthodontist*, vol. 70, pp. 415–423, 2000.

[11] Y. Shapira, M. M. Kuftinec, and D. Stom, "Maxillary canine-lateral incisor transposition—orthodontic management," *American Journal of Orthodontics and Dentofacial Orthopedics*, vol. 95, no. 5, pp. 439–444, 1989.

[12] H. S. Orton, M. T. Garvey, and M. H. Pearson, "Extrusion of the ectopic maxillary canine using a lower removable appliance," *American Journal of Orthodontics and Dentofacial Orthopedics*, vol. 107, no. 4, pp. 349–359, 1995.

[13] Y. Göyenç, A. I. Karaman, and A. Gökalp, "Unusual ectopic eruption of maxillary canines," *Journal of Clinical Orthodontics*, vol. 29, no. 9, pp. 580–582, 1995.

[14] S. Ericson and J. Kurol, "Radiographic examination of ectopically erupting maxillary canines," *American Journal of Orthodontics and Dentofacial Orthopedics*, vol. 91, no. 6, pp. 483–492, 1987.

[15] S. Ericson and J. Kurol, "Early treatment of palatally erupting maxillary canines by extraction of the primary canines," *European Journal of Orthodontics*, vol. 10, no. 1, pp. 283–295, 1988.

[16] B. Falahat, S. Ericson, R. Mak D'Amico, and K. Bjerklin, "Incisor root resorption due to ectopic maxillary canines: a long-term radiographic follow-up," *The Angle Orthodontist*, vol. 78, no. 5, pp. 778–785, 2008.

[17] S. Ericson and J. Kurol, "Incisor resorption caused by maxillary cuspids. A radiographic study," *The Angle Orthodontist*, vol. 57, pp. 332–346, 1987.

[18] D. G. Garib, G. Janson, T. D. O. Baldo, and P. B. D. SantosDos, "Complications of misdiagnosis of maxillary canine ectopic eruption," *American Journal of Orthodontics and Dentofacial Orthopedics*, vol. 142, no. 2, pp. 256–263, 2012.

[19] S. E. Bishara and D. Ortho, "Impacted maxillary canines: a review," *American Journal of Orthodontics and Dentofacial Orthopedics*, vol. 101, no. 2, pp. 159–171, 1992.

[20] D. N. Remington, D. R. Joondeph, J. Artun, R. A. Riedel, and M. K. Chapko, "Long-term evaluation of root resorption occurring during orthodontic treatment," *American Journal of Orthodontics and Dentofacial Orthopedics*, vol. 96, no. 1, pp. 43–46, 1989.

[21] A. Becker and B. Chaushu, "Long-term follow-up of severely resorbed maxillary incisors after resolution of an etiologically associated impacted canine," *American Journal of Orthodontics and Dentofacial Orthopedics*, vol. 127, no. 6, pp. 650–654, 2005.

Permissions

All chapters in this book were first published by Hindawi Publishing Corporation; hereby published with permission under the Creative Commons Attribution License or equivalent. Every chapter published in this book has been scrutinized by our experts. Their significance has been extensively debated. The topics covered herein carry significant findings which will fuel the growth of the discipline. They may even be implemented as practical applications or may be referred to as a beginning point for another development.

The contributors of this book come from diverse backgrounds, making this book a truly international effort. This book will bring forth new frontiers with its revolutionizing research information and detailed analysis of the nascent developments around the world.

We would like to thank all the contributing authors for lending their expertise to make the book truly unique. They have played a crucial role in the development of this book. Without their invaluable contributions this book wouldn't have been possible. They have made vital efforts to compile up to date information on the varied aspects of this subject to make this book a valuable addition to the collection of many professionals and students.

This book was conceptualized with the vision of imparting up-to-date information and advanced data in this field. To ensure the same, a matchless editorial board was set up. Every individual on the board went through rigorous rounds of assessment to prove their worth. After which they invested a large part of their time researching and compiling the most relevant data for our readers.

The editorial board has been involved in producing this book since its inception. They have spent rigorous hours researching and exploring the diverse topics which have resulted in the successful publishing of this book. They have passed on their knowledge of decades through this book. To expedite this challenging task, the publisher supported the team at every step. A small team of assistant editors was also appointed to further simplify the editing procedure and attain best results for the readers.

Apart from the editorial board, the designing team has also invested a significant amount of their time in understanding the subject and creating the most relevant covers. They scrutinized every image to scout for the most suitable representation of the subject and create an appropriate cover for the book.

The publishing team has been an ardent support to the editorial, designing and production team. Their endless efforts to recruit the best for this project, has resulted in the accomplishment of this book. They are a veteran in the field of academics and their pool of knowledge is as vast as their experience in printing. Their expertise and guidance has proved useful at every step. Their uncompromising quality standards have made this book an exceptional effort. Their encouragement from time to time has been an inspiration for everyone.

The publisher and the editorial board hope that this book will prove to be a valuable piece of knowledge for researchers, students, practitioners and scholars across the globe.

List of Contributors

Fatima Ezzahra Zidane and Mustapha El Alloussi
College of Health Sciences, International Faculty of Dental Medicine, BioMed Unit, International University of Rabat, Technopolis Parc, Rocade of Rabat-Salé, Sala-Al Jadida 11100, Morocco

Pier Paolo Poli and Silvia Pieriboni
Department of Biomedical, Surgical and Dental Sciences, University of Milan, Via Commenda 10, 20122 Milan, Italy

Luca Creminelli, Emma Grecchi and Gregorio Menozzi
Oral Surgery Department, Maxillofacial Surgery and Odontostomatology Unit, Fondazione IRCCS Cà Granda Maggiore Policlinico Hospital, University of Milan, Via Commenda 10, 20122 Milan, Italy

Carlo Maiorana
Oral Surgery and Implantology Departments, Maxillofacial Surgery and Odontostomatology Unit, Fondazione IRCCS Cà Granda Maggiore Policlinico Hospital, University of Milan, Via Commenda 10, 20122 Milan, Italy

Naji Kharouf
Inserm UMR_S 1121, Biomaterials and Bioengineering, Strasbourg University, 11 Rue Humann, 67085 Strasbourg, France

Youssef Haïkel and Davide Mancino
Faculty of Dental Medicine, Department of Endodontics, Strasbourg University, 8 Rue Sainte Elisabeth 67000 Strasbourg, France

Anita Thakur and Seema Thakur
Department of Pediatric and Preventive Dentistry, H.P Government Dental College and Hospital Shimla, Himachal Pradesh, India

Ammar Belal
Master's Degree, Clinical Instructor, School of Dentistry, Hama University, Removable prosthodontic Department, Hama, Syria

Bassil Monther
Professor, Doctorate, School of Dentistry, Hama University, Removable prosthodontic Department, Hama, Syria

Wael Alzarif
Oral and Maxillofacial Surgery, Syrian Board of Medical Specialties, Head of Oral and Maxillofacial Surgery, National Hospital of Hama, Hama, Syria

Zahra Mohammadi, Hadi Assadian, Behnam Bolhari, Mohammadreza Sharifian, Mehrfam Khoshkhounejad and Nazanin Chitsaz
Department of Endodontics, School of Dentistry, Tehran University of Medical Sciences (TUMS), Iran

Andrea Gómez-González, Miguel Ángel Rosales-Berber, Paola De Ávila-Rojas, Amaury Pozos-Guillén and Arturo Garrocho-Rangel
Pediatric Dentistry Postgraduate Program, Faculty of Dentistry, San Luis Potosi University, SLP, San Luis Potosi, Mexico

Malaz M. Mustafa, M. Zakirulla, Ibrahim AlShahrani, Rafi A. Togoo, Zuhair M. Alkahtani and Tasneem S. Ain
Department of Pediatric Dentistry & Orthodontic Sciences, College of Dentistry, King Khalid University, Abha, Saudi Arabia

Dorsaf Touil, Rahma Bouhouch, Raoua Belkacem Chebil, Lamia Oualha and Nabiha Douki
University of Monastir, Dental Faculty of Monastir, Research Laboratory LR12ES11, Tunisia

Claudio Novelli
DENS Centro Medico Lombardo, Milan 20124, Italy

Maurizio Pascadopoli and Andrea Scribante
DENS Centro Medico Lombardo, Milan 20124, Italy
Unit of Orthodontics and Pediatric Dentistry, Section of Dentistry, Department of Clinical, Surgical, Diagnostic and Pediatric Sciences, University of Pavia, 27100 Pavia, Italy

Ubiracy Gaião
Positivo University, Curitiba, Brazil

Ana Carolina Portes Pasmadjian, Gabriela Resende Allig, Liliana Vicente Melo de Lucas Rezende, Vitória Beatriz Souza da Silva and Leonardo Fernandes da Cunha
Department of Dentistry, School of Health Sciences, University of Brasília, DF, Brazil

Michele M. Figliuzzi, Maria Altilia, Amerigo Giudice and Leonzio Fortunato
School of Dentistry, Department of Periodontics and Oral Sciences, Magna Græcia University, Catanzaro, Italy

Simone Altilia
School of Dentistry, Department of Periodontics and Oral Sciences, Magna Græcia University, Catanzaro, Italy
Dentistry School, Tor Vergata University of Rome, Rome, Italy

Wisam Al-Hathlol and Raed Bokhari
Department of Pediatrics, National Guard Hospital, Dammam, Saudi Arabia

Nada Alzahrani and Elaf Alkuwaiti
College of Dentistry, Imam Abdulrahman Bin Faisal University, Dammam, Saudi Arabia

Ngoc Bao Vu
Dental Biomaterials Science Program, Graduate School, Chulalongkorn University, Bangkok 10330, Thailand
Department of Maxillofacial and Plastic Surgery, Hanoi National Hospital of Odonto-Stomatology, Hanoi 100000, Vietnam

Ngoc Tuyen Le
Department of Maxillofacial Reconstructive Surgery, Hanoi National Hospital of Odonto-Stomatology, Hanoi 100000, Vietnam

Risa Chaisuparat
Department of Oral Pathology, Faculty of Dentistry, Chulalongkorn University, Bangkok 10330, Thailand

Pasutha Thunyakitpisal
Research Unit of Herbal Medicine, Biomaterial, And Material for Dental Treatment, Department of Anatomy, Faculty of Dentistry, Chulalongkorn University, Bangkok 10330, Thailand

Ngoc Minh Tran
Department of Pathology, Hanoi Medical University, Hanoi 100000, Vietnam

Tania Saskianti, Udijanto Tedjosaongko, Regina Ayu Pramudita, Nita Naomi and Alit Rahma Restu
Department of Pediatric Dentistry, Faculty of Dentistry, Airlangga University, Surabaya 60132, Indonesia

Jean-Claude Abou Chedid and Michel Salameh
Department of Pediatric Dentistry, Faculty of Dental Medicine, Saint-Joseph University, Beirut, Lebanon

Abbass El-Outa
Private Practice of Oral Medicine and Restorative Dentistry, Beirut, Lebanon

Ziad E. F. Noujeim
Department of Oral Medicine and Maxillofacial Radiology and Imaging, Faculty of Dental Medicine, Lebanese University, Beirut, Lebanon

Hasan Sabah Hasan
Orthodontic Department, Khanzad Teaching Center, General Directorate of Hawler-Ministry of Health, Erbil, Iraq

Ayshan Kolemen
Orthodontic Department, Al-Mustaqbal University College, Babel, Iraq

Mohamed Elkolaly
Orthodontic Department, Royal Dental Center, Alexandria, Egypt

Anand Marya
Section of Orthodontics, University of Puthisastra, Phnom Penh, Cambodia

Shreyas Gujjar
Sri Balaji Dental College, Moinabad, Telangana, India

Adith Venugopal
Section of Orthodontics, University of Puthisastra, Phnom Penh, Cambodia
Department of Orthodontics, Saveetha Dental College, Saveetha Institute of Medical and Technical Sciences, Saveetha University, Chennai, India

V. Vinothini
Vinu Dental Clinic, Erode 638 452, Gobichettipalayam, India

A. Sanguida, A. Selvabalaji, G. S. Prathima and M. Kavitha
Department of Paedodontics and Preventive Dentistry, Indira Gandhi Institute of Dental Sciences, Sri Balaji Vidyapeeth, Pillaiyarkuppam, Puducherry 607 402, India

Carlos-Martín Ardila and Efraín Álvarez-Martínez
Universidad de Antioquia, Medellín, Colombia

Nazanin Chitsaz, Mehrfam Khoshkhounejad, Hadi Assadian, Behnam Bolhari, Mohammadreza Sharifian and Zahra Mohammadi
Department of Endodontics, School of Dentistry, Tehran University of Medical Sciences (TUMS), Tehran, Iran

Damian Chybicki, Alicja Popielarczyk, Wojciech Markowski, Gaja Torbicka and Anna Janas-Naze
Department of Oral Surgery, Central Clinical Hospital, Medical University of Lodz, Poland

Conor Carroll, Mishaal Gill, Eleanor Bowden, John Ed O'Connell and Chris Sweet
Department of Oral and Maxillofacial Surgery, Alder Hey Children's NHS Foundation Trust, East Prescot Road, Liverpool L14 5AB, UK

Rajeev Shukla
Department of Pathology, Alder Hey Children's NHS Foundation Trust, East Prescot Road, Liverpool L14 5AB, UK

N. Ismail
Centre for Paediatric Dentistry & Orthodontics Studies, Faculty of Dentistry, Universiti Teknologi MARA, Sungai Buloh Campus, Jalan Hospital, 47000 Sungai Buloh, Selangor, Malaysia
Ministry of Health, Malaysia

S. H. Hamzah
Centre for Paediatric Dentistry & Orthodontics Studies, Faculty of Dentistry, Universiti Teknologi MARA, Sungai Buloh Campus, Jalan Hospital, 47000 Sungai Buloh, Selangor, Malaysia

I. Wan Mokhtar
Centre for Paediatric Dentistry & Orthodontics Studies, Faculty of Dentistry, Universiti Teknologi MARA, Sungai Buloh Campus, Jalan Hospital, 47000 Sungai Buloh, Selangor, Malaysia
Centre for Comprehensive Care Studies, Faculty of Dentistry, Universiti Teknologi MARA. Sungai Buloh Campus, Jalan Hospital, 47000 Sungai Buloh, Selangor, Malaysia

G. Solinas and R. Strinna
RDH, Independent Researcher in Sassari, Italy

V. Grabesu
DDS and SLP, Independent Researcher in Sassari, Italy

M. Lattari
RDH, Independent Researcher in Pavia, Italy

N. Arnould
DDS, Independent Researcher in Sassari, Italy

A. A. Amodeo
RDH DHA, Adjunct Professor Degree Course Dental Hygiene University of Milan Department of Biomedical, Surgical and Dental Sciences, Italy
RDH DHA, Foundation IRCCS Ca' Granda Ospedale Maggiore Policlinico, Italy

Abbas O. Al-Ahmadi
Specialized Dental Centre, King Fahad Hospital, Medina, Saudi Arabia

Ali A. Assiry and Siraj D. A. A. Khan
Pediatric Dentistry, Faculty of Dentistry, Najran University, Saudi Arabia

Anand Marya
Department of Orthodontics, Faculty of Dentistry, University of Puthisastra, Phnom Penh, Cambodia
Department of Orthodontics, Saveetha Dental College, Saveetha Institute of Medical and Technical Sciences, Saveetha University, Chennai, India

Adith Venugopal
Department of Orthodontics, Saveetha Dental College, Saveetha Institute of Medical and Technical Sciences, Saveetha University, Chennai, India

Mohmed Isaqali Karobari
Conservative Unit, School of Dental Sciences, Universiti Sains Malaysia, Health Campus, Kubang Kerian, 16150 Kota Bharu, Kelantan, Malaysia

Kamis Gaballah
Department of Oral and Craniofacial Health Sciences, College of Dental Medicine, University of Sharjah, UAE

Sami Kenz
Rashid Centre for Diabetes & Research, Ajman, UAE

Raeefa Anis
Ajman University, UAE

Omar Kujan
UWA Dental School, The University of Western Australia, Perth WA6009, Australia

Farah Chouchene, Wassim Ben Ameur, Maissa Bouenba, Fatma Masmoudi, Ahlem Baaziz, Fethi Maatouk and Hichem Ghedira
Pediatric and Preventive Dentistry Department, Faculty of Dental Medicine of Monastir, Laboratory of Biological, Clinical and Dento-Facial Approach, University of Monastir, Monastir, Tunisia

Habib Hamdi
Dental Surgery Department, Faculty of Dental Medicine of Monastir, Monastir, Tunisia

Salah Afraa, Hashim Raghad and Hamid Aeshah
Growth and Development Department, Ajman University, UAE

Khalid Ayam
Basic Science Department, Ajman University, UAE

Alberto De Stefani, Giovanni Bruno, Martina Barone and Antonio Gracco
Department of Neuroscience, School of Dentistry, University of Padua, 35100 Padua, Italy

Niusha Abazarian
Department of Pediatric Dentistry, Dental School, AJA University of Medical Sciences, Tehran, Iran

Shabnam Milani and Marzieh Salehi Shahrabi
Department of Pediatric Dentistry, Tehran University of Medical Sciences, Tehran, Iran

Moahammad Hassan Hamrah
Department of Pediatric Dentistry, School of Dentistry, Tehran University of Medical Sciences Tehran, Iran

Makoto Yanoshita, Naoto Hirose, Azusa Onishi, Sayuri Nishiyama, Naoki Kubo, Daiki Kita and Kotaro Tanimoto
Department of Orthodontics and Craniofacial Developmental Biology, Hiroshima University Graduate School of Biomedical and Health Sciences, Kasumi 1-2-3 Minami-ku, Hiroshima-shi, Hiroshima Prefecture, Japan

Index

Printed in the USA
CPSIA information can be obtained
at www.ICGtesting.com
JSHW051908080424
60792JS00005B/63

9 798887 406527